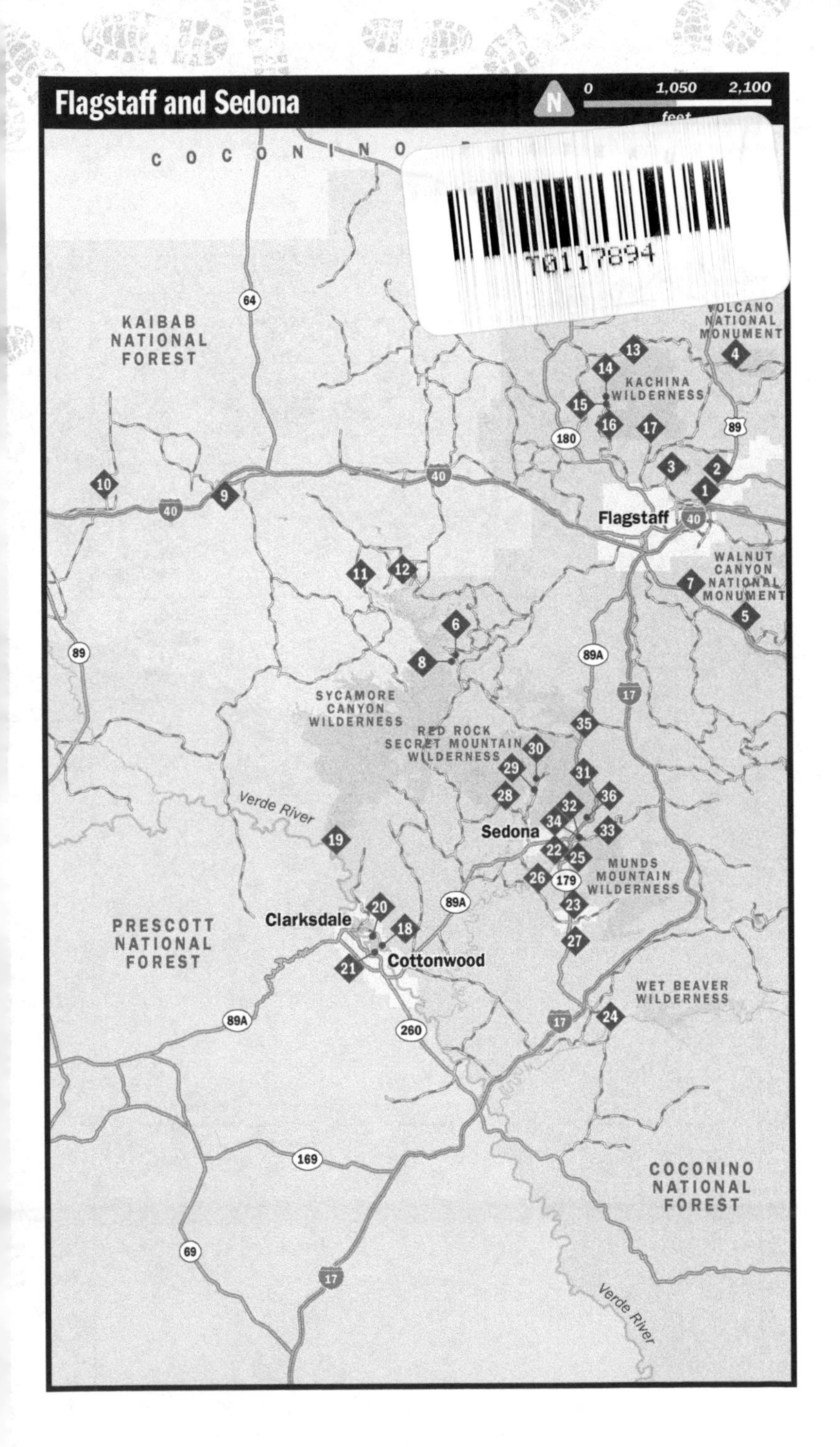
Flagstaff and Sedona
0
1,050
2,100
feet
COCONINO
KAIBAB NATIONAL FOREST
VOLCANO NATIONAL MONUMENT
KACHINA WILDERNESS
Flagstaff
WALNUT CANYON NATIONAL MONUMENT
SYCAMORE CANYON WILDERNESS
RED ROCK SECRET MOUNTAIN WILDERNESS
Verde River
Sedona
MUNDS MOUNTAIN WILDERNESS
Clarksdale
Cottonwood
PRESCOTT NATIONAL FOREST
WET BEAVER WILDERNESS
COCONINO NATIONAL FOREST
Verde River

Map Legend

Trailhead

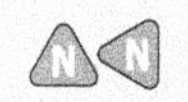

North Indicator

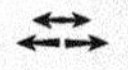
Path Direction

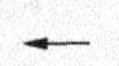
Off map
or pinpoint

Capital, Cities
and towns

Interstate highways

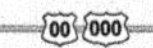

U.S. highways

00 000
State roads

FS 0 CR 00
Other roads

Unpaved roads

Featured trail

Alternate trail

Boardwalk or stairs

Powerline

Railroads

River or stream

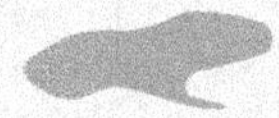
Water body

Marsh

STATE
PARK

Preserve or
other public land

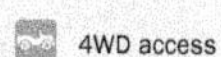

- 4WD access
- Airport
- Amphitheater
- Bench
- Bridge
- Campground
- Church
- Gate
- General Point of Interest
- Information
- Interpretive sign
- Lookout tower
- Mine/quarry
- Monument
- Motor bike access
- Overlook
- Parking
- Peak
- Picnic
- Ranger station
- Restrooms
- Scenic viewpoint
- Ski area
- Spring
- Swimming
- Tunnel
- Wall
- Waterfall

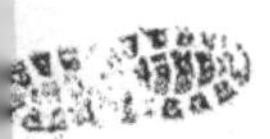

Overview Map Key

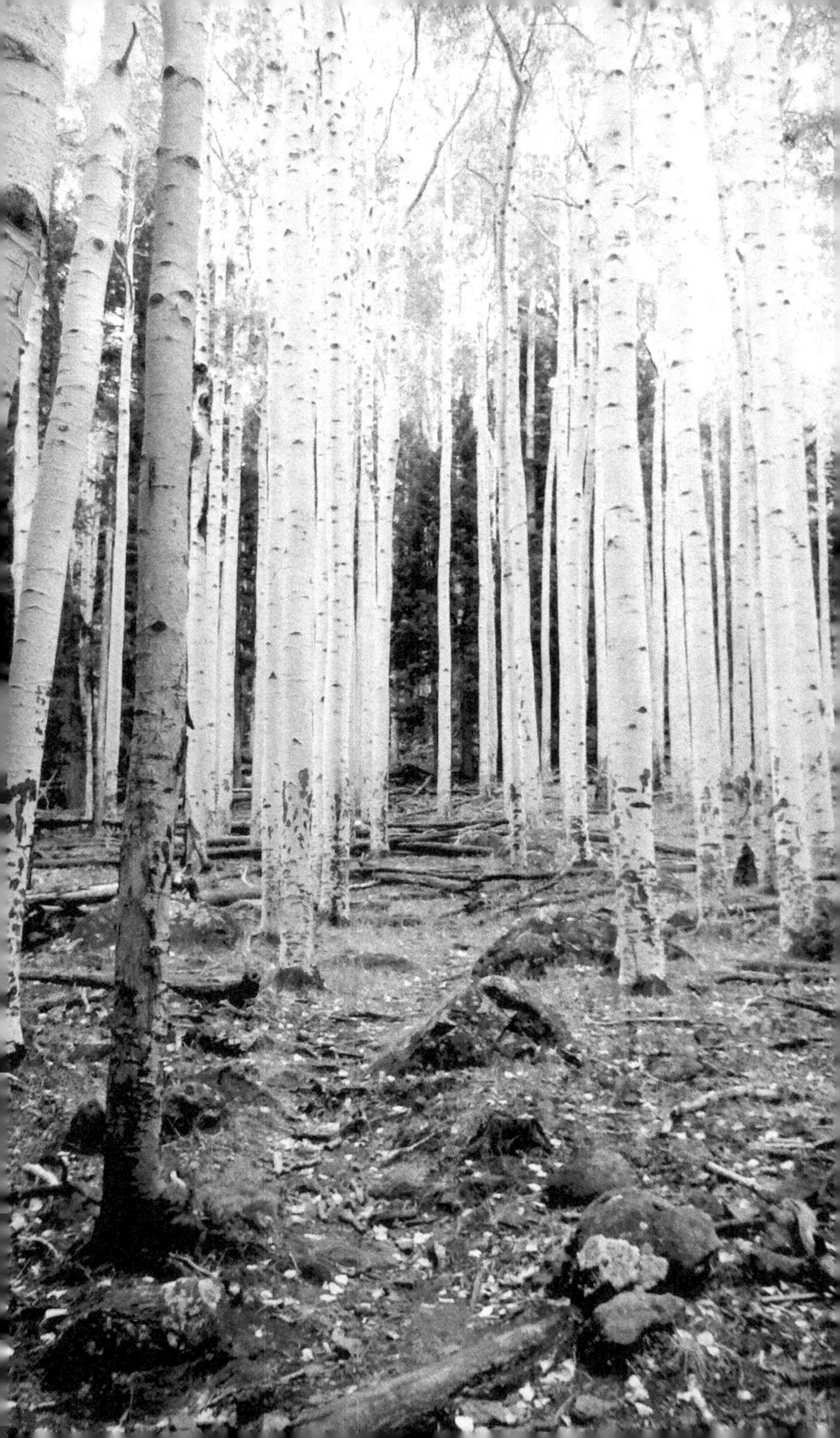

Five-Star Trails

Flagstaff & Sedona

Your Guide to the Area's Most Beautiful Hikes

Tony Padegimas

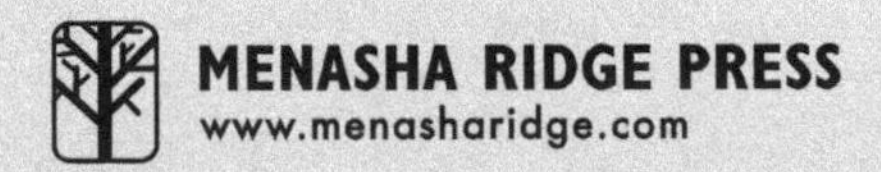

Five-Star Trails: Flagstaff & Sedona
Your Guide to the Area's Most Beautiful Hikes

Published by Menasha Ridge Press
Distributed by Publishers Group West
Printed in the United States of America
First edition, second printing

Cover design by Scott McGrew
Frontispiece: Aspens at Abineau–Bear Jaw Loop
Text design by Annie Long
Cover photograph of Brins Mesa–Soldier Pass Loop and back cover photograph of Bell Trail by Tony Padegimas
Author photograph by Penny Padegimas
Photograph on page 185 by Roxann Adamsen
All other interior photographs by Tony Padegimas
Cartography and elevation profiles by Tony Padegimas and Scott McGrew

Library of Congress Cataloging-in-Publication Data

Padegimas, Tony.
Five-star trails Flagstaff and Sedona : your guide to the area's most beautiful trails / Tony Padegimas.
p. cm.
Includes index.
ISBN-13: 978-0-89732-927-9
ISBN-10: 0-89732-927-9
1. Hiking--Arizona--Flagstaff Region--Guidebooks. 2. Hiking--Arizona--Sedona Region--Guidebooks. 3. Trails--Arizona--Flagstaff Region--Guidebooks. 4. Trails--Arizona--Sedona Region--Guidebooks. 5. Flagstaff Region (Ariz.)--Guidebooks. 6. Sedona Region (Ariz.)--Guidebooks. I. Title.
GV199.42.A72F537 2012
917.91'33--dc23

2011019146

Menasha Ridge Press, an imprint of AdventureKEEN
2204 First Ave. S., Suite 102
Birmingham, AL 35233
menasharidgepress.com

DISCLAIMER
This book is meant only as a guide to select trails in Flagstaff and Sedona, Arizona. This book does not guarantee hiker safety in any way—you hike at your own risk. Neither Menasha Ridge Press nor Tony Padegimas is liable for property loss or damage, personal injury, or death that result in any way from accessing or hiking the trails described in the following pages. Please be especially cautious when walking in potentially hazardous terrains with, for example, steep inclines or drop-offs. Do not attempt to explore terrain that may be beyond your abilities. Please read carefully the introduction to this book as well as further safety information from other sources. Familiarize yourself with current weather reports and maps of the area you plan to visit (in addition to the maps provided in this guidebook). Be cognizant of park regulations and always follow them. Do not take chances.

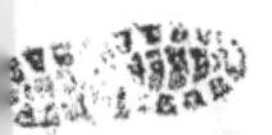

Contents

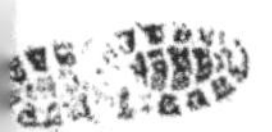

Dedication

For my family, who let me do this again, even though they certainly knew better, and especially my son, Ben, who never quit on a trail.

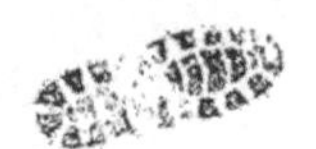

Acknowledgments

I would like to gratefully thank all the various companions on the various hikes, even those whose names I did not know:

The fine folks working for the Coconino and Kaibab national forests, who were always as helpful as regulations allowed, especially the two watchtower attendants I met.

The waitstaff at the Snowbowl Ski Lift Lodge for their unexpected generosity.

The gang at **HikeAZ.com,** the online source community for hiking information in this state.

Adam Schneider, the creator of GPS Visualizer (**gpsvisualizer.com**), a great, free resource for turning the piles of data in your GPS into a usable map.

And, most of all, the people in and around Sedona and Flagstaff who have generously allowed the rest of us to wander around what would otherwise be their backyards.

Preface

I am not some wilderness expert who drops into the remote badlands from a helicopter to fight his way out to civilization with only a knife, three sticks of gum, and a camera crew. I have had 30 different jobs over my life, but none of them was forester or guide or any other outdoor profession (unless you count camp counselor—and I do not). I am a writer, mostly of magazine articles, who likes to hike.

For whatever reason, I have always been able to march off into the boonies with no fear of getting lost. Consequently, I get lost—a lot. This book provides you with the opportunity to learn from my mistakes.

Much of what is cool to do in hiking boots in Arizona can be found within an hour's drive of either Flagstaff or Sedona. *Cool* has two meanings here: not just fun, but also not always in the deep desert.

In fact, Flagstaff sits on the pine-covered slopes of the San Francisco Peaks, the tallest mountains in the state. Sedona, even more famously, occupies the foot of red-rocks country, home to spiritual vortexes or, more tangibly, swimming holes, deep canyons, and stunning geology.

A hundred years ago, these lands were settled, to a point, by a loose collection of cowboys and lumberjacks. Seven hundred years ago, the Sinaguan people saw their civilization rise and fall across this region. A million years ago, the volcanoes that would become the San Francisco Peaks and Sunset Crater were violently landscaping the tops of the plateaus. More than 200 million years ago, this area was the shore of a shallow sea. All of this history and more can be seen from the trails described within.

The scenery is world-famous for a reason, and postcards are just not the same. Live in Phoenix long enough, and you will stop noticing the surrounding mountains. Yet every time you look up in either Flagstaff or Sedona, the light or the clouds are doing

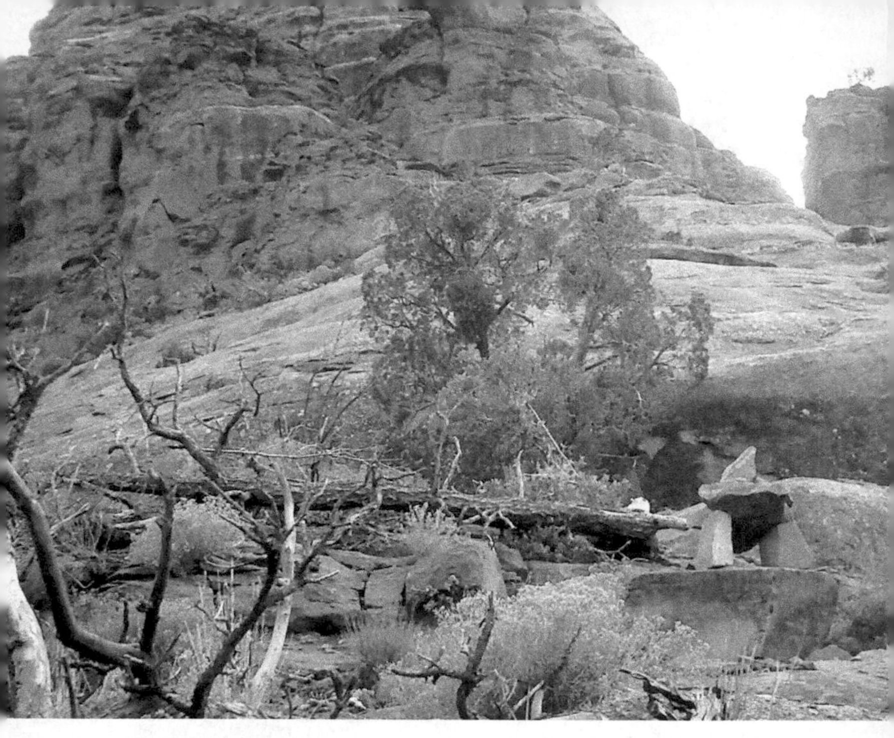

CAIRNS AT BELL ROCK

something startling across the surrounding slopes. You will never stop being amazed by what you see when you look up. At least, I haven't stopped.

Hundreds of trails wander across this region, and almost all of them are enjoyable to some extent. Narrowing that down to 36 for this guidebook took some hard thinking. I could have gone to at least 50 before the quality started to fade.

The publisher designed this book to be as helpful to as many hikers as possible. I then chose hikes for this guide with an eye to variety and quality, both in terrain type and difficulty. What all of the routes have in common is that they are day hikes. They are more than walks: Even the easiest will take at least an hour. They are less than expeditions: Even the most strenuous can be done in a day (assuming you get an early start). Hardened adventurers might find the hike descriptions remedial, though they may appreciate the maps and the GPS coordinates. Novice hikers might be overwhelmed by the more aggressive hikes, so I've identified easy turnaround points wherever reasonable.

These hikes will take you all over the place. They climb frigid mountain peaks and drop down to desert-canyon swimming holes. They traverse stark desert and alpine tundra, and every strata of mixed conifers in between. They visit the remnants of cowboys and Native Americans alike. They wander around pillars of sculpted sandstone and piles of blasted lava. They stretch along open prairies and tunnel through deep forests. They lead to archways and sinkholes, springs and caves, spires and vortices, and thousand-foot cliffs where the history of a geologic era is displayed in brightly colored sandstone.

In some places you share these trails with deer, javelina (sometimes called peccary [but not in Arizona]), or even black bears and rattlesnakes. If you do every hike in this book, I guarantee that you'll encounter at least one rattlesnake. I did. Mostly, though, you will share the trails with other people. Sedona and Flagstaff see nearly 4 million visitors a year, many of whom merge with the large and active local hiking community on the trails. There was only one hike where I did not encounter at least one other person. That was where I met the rattlesnake.

Other hikers were, for the most part, friendly—many extremely so. Why not? They've made the journey for the same reason you will: because the view beyond the parking lot is absolutely worth it.

Hike safely. Have fun. And try not to get lost—that's my job.

Recommended Hikes

Best Hikes for Scenery

Best Hikes for Wildlife

Best Hikes for Seclusion

Best Hikes for Kids

Best Hikes for Dogs

Best History Hikes

Best Geology Hikes

Best Hikes for Wildflowers

Best for Fall Leaves

Best Vortex Hikes

Best Arizona Trail Segments

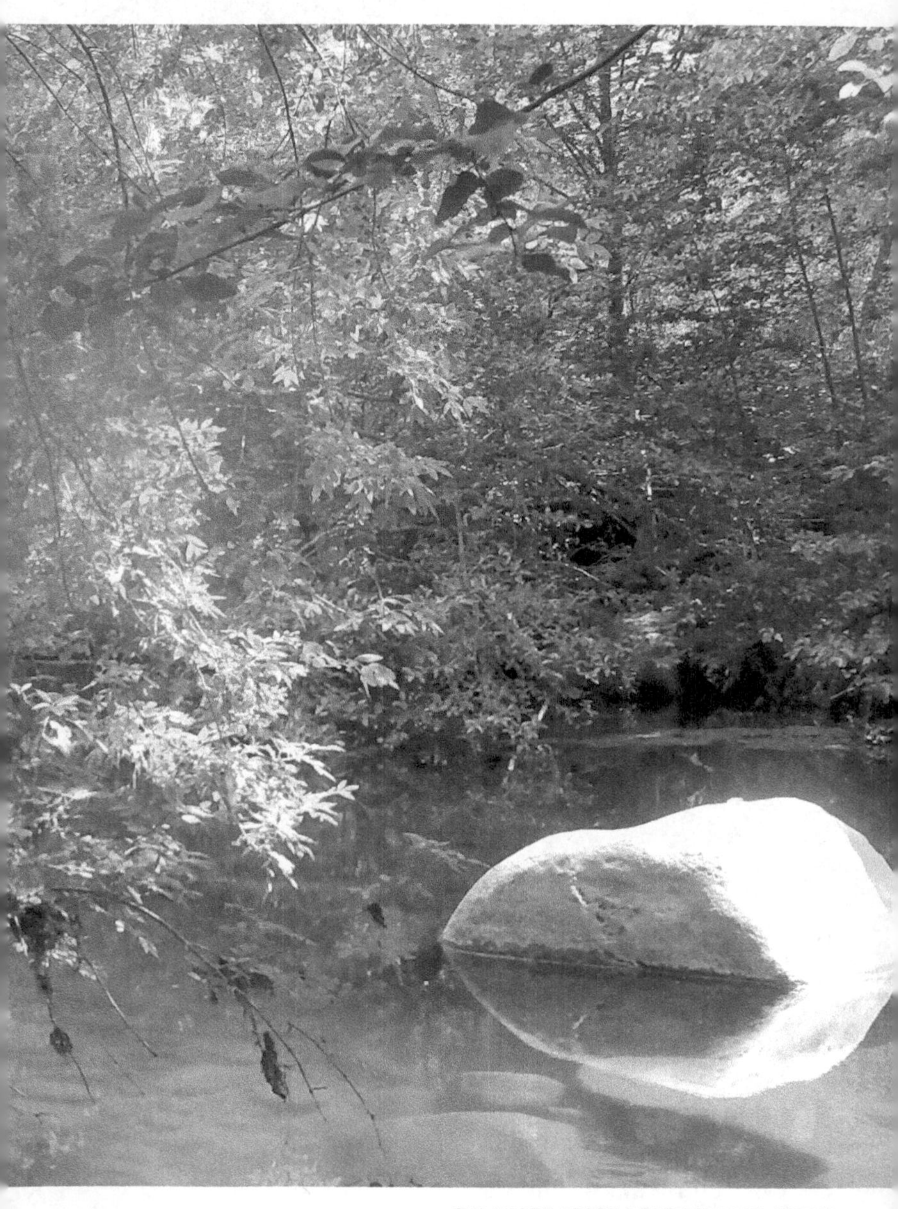

SYCAMORE CREEK NEAR PARSONS SPRING

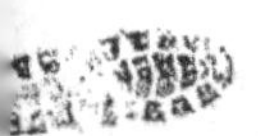

Introduction

About This Book

Sedona and Flagstaff are two small cities (Sedona is really just a town) in north-central Arizona. Though they are less than 30 miles apart, they are very different in terms of population, geography, and culture. What they have in common, though, is a high volume of tourist traffic, active outdoor communities, and extensive networks of trails branching into the surrounding mountains and wilderness. (Most of the trails are maintained by the U.S. Forest Service.) An hour's drive from either Sedona or Flagstaff can cover a lot of diverse geography, so in addition to dividing the book in half by city, each city is divided into regions as well.

Flagstaff

At an elevation of 7,000 feet, along the base of the San Francisco Peaks, Flagstaff is one of the highest cities in the United States. It has long been the center of commerce in northern Arizona, being a junction point of railroads and highways for most of its existence as a settled place. In July 1876 a party of settlers made an extended stopover in what is now Thorpe Park, and they fashioned a flagpole out of a stripped pine tree to celebrate the Fourth of July. That landmark, which stood for years afterwards, gave the settlement its name. The railroad, which reached the town in 1882, gave the settlement an economic purpose.

Flagstaff is now a small city, with a population of around 50,000, a major state university, a shopping mall, a ski resort, the county seat, and an Old Town district jammed with gift shops, restaurants, and bars—lots of bars. As a waiter explains, "We are a drinking town with a college problem."

In sober daylight, however, residents and visitors alike can explore the surrounding forests, peaks, canyons, and cinder cones. Flagstaff has three national monuments near or within city limits, and is surrounded by the Coconino and Kaibab national forests. On top of it all, literally, is the Kachina Wilderness, encapsulating the top of the San Francisco Peaks, the towering remnants of the largest of many volcanoes that burst forth from the top of the plateau as recently as 10,000 years ago.

In the summer of 2010 (as this book was being written), the Schultz Fire, named for the Schultz Pass site of the unattended campfire that started the blaze, incinerated more than 15,000 acres of forest along the north slopes of the Eldens (Little Elden and Mount Elden) and the southern and western slopes of the San Francisco Peaks. While no lives were lost and little property directly burned, the aftereffects will go on for decades. Homes spared from flames were flooded instead, as rainwater rushed unimpeded down the now-naked slopes. Lost for the season were signature hikes such as Inner Basin. Lost for a generation were good trails such as Little Bear, southern Water Line, and, of course, Schultz Pass.

CENTRAL FLAGSTAFF: Mount Elden is the tallest of several closely related peaks on the north edge of Flagstaff. Three of the trails in this section (Fatman's Loop, Little Elden Springs, and Mount Elden Loop) explore these slopes. A bit farther north, O'Leary Peak rises between Sunset Crater and Wupatki national monuments. Climbing to the top of the service road to that peak (which also houses a forest lookout station) offers panoramas from a different perspective.

SOUTH OF FLAGSTAFF: Sandys and Walnut canyons wind along the south edge of city limits, while Anderson Mesa juts up across the road from Lake Mary, all accessible from Lake Mary Road. Winter Cabin and Kelsey Springs loops, formed from a web of trails wandering through Sycamore Canyon, can only be reached by rough forest roads.

WILLIAMS: From its founding as a railroad work camp, Williams was the Wild West, as in drunken-gunfights-outside-the-brothel Wild West. It has tamed down to become a tourist spot—it's one of the last remaining towns on historic Route 66, and one of the last stops for gas and groceries on the way to the Grand Canyon.

Bill Williams Mountain offers steep climbs through old timbers. The Sycamore Rim Loop explores the north edge of Sycamore Canyon and is bisected by the historical Overland Trail, once the pack route between Flagstaff and Jerome. Farther west, you can explore the abandoned Johnson Canyon section of the Santa Fe Railroad, including the infamous tunnel that finally drove railroad planners to search out a more level approach.

THE SAN FRANCISCO PEAKS: Some peaks in the Cascades of the Pacific Northwest still dwarf this highest Arizona range, but it is tall enough here. It is the only spot in the state where you can hike above tree line. Three trails, Abineau–Bearjaw Loop, Weatherford Trail, and Humphreys Trail (leading to the highest point on the mountain) will get you there. The Kachina Trail is a gentler hike around the base of the peaks, while the Veit Springs Loop is a kid-friendly romp through springs and old cabins and tall trees.

Sedona

The town of Sedona lies at the mouth of Oak Creek Canyon as it carves into the face of the Mogollon Rim, the southern boundary of the Colorado Plateau, an uplift that covers portions of five states. Erosion and faulting have revealed the red, orange, and white sandstone cliffs and formations that have made the area world-renowned.

The Coconino National Forest, specifically the Red Rock Ranger District, surrounds Sedona. Three major wilderness areas are within sight of the town. The town itself is the center of a web of trails going up the hills, around the buttes, and into the canyons. The U.S. Forest Service maintains a major visitor center south of town on AZ 179 and also posts a representative in the Chamber of Commerce Visitor Center in uptown Sedona.

Sedona is composed of three distinct districts: West Sedona, Uptown Sedona, and the nearby Village of Oak Creek. West Sedona is the functional portion of the town, while Uptown Sedona consists primarily of resorts, restaurants, gift shops, and galleries. The Village of Oak Creek, about 4 miles south of Sedona, offers similar—if slightly lower-end—services.

The town has all the necessary amenities, but outside of gas and basic groceries, you should expect to pay a premium, especially for lodging. Many stores offer outdoor supplies, but mostly higher-end stuff at gift-store prices. Your nearest big-box retailer (for cheap stuff) is in Cottonwood. You can also shop for New Age–related books and paraphernalia and western and New Age–themed art at any number of shops and galleries.

The center of town is "The Y," the intersection of AZ 179 and AZ 89A. Actually a roundabout, this junction is north of the bridge crossing Oak Creek on AZ 179 and south of uptown Sedona on AZ 89A. It is worth locating on a map, as many of the directions in this guide (and many other published sources) proceed from this point.

The 10,000-plus residents of Sedona are collectively older and wealthier than the U.S. average. Along with the tourists, they support deep and thriving artistic and New Age communities, whose works are represented in galleries and gift shops all across town. A library, an airport, and an outpatient medical center complete the town setting. The nearest hospital is 20 minutes south in Cottonwood.

J. J. Thompson is credited as the first homesteader in the area, in Oak Creek Canyon. In 1876 he redeveloped gardens left by the Apaches, whom the U.S. Army had chased out a few years earlier. Other settlers followed, growing fruit and raising cows and horses. Their names—Scheurman, Wilson, Lee, and Schnebly, among many—identify local landmarks. By 1902 the residents grew weary of retrieving mail from Flagstaff, and they established a post office. The name they settled on was the first name of the new postmaster's wife: Sedona Schnebly.

Sedona remained a small farming community through most of the 20th century. Though several western films were shot in the area, the town did not become the tourist nexus that it is today until better roads were laid down in the 1970s. The community was not incorporated until 1988—after which the local merchants began more aggressively promoting themselves. If they seem overwhelmed by visitors, they really have no one to blame but themselves.

I have organized the Sedona-area hikes into four sections: Cottonwood, Southeast Sedona, Dry Creek, and Oak Creek Canyon.

COTTONWOOD: This Sedona-area community is a relatively normal small city about a 20-minute drive south of Sedona. Though the residents try to bring in tourists, their economy is not dependent on them. Cottonwood is, and always has been, easier to get to than most of the neighboring towns, so it is the center of commerce. In modern terms, this means that it has the hospital, the Home Depot, and the Walmart.

The two Verde River Greenway hikes follow the water as it flows near the downtown Cottonwood area and near Dead Horse Ranch State Park, which lies essentially in town. The Parsons Trail follows the lower mouth of Sycamore Canyon about 20 miles to the west. Lime Kiln Trail follows the historical wagon route that once connected Sedona to Cottonwood.

Cottonwood lies at about 3,500 feet, significantly lower and warmer than Sedona, so summer hikes should be considered with care. Parsons Spring and the Verde River Greenway hikes offer swimming holes, but Lime Kiln can be a long march in the sun if tried in its entirety at the height of summer.

SOUTHEAST SEDONA: Five hikes in this section are south and a little east of Sedona proper. (Airport Mesa Loop, which is actually within city limits, in West Sedona, is an exception.)

All of these hikes are heavily traveled except the Woods Canyon Trail. While it departs from the always-busy U.S. Forest Service Visitor Center just south of the Village of Oak Creek, it soon becomes relatively abandoned once that parking lot is out of sight. Four of these hikes are within sight of civilization. The most remote one, Bell Trail, explores the Wet Beaver Creek Wilderness, about 30 miles southeast of town, just across I-17.

DRY CREEK: Dry Creek Road (Forest Road 152) runs north from Sedona, roughly splitting the Red Rock portion from the Secret Mountain portion of the wilderness area, though administratively they are combined. This rough but passable dirt road provides access to three trails: Brins Mesa, Vultee Arch, and the Secret Canyon–Bear Sign Canyon Loop. Boynton Canyon, while in roughly the same direction, can be reached without leaving pavement, which only adds to its popularity.

OAK CREEK CANYON: This is the showcase for Sedona. Without the perennial Oak Creek cutting a canyon through the red rocks, Sedona would be just another dusty farming village—if it existed at all. Towering over this canyon is Wilson Mountain, the highest point in the region and the only serious climb in the Sedona half of the guide.

Three of the hikes in the Oak Creek Canyon section form a loop that runs from Oak Creek toward Schnebly Hill (that is Hike 32, Huckaby Trail), up Bear Wallow Canyon (Hike 33, Munds Wagon Trail), across the Cow Pies and Mitten Ridge and then back down to Oak Creek (Hike 34, Mitten Ridge).

The jewel in the crown, of course, is West Fork Trail, up the West Fork of Oak Creek, one of the most scenic hikes in the state, if not the country. It's crowded, expensive ($10 for parking), and still worth it.

How to Use This Guidebook

The following information walks you through this guidebook's organization to make it easy and convenient for you to plan great hikes in the Flagstaff-Sedona area.

Overview Map, Overview Map Key, and Map Legend

The overview map on the inside front cover depicts the location of the primary trailhead for all 36 hikes in this book. The numbers shown on the overview map pair with the map key on the first page. Each hike's number remains with that hike throughout the book. Thus, if you spot an appealing hiking area on the overview map, you can flip through the book and find those hikes easily by their numbers at the top of each profile page.

Trail Maps

In addition to the overview map on the inside cover, a detailed map of each hike's route appears with its profile. On this map, symbols indicate the trailhead, the complete route, significant features, facilities, and topographic landmarks such as creeks, overlooks, and peaks. A legend identifying the map symbols used throughout the book appears on the inside back cover.

To produce the highly accurate maps in this book, I used a handheld GPS unit to gather data while hiking each route, and then sent that data to the publisher's expert cartographers. Most of these hikes were done holding a Garmin GPSmap 60CSx, which is a fine unit but can still be off by up to 70 feet or so, especially in a deep canyon. Your GPS is not really a substitute for sound, sensible navigation according to conditions on the ground. Most of the trails in this book are actually quite easy to follow, so where they differ from our imaginary lines, stay on the trail.

Further, despite the high quality of the maps in this guidebook, the publisher and I strongly recommend that you always carry an additional map, such as the ones noted in each hike profile's introductory listing for "Maps."

Elevation Profile (diagram)

For all featured trails, the hike description will include this graphic profile. Also, each entry will list the elevation at the hike ***trailhead,*** and it will list the elevation ***peak*** if there is any notable elevation change for that trail. Otherwise, it will simply indicate the trailhead elevation.

The elevation diagram represents the rises and falls of the trail as viewed from the side, over the complete distance (in miles) of that trail. On the diagram's vertical axis, or height scale, the number of feet indicated between each tick mark lets you visualize the climb. To avoid making flat hikes look steep and steep hikes appear flat, varying height scales provide an accurate image of each hike's climbing difficulty. For example, one hike's scale might rise to 3,500 feet, while another goes to 13,000 feet.

The Hike Profile

This book contains a concise and informative narrative of each hike from beginning to end. The text will get you from a well-known road or highway to the trailhead, to the twists and turns of the hike route, back to the trailhead, and to notable nearby attractions, if there are any. Each profile opens with the route's star ratings, GPS trailhead coordinates, and other key information. Below is an explanation of the introductory elements that give you a snapshot of each of this book's 36 routes.

Star Ratings

Five-Star Trails is the Menasha Ridge Press series title of guidebooks geared to specific cities across the United States, such as this one for Flagstaff and Sedona. Following is the explanation for the rating system of one to five stars in each of the five categories.

FOR SCENERY:

★★★★★ Unique, picturesque panoramas
★★★★ Diverse vistas
★★★ Pleasant views
★★ Unchanging landscape
★ Not selected for scenery

Author's note: Every hike in this guide was, at some level, selected for scenery.

FOR TRAIL CONDITION:

★★★★★ Consistently well maintained
★★★★ Stable, with no surprises
★★★ Average terrain to negotiate
★★ Inconsistent, with good and poor areas
★ Rocky, overgrown, or often muddy

Author's note: With a few exceptions, all the trails in this guide are in good condition.

FOR CHILDREN:

★★★★★ Babes in strollers are welcome
★★★★ Fun for anyone past the toddler stage
★★★ Good for young hikers with proven stamina
★★ Not enjoyable for children
★ Not advisable for children

Author's note: I have been spoiled by my own children and rate a child's abilities with a fair bit of optimism. If your young companions do not hike regularly, you may want to adjust my ratings down one notch.

FOR DIFFICULTY:

★★★★★ Grueling
★★★★ Strenuous
★★★ Moderate (won't beat you up—but you'll know you've been hiking)
★★ Easy with patches of moderate
★ Good for a relaxing stroll

FOR SOLITUDE:

★★★★★ Positively tranquil
★★★★ Spurts of isolation
★★★ Moderately secluded
★★ Crowded on weekends and holidays
★ Steady stream of individuals and/or groups

Author's note: As I hinted in the "Preface," hikes in this region do not offer a great deal of solitude.

GPS Trailhead Coordinates

As noted previously in "Trail Maps," I used a handheld GPS unit to obtain geographic data and sent that information to the publisher's cartographers. For each hike profile, I have provided the intersection of the latitude (north) and longitude (west) coordinates to orient you at the trailhead. In some cases, you can drive within viewing distance of a trailhead. Other hikes require a short walk to reach the trailhead from a parking area. Either way, the trailhead coordinates are given from the trail's actual head—its point of origin. You will also note that this guidebook uses the degree–decimal minute format for presenting the GPS coordinates.

The latitude–longitude grid system is likely quite familiar to you, but here is a refresher, pertinent to visualizing the GPS coordinates:

Imaginary lines of latitude—called parallels and approximately 69 miles apart from each other—run horizontally around the globe. Each parallel is indicated by degrees from the equator (established to be 0°): up to 90°N at the North Pole, and down to 90°S at the South Pole.

Imaginary lines of longitude—called meridians—run perpendicular to latitude lines. Longitude lines are likewise indicated by degrees: Starting from 0° at the Prime Meridian in Greenwich, England, they continue to the east and west until they meet 180° later at the International Date Line in the Pacific Ocean. At the equator, longitude lines also are approximately 69 miles apart, but that distance narrows as the meridians converge toward the North and South poles.

To convert GPS coordinates given in degrees, minutes, and seconds to the format in degrees–decimal minutes, the seconds are divided by 60. For more on GPS technology, visit **usgs.gov.**

Distance & Configuration

The distance shown is for the hike from start to finish, as recorded with the GPS unit. There may be options to shorten or extend the hike, but the mileage corresponds to the hike described. The configuration defines the trail as a loop, an out-and-back (taking you in and out via the same route), a figure-eight, or a balloon. As the mileage is for the total hike, it is measured round-trip.

Hiking Time

Unlike distance, which is a real, measured number, hiking time is an estimate. Every hiker has a different pace. Mine is about 2 miles per hour (when taking notes and pictures), and that is the standard for most of the hike times. I made some adjustment for steepness, rough terrain, and high elevation. There is some time built in for a quick breather here and there, but hikers should consider that any prolonged break (such as lunch or swimming) will add to the hike time.

Highlights

The author provides a capsule list of the main attractions, such as a waterfall or a historical site, that draw hikers to this trail.

Elevation

At the beginning of each hike's profile, you will see the elevation at the trailhead and another figure for the peak height on that route. Because most of these routes entail significant inclines and declines, the full hike profile will also include a complete elevation profile diagram (see page 7).

Access

Fees or permits needed to hike the trail are indicated here, and I note if there are none.

Maps

U.S. Geological Survey maps serve as the basis for maps within this book. I also recommend the Beartooth Maps, which are available for both Flagstaff and Sedona and are specific to hiking. U.S. Forest Service (USFS) maps, particularly the one for Coconino National Forest, contain the best rendering of forest roads. All of these maps are available at any local outdoor retailer and at the USFS visitor centers in Sedona, Flagstaff, or Williams.

Facilities

For planning a hike, it's helpful to know what to expect at the trailhead or nearby in terms of restrooms, phones, water, and other niceties.

Wheelchair Access

For each hike, you will readily see whether or not it is feasible for the enjoyment of outdoor enthusiasts who use a wheelchair.

Comments

Here you will find assorted nuggets of information, such as whether or not your dog is allowed on the trails.

Contacts

To check trail conditions or to answer other questions, you'll find phone numbers and websites here.

Overview, Route Details, Nearby Attractions, and Directions

Each profile contains a complete narrative of the hike: "Overview" gives you a quick summary of what to expect on that trail. "Route Details" guides you on the hike, start to finish. "Nearby Attractions" suggests other area sites that you might like, such as restaurants, museums, or other trails. "Directions" will get you to the trailhead from a well-known road or highway.

Weather

Sedona occupies a sweet spot in terms of climate. Afternoon temperatures will touch 100°F in the summer, but they won't stay there week after week as they will in the lower deserts. There will be a dusting of snow in the winter, but the town won't be buried by it week after week as happens on top of the Mogollon Rim.

Flagstaff, because of its elevation, often mimics the weather of points farther north. Summer highs rarely break out of the 80s, while winter can bury the slopes in snow, shortening the hiking season to late spring through early autumn. Many of the locals will tackle these trails with parkas and snowshoes, but that is outside the coverage of this guide.

Two annual events influence hiking conditions of both regions every year. First is the spring runoff that will turn otherwise-dry washes into roaring creeks. The other is the monsoon season. From about mid-July through late September, storm systems will flow up from the Sea of Cortez and across the state. This means that every afternoon for about 2 months, there is a standing threat of rain. While this is little more than a nuisance in Sedona, it could be a hazard on the high slopes of Flagstaff, where the rain turns cold and the storm comes with plenty of lightning.

As a general rule, wildflowers bloom first in the lower deserts, and the color works uphill through spring to the high-slope prairies around Flagstaff in early summer. The more rain and snow in the previous winter, the more the flowers will bloom. Fall leaves, conversely, start turning in the Flagstaff area as early as September, while trees in the lowlands around Cottonwood might stay green well into November.

The following charts list average temperatures and precipitation by month for both regions. "Hi Temp" is the average daytime high, and "Lo Temp" is the average nighttime low for that month. "Rain" lists average precipitation for that month, be it rain or snow.

FLAGSTAFF			
MONTH	HI TEMP	LO TEMP	RAIN
January	42°F	15°F	2.0"
February	45°F	17°F	2.1"
March	49°F	21°F	2.6"
April	57°F	26°F	1.5"
May	67°F	33°F	0.7"
June	78°F	41°F	0.4"
July	81°F	50°F	2.8"
August	79°F	48°F	2.8"
September	73°F	41°F	2.0"
October	63°F	31°F	1.6"
November	51°F	22°F	2.0"
December	43°F	15°F	2.4"

SEDONA			
MONTH	HI TEMP	LO TEMP	RAIN
January	56°F	30°F	2.0"
February	60°F	33°F	1.9"
March	65°F	36°F	2.1"

SEDONA			
MONTH	HI TEMP	LO TEMP	RAIN
April	73°F	42°F	1.1"
May	82°F	49°F	0.6"
June	92°F	58°F	0.4"
July	96°F	65°F	1.7"
August	93°F	64°F	2.1"
September	88°F	58°F	1.7"
October	78°F	49°F	1.5"
November	65°F	37°F	1.4"
December	57°F	31°F	1.5"

Water

How much is enough? A hiker walking steadily in 90°F heat needs approximately 10 quarts of fluid per day. That's 2.5 gallons. A good rule of thumb is to hydrate prior to your hike, carry (and drink) 6 ounces of water for every mile you plan to hike, and hydrate again after the hike. If you are hiking in the desert in the summer (any hike in the Southeast Sedona or Cottonwood section qualifies), you should double this formula. For most people, the pleasures of hiking make carrying water a relatively minor price to pay to remain safe and healthy. So pack more water than you anticipate needing even for short hikes. Only a handful of hikes in this guide pass by reliable water sources.

If you are tempted to drink "found water," do so with extreme caution. Every water source in these regions drain through cattle country, leaving what water can be found a prime threat for giardia parasites. Painful intestinal giardiasis can last for weeks after ingestion. For information, visit the Centers for Disease Control website at **cdc.gov/parasites/giardia.**

In any case, effective treatment is essential before using any water source found along the trail. Boiling water for 2–3 minutes is always a safe measure for camping, but day hikers can consider iodine tablets, approved chemical mixes, filtration units rated for giardia, and UV filtration. Some of these methods (for example, filtration with an added carbon filter) remove bad tastes typical in stagnant water, while others add their own taste. Carry a means of purification to help in a pinch and if you realize you have underestimated your consumption needs.

Clothing

Weather, unexpected trail conditions, fatigue, extended hiking duration, and wrong turns can individually or collectively turn a great outing into a very uncomfortable one at best—and a life-threatening one at worst. Thus, proper attire plays a key role in staying comfortable and, sometimes, staying alive. Here are some helpful guidelines:

- ★ Choose silk, wool, or synthetics for maximum comfort in all of your hiking attire—from hats to socks and in between. Cotton is fine if the weather remains dry and stable, but you won't be happy if it gets wet.
- ★ Always wear a hat, or at least tuck one into your day pack or hitch it to your belt. Hats offer all-weather sun and wind protection as well as warmth if it turns cold.
- ★ Be ready to layer up or down as the day progresses and the mercury rises or falls. Today's outdoor wear makes layering easy, with such designs as jackets that convert to vests and zip-off or button-up legs.
- ★ Wear hiking boots or sturdy hiking sandals with toe protection. Flip-flopping on a paved path in an urban botanical garden is one thing, but never hike a trail in open sandals or casual sneakers. Your bones and arches need support, and your skin needs protection.
- ★ Pair that footwear with good socks! If you prefer not to sheathe your feet when wearing hiking sandals, tuck the socks into your day pack; you may need them if the weather plummets or if you hit rocky turf and pebbles begin to irritate your feet. And in an emergency, if you have lost your gloves, you can adapt the socks into mittens.
- ★ Don't leave rainwear behind, even if the day dawns clear and sunny (especially in August). Tuck into your day pack, or tie around your waist, a jacket that is breathable and either water-resistant or waterproof. Investigate different choices at your local outdoors

retailer. If you are a frequent hiker, ideally you'll have more than one rainwear weight, material, and style in your closet to protect you in all seasons in your regional climate and hiking microclimates.

Essential Gear

Today you can buy outdoor vests that have up to 20 pockets shaped and sized to carry everything from toothpicks to binoculars. Or, if you don't aspire to feel like a burro, you can neatly stow all of these items in your day pack or backpack. The following list showcases never-hike-without-them items:

- *Water:* As emphasized more than once in this book, bring more than you think you will drink. Two small containers are better than one huge one. That way, if one leaks all over your extra clothes, you are inconvenienced, not doomed. Depending on your destination, you may want to bring a water bottle and iodine or filter for purifying water in the wilderness in case you run out.
- *Map and high-quality compass:* Even if you know the terrain from previous hikes, don't leave home without these tools. As noted earlier, you should always carry more than one map.
- *A pocketknife* and/or multitool.
- *Flashlight or headlamp* with extra bulb and batteries.
- *Windproof matches* and/or a lighter, as well as a fire starter.
- *Extra food:* Trail mix, granola bars, or other high-energy foods.
- *Extra clothes:* Raingear, warm hat, gloves, and change of socks and shirt.
- *Whistle:* You can only shout so loud and for so long. As anyone with children knows, though, you can blow a whistle forever.
- *Duct tape:* One of those small rolls you get at the drugstore will do. Not just for holding gear together after it has fallen apart, duct tape is also good for blisters if you apply it to the swelling early enough.
- *Sunscreen:* The desert sun will burn you red within an hour. Note the expiration date on the tube or bottle; it's usually embossed on the top.
- *Insect repellent:* For some areas and seasons, this is extremely vital. See "Mosquitoes," page 20.

First-aid Kit

In addition to the items above, those below may appear overwhelming for a day hike. But any paramedic will tell you that the products listed here, in alphabetical order, are just the basics. The reality of hiking is that you can be out for a week of backpacking and acquire only a mosquito bite—or you can hike for an hour, slip, and suffer a bleeding abrasion or broken bone. Fortunately, these items will collapse into a very small space, and convenient, prepackaged kits are available at your pharmacy and online.

Consider your intended terrain and the number of hikers in your party before you exclude any article listed below. A botanical-garden stroll may not inspire you to carry a complete kit, but anything beyond that warrants precaution. When hiking alone, you should always be prepared for a medical need. And if you are a twosome or with a group, one or more people in your party should be equipped with first-aid material.

- Ace bandages or Spenco joint wraps
- Antibiotic ointment (Neosporin or the generic equivalent)
- Athletic tape
- Band-Aids
- Benadryl or the generic equivalent, diphenhydramine (in case of allergic reactions)
- Blister kit (such as moleskin/Spenco Second Skin)
- Butterfly-closure bandages
- Epinephrine in a prefilled syringe (for people known to have severe allergic reactions to such things as bee stings, usually by prescription only)
- Gauze (one roll and a half dozen 4-by-4-inch pads)
- Hydrogen peroxide or iodine
- Ibuprofen or acetaminophen

General Safety

Mother Nature has no sympathy for the foolish or unlucky. If you are to journey beyond sight of your car, take these sensible precautions:

- ★ *Always let someone know where you will be hiking and how long you expect to be gone.* It's a good idea to give that person a copy of your route, particularly if you are headed into any isolated area. Let them know when you return.
- ★ *Always sign in and out of any trail registers provided.* Don't hesitate to comment on the trail condition if space is provided; that's your opportunity to alert others to any problems you encounter.
- ★ *Do not count on a cell phone for your safety.* Reception may be spotty or nonexistent on the trail, even on an urban walk embraced by towering trees.
- ★ *Always carry food and water, even for a short hike.* And bring more water than you think you will need. (I cannot say this often enough!)
- ★ *Stay on designated trails.* Even on the most clearly marked trails, there is usually a point where you have to stop and consider in which direction to head. If you become disoriented, don't panic. As soon as you think you may be off-track, stop, assess your current direction, and then retrace your steps to the point where you went astray. Using a map, a compass, and this book, and keeping in mind what you have passed thus far, reorient yourself and trust your judgment on which way to continue. If you become absolutely unsure of how to continue, return to your vehicle the way you came in. Should you become completely lost and have no idea how to return to the trailhead, remaining in place along the trail and waiting for help is most often the best option for adults and always the best option for children.
- ★ *Always carry a whistle.* It may be a lifesaver (or at least a major stress-reducer) if you do become lost or sustain an injury.
- ★ *Be especially careful when crossing streams.* Whether you are fording the stream or crossing on a log, make every step count. If you have any doubt about maintaining your balance on a log, ford the stream instead: Use a trekking pole or stout stick for balance, and face upstream as you cross. If a stream seems too deep to ford, turn back. Whatever is on the other side is not worth risking your life.

- *Be careful at overlooks.* While these areas may provide spectacular views, they are potentially hazardous. Stay back from the edge of outcrops, and be absolutely sure of your footing; a misstep can mean a nasty and possibly fatal fall.
- *Standing dead trees and storm-damaged living trees pose a real hazard to hikers.* These trees may have loose or broken limbs that could fall at any time. While walking beneath trees and when choosing a spot to rest or enjoy your snack, look up!
- *Know the symptoms of hypothermia.* Shivering and forgetfulness are the two most common indicators of this stealthy killer. Hypothermia can occur at any elevation, even in the summer, especially when the hiker is wearing lightweight cotton clothing. If symptoms present themselves, get to shelter, hot liquids, and dry clothes ASAP.
- *Know the symptoms of heat exhaustion (hyperthermia).* Lightheadedness and loss of energy are the first two indicators. If you feel these symptoms, find some shade, drink your water, remove as many layers of clothing as practical, and stay put until you cool down. Marching through heat exhaustion leads to heatstroke—which can be fatal. If you should be sweating and you're not, that's the signature warning sign. Your hike is over at that point—heatstroke is a life-threatening condition that can cause seizures, convulsions, and eventually death. If you or a companion reaches that point, do whatever can be done to cool the victim down and seek medical attention immediately.
- *Ask questions.* U.S. Forest Service and park service employees are there to help. Also, most of the local hikers are friendly and happy to show off what they know. It's a lot easier to ask advice beforehand, and it will help you avoid a mishap away from civilization when it's too late to amend an error.
- *Most important of all, take along your brain.* A cool, calculating mind is the single most important asset on the trail. Think before you act. Watch your step. Plan ahead. Avoiding accidents before they happen is the best way to ensure a rewarding and relaxing hike.

Watchwords for Flora & Fauna

Here is some specific advice about dealing with the various hazards that come with wandering through the ecosystem. They are listed in approximate order of likelihood while hiking in the Flagstaff-Sedona area.

SNAKES: Rattlesnakes are found in Arizona elevations as high as 9,000 feet, though they will hibernate from October into April. However, the snakes you will most likely see while hiking will be nonvenomous species and subspecies. The best rule is to leave all snakes alone, give them a wide berth as you hike past, and make sure that any hiking companions (including dogs) do the same.

When hiking, stick to well-used trails and wear over-the-ankle boots and loose-fitting long pants. Rattlesnakes like to bask in the sun and won't bite unless threatened. Do not step or put your hands where you cannot see, and avoid wandering around in the dark. Step onto logs and rocks, never over them, and be especially careful when climbing rocks. Always avoid walking through dense brush or thickets.

POISON IVY, OAK, & SUMAC: Recognizing and avoiding poison ivy, oak, and sumac are the most effective ways to prevent the painful, itchy rashes associated with these plants. Poison ivy occurs as a vine or ground cover, 3 leaflets to a leaf; poison oak occurs as either a vine or shrub, also with 3 leaflets; and poison sumac flourishes in swampland, each leaf having 7–13 leaflets. Urushiol, the oil in the sap of these plants, is responsible for the rash.

Within 14 hours of exposure, raised lines and/or blisters will appear on the affected area, accompanied by a terrible itch. Refrain from scratching because bacteria under your fingernails can cause an infection. Wash and dry the affected area thoroughly, applying calamine lotion to help dry out the rash. If itching or blistering is severe, seek medical attention. If you do come into contact with one of these plants, remember that oil-contaminated clothes, pets, or hiking gear can easily cause an irritating rash on you or someone else, so wash not only any exposed parts of your body but also clothes, gear, and pets if applicable.

MOSQUITOES: Insect repellent and/or repellent-impregnated clothing are the only simple methods to ward off these pests. In some areas, including central Arizona, mosquitoes are known to carry the West Nile virus, so all due caution should be taken to avoid their bites.

TICKS: Ticks are often found on brush and tall grass, where they seem to be waiting to hitch a ride on a warm-blooded passerby. Adult ticks are most active April into May and again October into November. Among the varieties of ticks, the black-legged tick, commonly called the deer tick, is the primary carrier of Lyme disease. Wear light-colored clothing so ticks can be spotted before they make it to the skin. And be sure to visually check your hair, back of neck, armpits, and socks at the end of the hike. During your posthike shower, take a moment to do a more complete body check. For ticks that are already embedded, removal with tweezers is best. Use disinfectant solution on the wound.

BLACK BEARS: Though attacks by black bears are virtually unheard of, the sight or approach of a bear can give anyone a start. Bears have not been seen in Sedona for decades, but they still inhabit the high slopes around Flagstaff and Williams. If you encounter a bear while hiking, remain calm and never run away. Make loud noises to scare off the bear and back away slowly. In primitive and remote areas, assume bears are present; in more-developed sites, check on the current bear situation before you hike. Most encounters are food-related, as bears have an exceptional sense of smell and not particularly discriminating tastes. While this is of greater concern to backpackers and campers, on a day hike you may plan a lunchtime picnic or munch on an energy bar or other snack from time to time. So remain aware and alert.

MOUNTAIN LIONS: Though seldom encountered, where there are deer, there will be mountain lions. Lion attacks on people are rare, with fewer than 12 fatalities in 100 years. All of those fatalities occurred with solo hikers, so the single best defense against mountain lions is hiking with friends. Should you encounter one of these predatory felines, stay calm, stop or back up slowly, talk firmly to the lion, and make yourself appear as large as possible. The lion will not attack unless it's convinced you are prey. Do not turn and run because that's what a deer would do. If the animal does attack, fight back and stay on your feet.

Hunting

Separate rules, regulations, and licenses govern the various hunting types and related seasons. Though there are generally no problems, hikers may wish to forgo their trips during the big-game seasons, when the woods suddenly seem filled with orange and camouflage.

In Arizona, the season is on for some species or other from September to March, but the heavy hunting starts in November. Most of the trails around Sedona are too close to city limits for this to be a concern, but the mountains and prairies around Flagstaff are heavily hunted throughout the late fall and winter.

The Arizona Department of Game and Fish regulates all hunting in the state. It has an encyclopedic website (**azgfd.gov/h_f/hunting.shtml**) and can be reached at (602) 942-3000.

Regulations

Following are requirements you'll need to observer while hiking in the state of Arizona:

- Dogs must be leashed throughout the national forests and other jurisdictions explored in this guide.
- Any hunting or fishing requires an appropriate Arizona license, which is available from the Arizona Game and Fish Department.

Many hikes are in wilderness areas, which have their own sets of rules:

- No wheels, including no mountain bikes.
- Nothing can be removed and nothing can be left behind. This means no souvenir collecting and no physical geocaching.
- You are also limited to 15 people in a group and/or 15 head of livestock, if that somehow concerns you.
- Ruins, particularly Native American ruins (which are found

throughout the region), are specifically protected by federal law, regardless of where they are encountered, and no portion may be removed or disturbed.

- Most campgrounds and camping areas have a 14-day-stay limit.
- The Coconino National Forest may impose fire restrictions, frequently starting in late May and extending into July. This means no campfires anywhere (except in designated campgrounds) and no smoking. Any stove must be able to be instantly extinguished, which leaves, for all practical purposes, only liquid-fuel stoves.
- In winter, the Kachina Wilderness Area on top of the San Francisco Peaks requires a backcountry permit (and snowshoes are a good idea, though they are not legally required).

Trail Etiquette

Always treat the trail, wildlife, and fellow hikers with respect. Here are some reminders.

- *Plan ahead in order to be self-sufficient at all times;* carry necessary supplies for changes in weather or other conditions. A well-executed trip is a satisfaction to you and to others.
- *Hike on open trails only.*
- *Respect trail and road closures, avoid possible trespassing* on private land, and obtain all permits and authorization as required. Also, leave gates as you found them or as noted by signs.
- *Be courteous to hikers, bikers, equestrians, and others* you encounter on the trails.
- *Never spook animals.* An unannounced approach, a sudden movement, or a loud noise startles most animals. A surprised animal can be dangerous to you, to others, and to itself. Give them plenty of space.
- *Observe the* YIELD *signs* that are displayed around the region's trailheads and backcountry. They advise hikers to yield to horses, and bikers to yield to both horses and hikers. A common courtesy on hills is that hikers and bikers yield to any uphill traffic. When encountering mounted riders or horse packers, hikers can courteously step off the trail, on the downhill side if possible. Speak to the riders before they reach you, and do not dart behind trees. You are less spooky if the

horse can see and hear you. Resist the urge to pet horses unless you are invited to do so.

- *Leave only footprints.* Be sensitive to the ground beneath you. This also means staying on the existing trail and not blazing any new trails.
- *Pack out what you pack in.* No one likes to see the trash someone else has left behind.

Tips on Hiking in the Flagstaff & Sedona Area

Visit the Coconino National Forest website, **www.fs.fed.us/r3/coconino,** for information about facilities, access, and occasionally fire and flood closures. Click on "Recreational Activities," then on the map for either Red Rock (for Sedona) or Peaks (for Flagstaff) District, and then "Trails" to find information on the various trails and trailheads. (You will find anything from a vague paragraph to a complete pamphlet, depending on the hike.)

For the Williams area west of Flagstaff, the Kaibab National Forest maintains a similar website: **fs.usda.gov/kaibab.**

You need a Red Rock Pass to park at many of the recreation sites and trailheads (or even the side of the road) near the Sedona area. A 1-day pass costs $5, a 7-day pass costs $15, and an annual pass costs $20. The passes are available at any ranger station and from a multitude of merchants in and around Sedona. They are also available through solar-powered vending machines at many trailheads (1-day passes only). These passes do not apply at most fee areas, including the more popular trailheads and campgrounds along Oak Creek.

The fee areas in or near Oak Creek Canyon are run by private concessionaires and do not accept Red Rock Passes. The sole exception is Slide Rock State Park, and they won't take a Red Rock Pass either. The fees are quite stiff and these places still fill quickly, so there is no point whining about the money. The concessionaires know that the guy behind you will pay if you do not. None of these places take credit cards. Some take checks. All of them take cash.

Of the trailheads listed in this book, only three are fee areas: Call of the Canyon (West Fork Trail), Grasshopper Point (Mitten Ridge Trail), and Dead Horse Ranch State Park near Cottonwood (Lime Kiln Trail). All of the other trailheads around Sedona require only a Red Rock Pass.

None of the trails around Flagstaff require a fee or pass. Not one. They are, however, subject to seasonal closure due to snow. Flagstaff gets enough snow at times to close the interstates. However, that snow gets plowed away quickly. Snow over a remote trailhead at the end of a forest road stays until it melts.

Forest roads are maintained on a need-to-use basis, which means that some are not maintained at all. Inquire about road conditions before setting out, particularly during or after rainfall. Several trailheads listed in this guide cannot be reached by wheeled conveyance following heavy rains. As mentioned above, many trailheads around Flagstaff may be unavailable from fall to spring due to snow. Sedona, in contrast, receives few snow closures, but many roads (Dry Creek Road in particular) are closed during heavy rains.

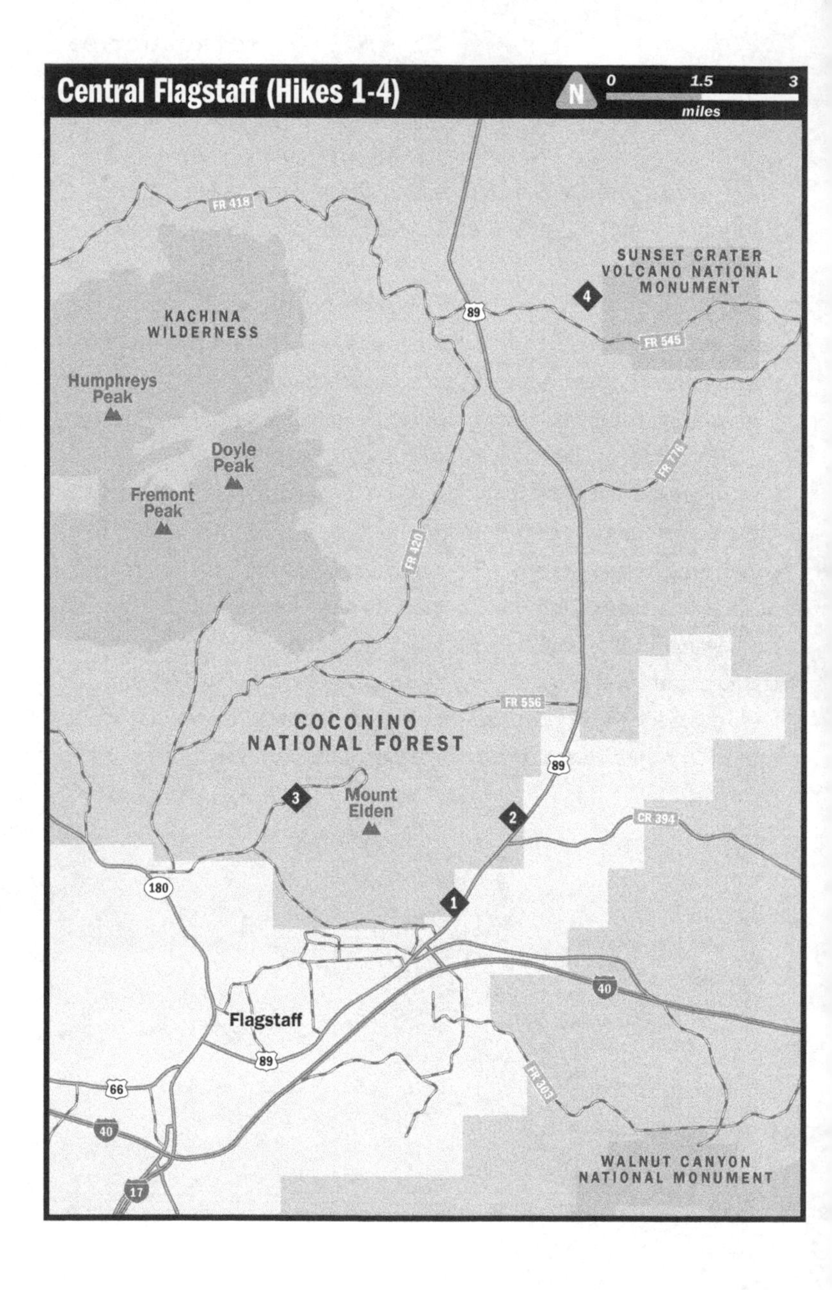

Central Flagstaff (Hikes 1-4)
N
0
1.5
3
miles
FR 418
SUNSET CRATER
VOLCANO NATIONAL
MONUMENT
4
89
KACHINA
WILDERNESS
FR 545
Humphreys
Peak
Doyle
Peak
FR 776
Fremont
Peak
FR 420
FR 556
COCONINO
NATIONAL FOREST
89
3
Mount
Elden
2
CR 394
180
1
40
Flagstaff
89
FR 303
66
40
WALNUT CANYON
NATIONAL MONUMENT
17

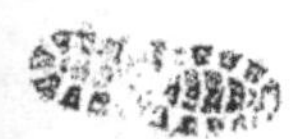

Central Flagstaff

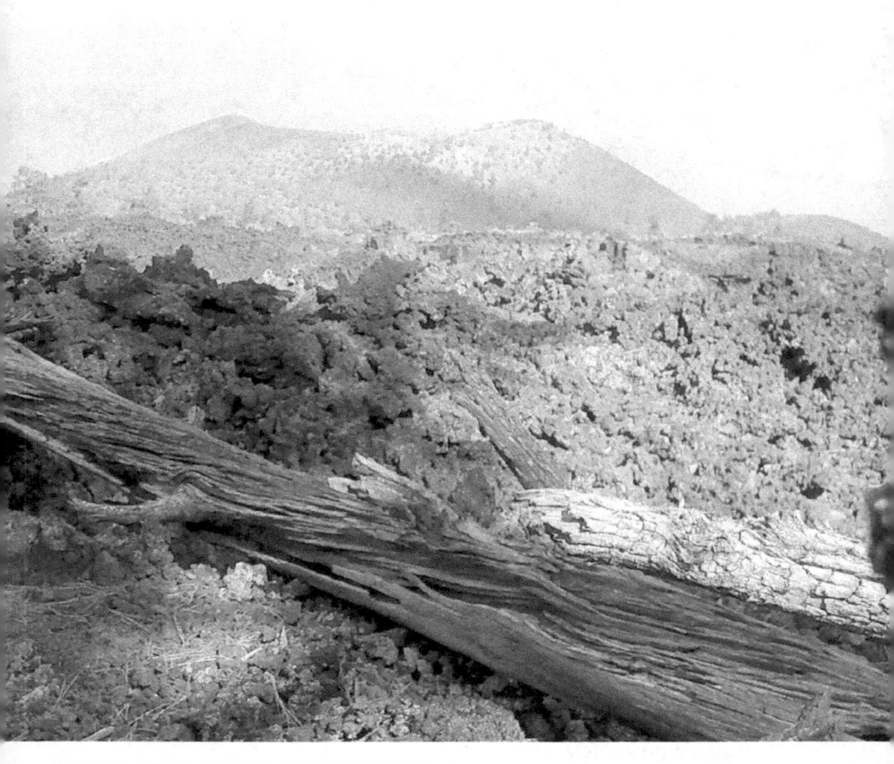

BONITO LAVA FLOW NEAR O'LEARY PEAK

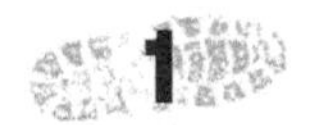

Fatman's Loop

SCENERY: ★★★★
TRAIL CONDITION: ★★★★
CHILDREN: ★★★
DIFFICULTY: ★★★
SOLITUDE: ★

FATMAN'S GAP

GPS TRAILHEAD COORDINATES: N35° 13.822' W111° 34.769'

DISTANCE & CONFIGURATION: 2.6-mile loop

HIKING TIME: 1.5 hours

HIGHLIGHTS: Vistas, geology, and foliage

ELEVATION: 6,918 feet at trailhead to 7,462 feet at top of loop

ACCESS: No fees or restrictions; open year-round

MAPS: USGS Flagstaff East

FACILITIES: None

WHEELCHAIR ACCESS: None

COMMENTS: No water available on trail. Popular with locals.

CONTACTS: Flagstaff Ranger District, 5075 N. AZ 89, Flagstaff, AZ 86004; (928) 526-0866; **www.fs.fed.us/r3/coconino/recreation/peaks/fatmans-loop-tr.shtml**

Overview

This short but strenuous hike loops up and down the face of Mount Elden, offering views of eastern Flagstaff. It presents a case study in the aftermath of a forest fire, as well as close encounters with volcanic geology. One such encounter is a squeeze between two boulders that lends the hike its name. The trail also provides a bit of a workout. These factors and the hike's proximity to town make it quite popular with the locals.

Route Details

Fatman's Loop 25 starts as a wide, easy track roughly northwest through the pine forest. A variety of plants dots these low slopes. Everything from squat prickly pear cacti to towering spruce trees greets your eye, but most of what you'll see is piñon, ponderosa pine, and some alligator juniper growing through the thick prairie grass.

The trail soon branches into a Y. There is no compelling advantage to either direction, but this hike description, for arbitrary reasons, assumes that you stay left (west) and take the loop clockwise.

Just past the Y, you come to a fence. The zigzag gate in the fence (called a deer maze) is, in fact, the tightest squeeze of the hike. An unofficial trail cuts to the right (east) to bypass the Y. Ignore it and press forward.

At 0.5 mile, you come to the junction with the Pipeline Trail 42, leading around the south slope of Mount Elden. Stay on Fatman's Loop 25. Soon after, you start to climb. The scrub closes in as you travel up the slope. The trail itself is well constructed, making the short climb more like a set of stairs and less like mountaineering.

After 0.25 mile of these steep switchbacks, views of northern Flagstaff will open up. It's hardly breathtaking. This is the industrial portion of the city, the landscape dominated by the Purina Tower and the bald remains of Sheep Hill. Beyond these sites (and sights), though, you can make out the assorted cinder cones of the eastern volcanic field, including Sunset Crater.

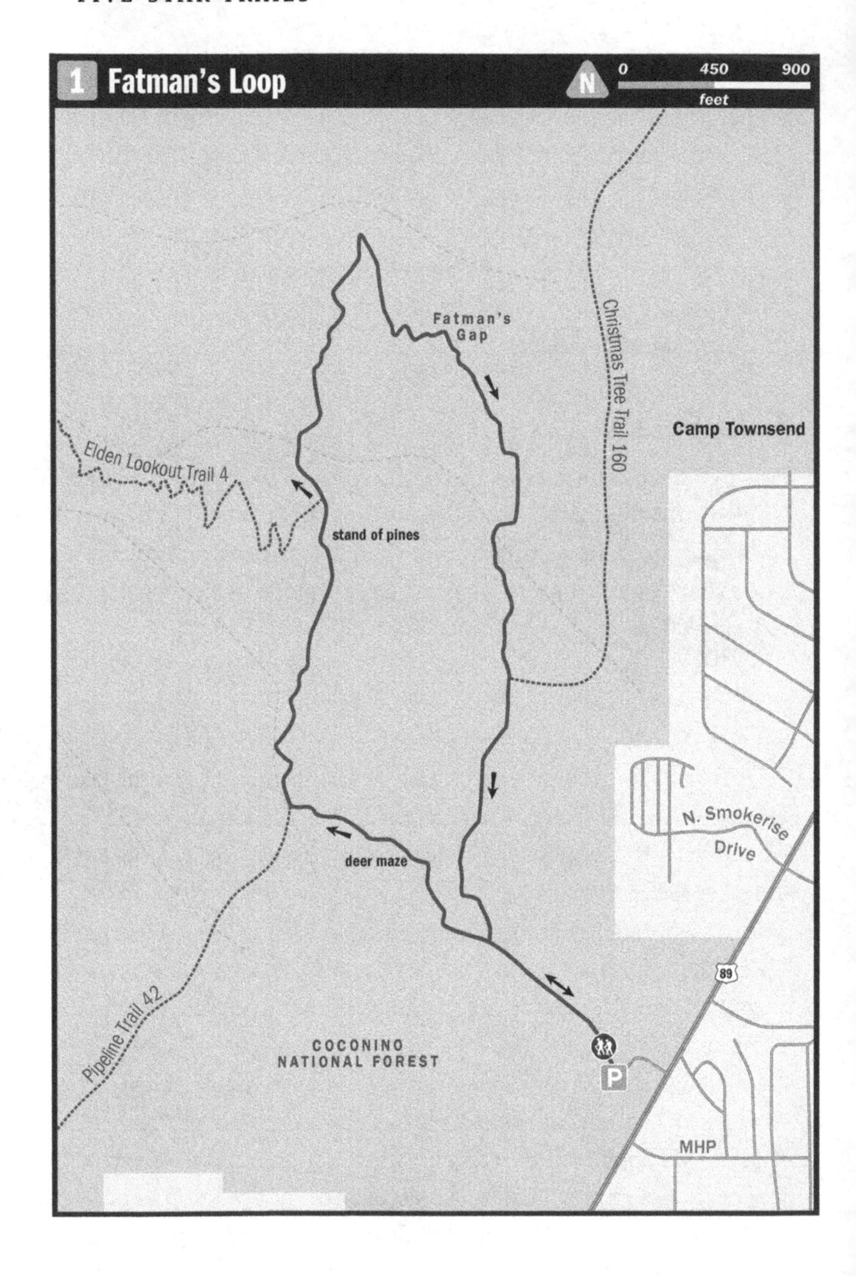
1 Fatman's Loop
N
0
450
900
feet
Fatman's Gap
Christmas Tree Trail 160
Camp Townsend
Elden Lookout Trail 4
stand of pines
N. Smokerise Drive
deer maze
89
Pipeline Trail 42
COCONINO NATIONAL FOREST
P
MHP

At 0.9 mile, a small stand of ponderosa pines grows stubbornly out of the steep slope, and the trail levels off for a while through here. To your left (northwest), Mount Elden towers steeply overhead, and another short climb brings you to the junction with the Elden Lookout Trail 4—just shy of your 1-mile mark.

Elden Lookout Trail 4 is the shortest route to the top of the mountain. This is because it goes straight up the near slope, with staircase-grade switchbacks that dare you to climb them and not die. On top of the peak are a fire lookout station and assorted transmission antennae, none of which are open to the public. This area is covered in more detail in the Mount Elden Loop hike profile (see page 38).

The trail flattens as it winds west, though you will still have a lot of little ups and downs. On the way, you pass through small stands of Gambel oaks and fields of boulders. At about 1.3 miles, the switchbacks start taking you down through this maze of scrub and rock.

At last, Fatman's Gap waits for you at the 1.5-mile mark. You have already navigated past a number of boulders crowding the trail, but the aptly named Fatman's Gap will not be mistaken. Even so, you'll fit. The squeeze is actually tighter between the Gambel oaks that immediately follow.

Past the gap, the trail continues to wind back south down the slopes. Farther down you will see boulders with little holes eroded out of them, and ancient alligator junipers large enough to house

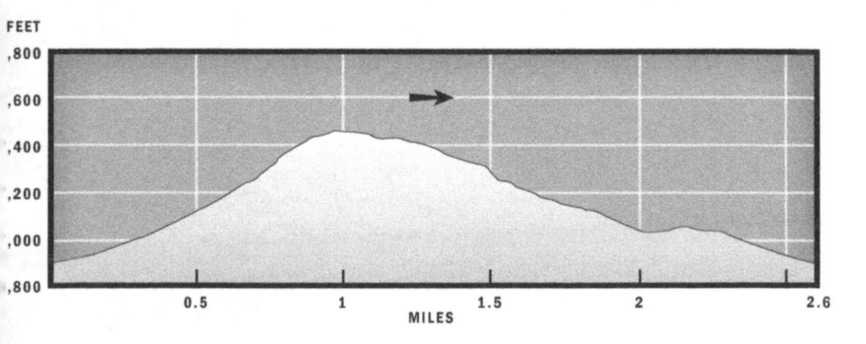

hobbits. Some of these junipers are old enough to have endured cinder fall from Sunset Crater 900 years ago.

Just beyond the 2-mile mark, you pass the junction with the Christmas Tree Trail 160, which winds westward around the mountain to eventually reach the Sandy Seep Trail 129 (see the next profile for Little Elden Springs). You, of course, stay on Fatman's. The next stop is the base of the loop. Return the way you came.

Nearby Attractions

Because this is not an all-day hike, take some time to explore downtown Flagstaff, a snug collection of bars, bookstores, retail outlets, and more bars. Among these you can find Charly's Pub & Grill in the Hotel Weatherford, a landmark that has been in business here since 1897 ([928] 779-1919; **weatherfordhotel.com**). Rooms run about $90 per night; some older rooms, with shared bath facilities, are cheaper. Charly's serves breakfast, lunch, and dinner; expect to pay $10–$25 a plate.

Directions

In Flagstaff, take AZ 89 north, past where US 66 splits off and past the Flagstaff Mall. Continue just past the Flagstaff Ranger District Office. The trailhead parking lot sits just off the north side of the street. There's a sign.

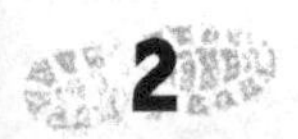

2 Little Elden Springs

SCENERY: ★★★★
TRAIL CONDITION: ★★★★
CHILDREN: ★★★
DIFFICULTY: ★★
SOLITUDE: ★★

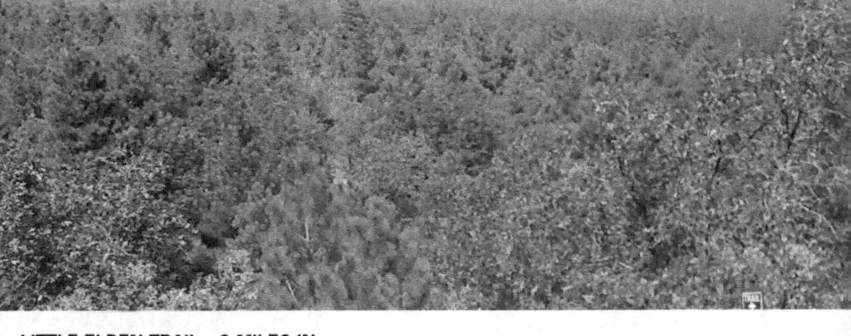

LITTLE ELDEN TRAIL—3 MILES IN

GPS TRAILHEAD COORDINATES: N35° 14.996' W111° 34.107'

DISTANCE & CONFIGURATION: 8 miles out-and-back; easy version is 3.4 miles out-and-back

HIKING TIME: 4 hours; easy hike is less than 2 hours

HIGHLIGHTS: Vistas, wildlife, and springs

ELEVATION: 6,900 feet at trailhead to 7,200 feet at Little Elden Springs

ACCESS: No fees or restrictions; open year-round

MAPS: USGS Sunset Crater West

FACILITIES: None

WHEELCHAIR ACCESS: None

COMMENTS: The easy hike turns around at Sandy Seep. The northern reaches of this hike were damaged in the 2010 Schultz Fire and may still be closed as this guide goes to press. Bring your own water.

CONTACTS: Flagstaff Ranger District, 5075 N. AZ 89, Flagstaff, AZ 86004; (928) 526-0866; **www.fs.fed.us/r3/coconino/recreation/peaks/sandy-seep-tr.shtml; www.fs.fed.us/r3/coconino/recreation/peaks/little-elden-tr.shtml**

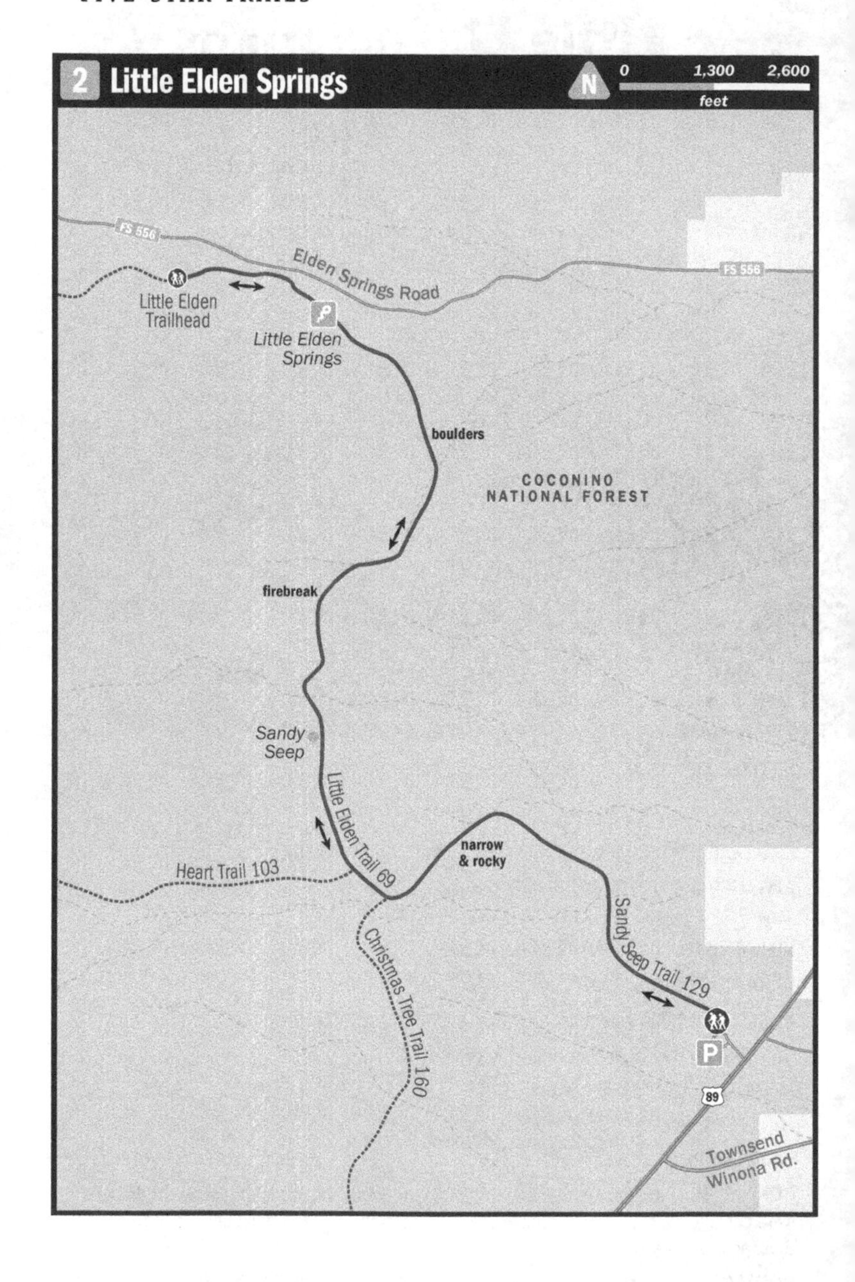
2 Little Elden Springs
N
0
1,300
2,600
feet
FS 556
Elden Springs Road
FS 556
Little Elden Trailhead
Little Elden Springs
boulders
COCONINO NATIONAL FOREST
firebreak
Sandy Seep
Little Elden Trail 69
narrow & rocky
Heart Trail 103
Christmas Tree Trail 160
Sandy Seep Trail 129
P
89
Townsend Winona Rd.

Overview

Following an abandoned jeep trail, this hike wanders through forested meadows and then around the east slopes of Little Elden Mountain. Along the way, it passes through old- and new-growth forests and the remains of the 1977 Radio Fire. The route leads you by two springs: the obscure Sandy Seep and the more developed Elden Springs near the end of the hike. This hike is part of the Arizona National Scenic Trail (AZT), a route stretching lengthwise more than 800 miles through the state from Utah to Mexico.

Route Details

Sandy Seep Trail 129 is the remnant of the old roadway that used to provide access to Sandy Seep and Elden Springs farther on. Now closed to vehicles and managed as a hiking trail, the wide, sandy track rolls through the tall grass, wildflowers, scrubby manzanitas, and towering pines that typify the lower slopes of Mount Elden and Little Elden Mountain.

Within sight of the trailhead, you cross the junction with the AZT Equestrian Bypass. There's a sign. North of this junction, Sandy Seep (and Little Elden Trail 69 beyond) becomes part of the AZT.

The trail through here is wide enough for two people to walk side by side. Ants have cleared huge circles in the surrounding grass,

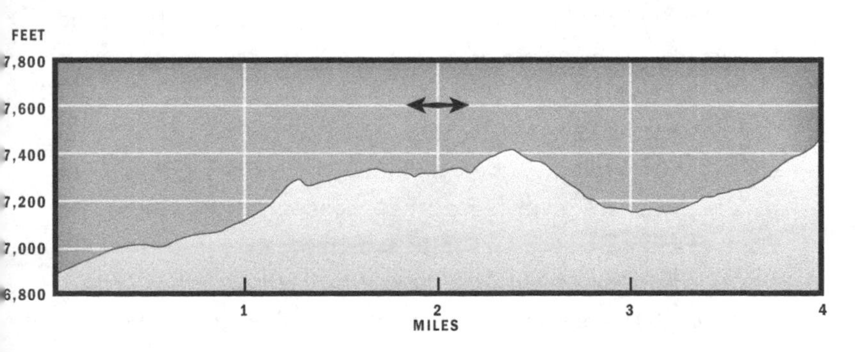

and birds soar about in the pines and oaks. In early morning and late evening, mule deer might be about, especially toward winter.

After 1 mile, the trail bends to the south as it climbs the slope, becoming narrower and rockier in the process. A few ancient, twisted alligator junipers and cliff roses line the slopes.

At the junction with the Christmas Tree Trail 160, about 1.5 miles in, Sandy Seep Trail 129 ends, and Little Elden Trail 69 takes over. Christmas Tree Trail 160 heads south from here, toward Fatman's Loop 25 (see page 28). Continue right (north) along Little Elden.

Within 0.2 mile, you will come to the junction with Heart Trail 103, which charges left (east) up the slopes. Stay straight (north).

Note: At press time Little Elden Trail 69 was closed per order of the U.S. Forest Service north of Heart Trail 103, meaning everything that follows in this description. It is expected that the portion described here will be open by the summer of 2012, but it could be as long as 2013. If in doubt, contact the Flagstaff Ranger District at (928) 526-0866.

Little Elden Trail 69 soon climbs over the low hills and into a sandy meadow stretching between two hills. In a depression near the base of the white-capped northern hill is Sandy Seep, which is sometimes a small pond but most often is a basin full of weeds and brush. Regardless, the attraction is the meadow itself, and this is the turnaround for the easy hike.

The trail continues north, crossing between the north hill and the slope of the mountain. At 0.5 mile past the seep, you encounter a wide dirt firebreak.

Here, after three decades, the boundary of the 1977 Radio Fire is still easy to determine. As is often the case, this loss of shade has been replaced by excellent views. From here, your vista takes in northern Flagstaff and the cinder cones of the eastern volcanic range beyond.

Look for the trail to continue past the firebreak. It soon makes a U through a ravine, and then heads downhill. At the 3-mile mark you turn sharply left (roughly northwest) and down into a wash.

Climb out of that wash and into a second wash, where you

will be greeted by car-sized pink boulders strewn about the bottom of the drainage. Beyond here, the trail will climb slightly as it bends northward around the base of the mountain. The stumpy forest of saplings gives way to older-growth mixed conifers as you climb.

At 3.6 miles, you reach Little Elden Springs, mostly indicated by a 15-foot-diameter dry concrete basin. Upslope from here, a hose runs down to a little metal canister (probably also dry) lying by the fence. The fence is there for cows, not people, so you can go beyond it, following the little trails to the base of the cliff. There you will find the green pool of water that flows from the spring proper. The other trail heading downhill from here goes to Forest Road 556.

Unless you have arranged a car shuttle at Little Elden Trailhead, this is the turnaround for the 8-mile out-and-back. If you opt to remain on Little Elden, it proceeds another 0.5 mile to its spur to the trailhead of the same name, and then 2.5 miles farther to Schultz Tank—or at least it used to.

North of the trailhead spur, Little Elden Trail 69 passes through areas torched by the 2010 Schultz Fire. The U.S. Forest Service closed the northern portions of this trail, which remain closed at the time this book goes to press, and they are likely to be troublesome and depressing well into the 2020s.

Return the way you came.

Directions

From downtown Flagstaff, take US 66 north, staying on AZ 89 north when US 66 splits east. Proceed north, past the Flagstaff Mall, to 0.5 mile north of the Townsend-Winona Road intersection (there's a traffic light). Turn onto FR 9139 on the west (left) side. This short road terminates at the trailhead.

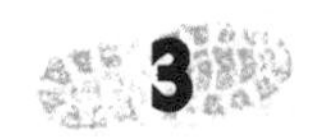

3 Mount Elden Loop

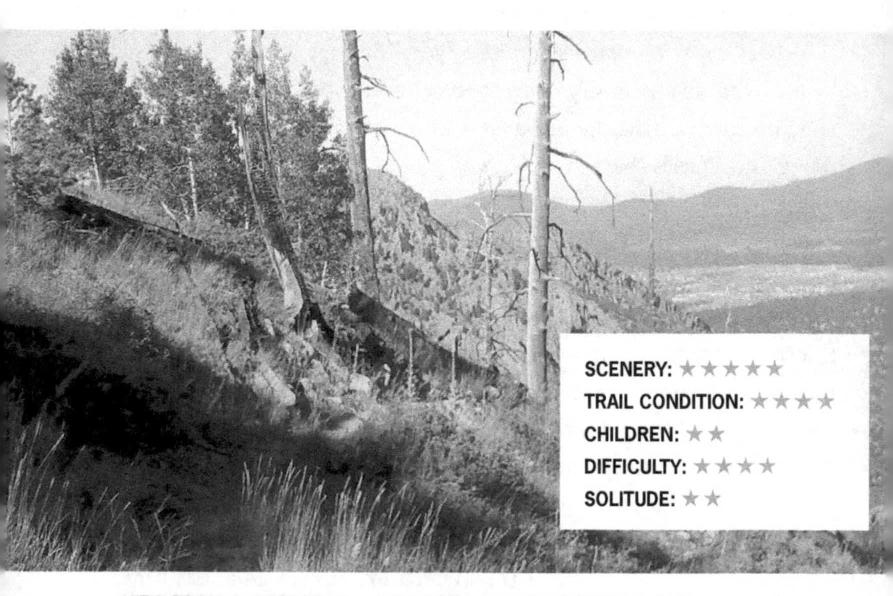

VIEW FROM SUNSET TRAIL—COURTESY OF THE 1977 RADIO FIRE

GPS TRAILHEAD COORDINATES: N35° 15.304' W111° 37.473'

DISTANCE & CONFIGURATION: 7.7-mile loop; add 2 miles for the Elden Lookout spur

HIKING TIME: 4.5 hours; add 1 hour for the Elden Lookout spur

HIGHLIGHTS: Expansive vistas, old-growth forest, wildlife, and lookout tower

ELEVATION: 7,758 feet at trailhead to 9,275 feet at the peak

ACCESS: No fees or restrictions; road may be closed after heavy snows

MAPS: USGS Humphreys and Sunset West

FACILITIES: None

WHEELCHAIR ACCESS: None

COMMENTS: Northern reaches of the Sunset Trail 23 may yet be closed due to the 2010 Schultz Fire. Mileages in the following description do *not* count the spur to Elden Lookout. If you take that spur, add 2 miles and about an hour.

CONTACTS: Flagstaff Ranger District, 5075 N. AZ 89, Flagstaff, AZ 86004; (928) 526-0866; **www.fs.fed.us/r3/coconino/recreation/peaks/oldham-tr.shtml; www.fs.fed.us/r3/coconino/recreation/peaks/sunset-tr.shtml; www.fs.fed.us/r3/coconino/recreation/peaks/brookbank-tr.shtml**

Overview

This loop takes the Upper Oldham Trail 1 up the west slope of Mount Elden to its junction with Sunset Trail 23. From there, you can head south to Elden Lookout, and/or north, across the ridgetops, passing through dense forests, open meadows, and commanding views of Flagstaff. Then follow Brookbank Trail 2 to wind back down to the trailhead.

Route Details

UP THE UPPER OLDHAM: From the roadside, Upper Oldham Trail 1 (not to be confused with either the regular or "easy" Oldham Trails farther down the slope to the west) immediately crosses a wash as it marches north through the mixed-conifer forest. The huge cluster of granite boulders to the right is a popular climbing spot. Where logs have fallen across the track, mountain bikers have fabricated improvised ramps. The footpath parallels the road for 0.2 mile until it forms a Y at the Brookbank junction. Stay right, on Upper Oldham, which will begin to bend east.

The trail now splits the ridge between the road and the wash. It will brush the road but never crosses it. Just past 0.5 mile in, you cross a spur heading straight up into the granite. This is for rock climbers—stay straight ahead.

After 1 mile, the trail curves south as it begins a sustained climb up a ravine. The grade isn't crushing by itself, but it is relentless and the cumulative effect can become challenging. It levels out after 0.33 mile, but the respite is short-lived.

Switchbacks lead you up the steep, grassy slopes for 0.5 mile, terminating at a wide field called Oldham Park. You have gone just more than 2 miles at this point. The trail crosses this wide meadow to meet the road at a little parking area for perhaps four to six vehicles. A 100-foot spur trail leads from the opposite side of the lot to the Sunset Trail 23 at its junction with the Heart Trail 103. The vista here is a taste of what remains to be witnessed.

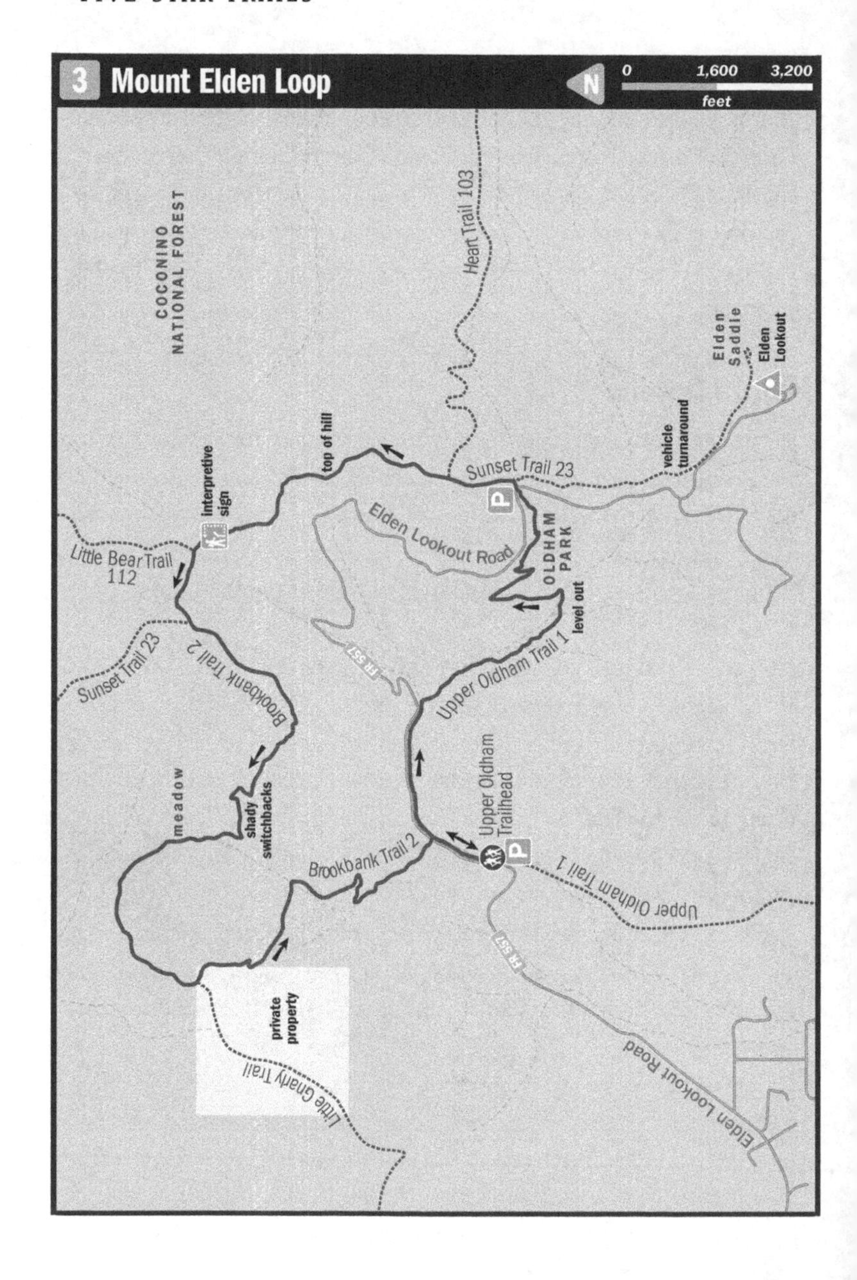
3 Mount Elden Loop
N
0
1,600
3,200
feet
COCONINO NATIONAL FOREST
Heart Trail 103
Elden Saddle
Elden Lookout
vehicle turnaround
top of hill
Sunset Trail 23
interpretive sign
Elden Lookout Road
OLDHAM PARK
level out
Little Bear Trail 112
Sunset Trail 23
Brookbank Trail 2
FR 557
Upper Oldham Trail 1
Upper Oldham Trailhead
meadow
shady switchbacks
Brookbank Trail 2
Upper Oldham Trail 1
FR 557
private property
Little Gnarly Trail
Elden Lookout Road

ELDEN LOOKOUT SPUR (OPTIONAL): For the optional side trip to Elden Lookout, take a right at this junction, following Sunset Trail 23 loosely southeast. This spur will add 2 miles round-trip.

From this vantage point, you can see what the 2010 Schultz Fire will look like in 30 years, for the 1977 Radio Fire ravaged these slopes. Most of the deadfall has tumbled down and the ground is covered with grass and saplings, holding the soil in place at last. While there is no shade, you will find good views. The altitude along here verges on 9,000 feet and climbing.

Sunset stays at or near the ridgetop, climbing through open prairie or pushing through thickets of Gambel oaks or aspen saplings. At 0.5 mile, it touches the road again at a vehicle turnaround. The road past here to the lookout is not generally open to public vehicles.

The footpath splits from the road on its way to the saddle to meet with the Elden Lookout Trail 4. If you want to go to the towers, you are just as well on the road because the top portion of Elden Lookout Trail 4 from the saddle to the peak is desperately steep.

Neither the U.S. Forest Service watchtower nor any of the other buildings and accompanying antennae are open to the public, but you can walk among them on your way around the peak. Doing so will reveal all of Flagstaff sprawled below. Know, though, that there are no restrooms, drinking water, or even a trash can. Just pretend the

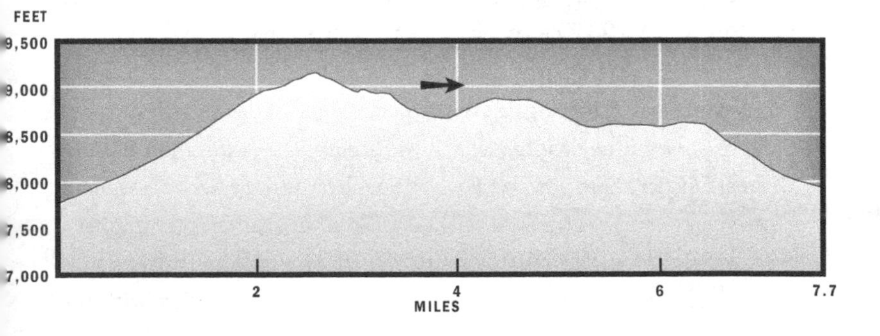

buildings aren't there and that the peak is barren. When satisfied, return to the Upper Oldham–Heart junction.

NORTH ON SUNSET: Sunset Trail 23 heads north from the Upper Oldham–Heart junction across the top of the ridge. The wide dirt track is fenced in by old-growth pines and spruces. At 2.8 miles, it starts climbing. Shutterbug trails head to the right through the rocks and logs, toward better vistas at the east edge of the ridge. At about the 3-mile mark (and 8,900 feet), you reach the top the hill, near a pile of boulders.

As you cross this hill and the ridges beyond, keep an eye out for mule deer and elk that are known to graze through here. A family of black bears lives on the slopes of Mount Elden, but you are unlikely to encounter these shy omnivores.

On the far side, the forest thins and you encounter a sign explaining the logic behind the controlled burn that diluted it. True to that logic, the trail winds through a green, grassy meadow interrupted by enormous old-growth pines and spruces. Seeing that, did you notice how the deadwood was almost waist-high up the hill?

The sandy singletrack continues through this picturesque forest. Birds will sing. Deer may prance. This is why you climbed up here.

At 3.5 miles, you come to the junction with the Little Bear Trail 112. In the first few years of this century, the then–newly constructed Little Bear Trail 112 was the five-star way up Little Elden Mountain to the Sunset Trail 23. The Schultz Fire incinerated that slope to the point that the U.S. Forest Service closed the trail in 2010, and it is unlikely to become fun to hike again for the next couple of decades. That is not just because of the deadfall, which will accumulate faster than the U.S. Forest Service could possibly clear it, but also the unavoidable evidence everywhere of what was lost to the flames of an abandoned campfire.

This far up, though, the forest remains pristine as Sunset bends west, climbing to the top of the next ridge and its junction with the Brookbank Trail 2 at 4.2 miles.

Sunset continues north toward Schultz Pass and the heart of

the fire damage that bears the pass's name, but it may be closed at its northern terminus for some time.

DOWN THE BROOKBANK: The Brookbank Trail 2 continues southwest along the top of the ridge for another 0.25 mile before bending northwest and winding down gently through the thick forest. At 1 mile past the junction, gentle winding becomes steeper switchbacks, but they soon level out in a small meadow.

From here, the Brookbank begins a long U (just over 1 mile) around the mountain to the north. On the far side, you come to a Y. To your right (west), the Little Gnarly Trail climbs over the low hill to the west as it cuts through a parcel of private property. Continuing straight and south, which is what you want, the trail winds along the side of the hill past some property-boundary markers posted above the ferns.

The trail more clearly betrays its origin as a road as it completes the southeast circuit down the hill and into the ravine. It follows this ravine all the way to the forest road. Immediately across this road is the junction with the Upper Oldham Trail 1 that you passed 7.25 miles ago. Return down that trail to the trailhead.

Directions

From downtown Flagstaff, take US 180 (also called Fort Valley Road) north, past the museums to Elden Lookout Road (FR 557). Follow this paved, then graded dirt road for about 3 miles to the pullouts by the trailhead. The trailhead has a sign and parking for about four to six vehicles, but no other services.

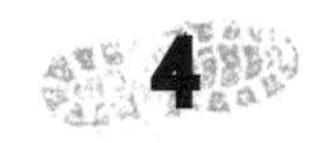

4 O'Leary Peak

SCENERY: ★★★★★
TRAIL CONDITION: ★★★★
CHILDREN: ★★
DIFFICULTY: ★★★★
SOLITUDE: ★★★★

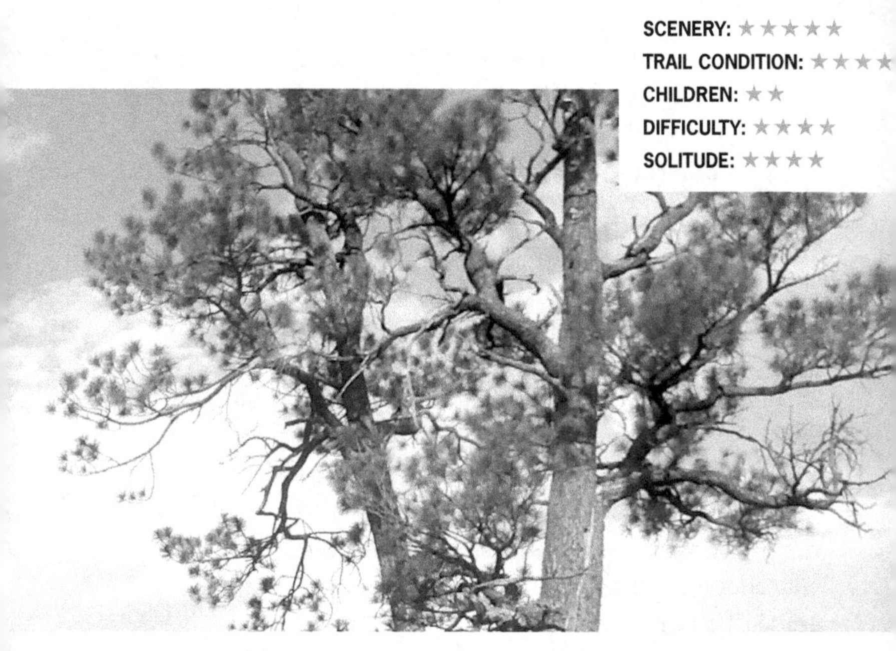

PONDEROSA PINE NEAR O'LEARY PEAK

GPS TRAILHEAD COORDINATES: N35° 22.306' W111° 32.479'

DISTANCE & CONFIGURATION: 10.2 miles out-and-back; easy hike is 5 miles out-and-back

HIKING TIME: 6 hours; easy hike is 2.5 hours

HIGHLIGHTS: Lava flow, scenic vistas, diverse geology, and lookout tower

ELEVATION: 6,890 feet at trailhead to 8,935 feet at the peak

ACCESS: No fees; trailhead is day-use only

MAPS: USGS O'Leary Peak

FACILITIES: None at trailhead; see comment in "Directions"

WHEELCHAIR ACCESS: None

COMMENTS: Hike follows an established roadway that is normally closed to nonofficial vehicles. The easy hike option turns around after the first switchback. The lookout tower atop the peak is a working facility, not a visitor center, and has no services available to the public.

CONTACTS: Flagstaff Ranger District, 5075 N. AZ 89, Flagstaff, AZ 86004; (928) 526-0866; **www.fs.fed.us/r3/coconino/recreation/peaks/oleary-peaks-tr.shtml**

Overview

The route follows Forest Service Road 545A past the Bonito Lava Flow within Sunset Crater National Monument, and then up the slopes of O'Leary Peak to terminate near the fire lookout tower on top of the mountain. Along the way are splendid examples of volcanic geology underfoot and scenic vistas all about. Go on a clear day and take a good camera.

Route Details

The gravel service road heading east from the trailhead is the trail. Black-lava gravel covers everything so that the scattered pine trees seem to be growing from some long-abandoned parking lot. The road soon turns more north. Now, to the right (east), the Bonito Lava Flow that covers much of Sunset Crater National Monument skirts the road. Above the 6- to 10-foot-tall pile of jagged basalt boulders, you can see Sunset Crater farther east and O'Leary Peak in the distance to the north. While a U.S. Forest Service description of this hike recommends exploring this lava flow, the National Park Service, on whose property most of the flow resides, actually prohibits hiking off-trail. If you were to climb to the top, you'd see that the jagged and nearly impassable field of lava extends for miles, like a black, stormy sea that had been suddenly fossilized.

The road cuts through a corner of the monument that is marked by a fence line. Just past this landmark, the road climbs 200 feet in 0.5 mile. That's steep enough to feel, but it's the easiest climb of the hike. As the road levels a bit, a trace road goes northwest through the lava gravel toward the slopes of nearby Robinson Mountain. Stay on the main road.

After 2 miles, the first big switchback starts. The grade is relatively gentle. Best of all, as the black slope drops to your south (left), the view opens up, revealing the Bonito Lava Flow and Sunset Crater beyond. At the first U-turn of the switchback, wire ropes guard a trace road, prohibiting vehicle use. (This road once joined with that

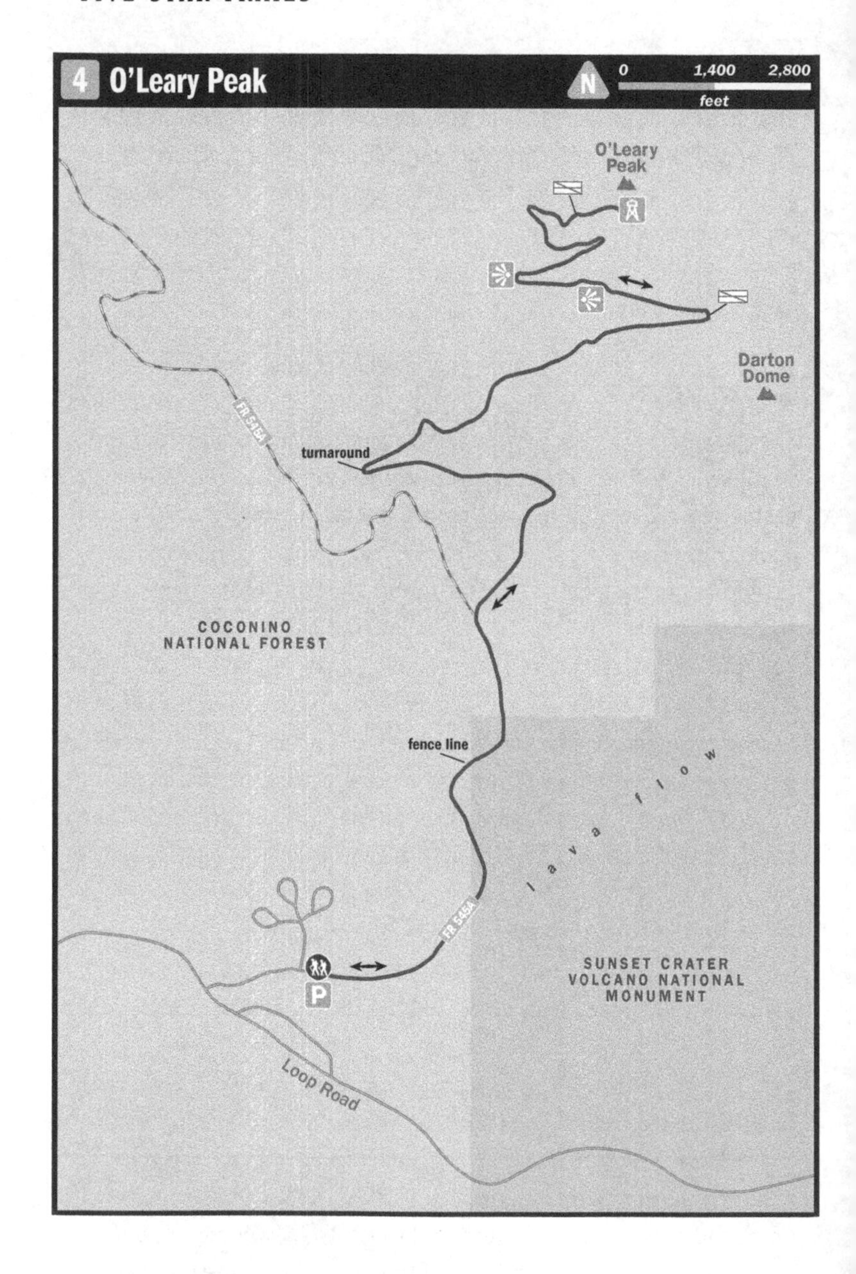
4 O'Leary Peak
0
1,400
2,800
feet
N
O'Leary Peak
Darton Dome
FR 545A
turnaround
fence line
COCONINO NATIONAL FOREST
lava flow
SUNSET CRATER VOLCANO NATIONAL MONUMENT
Loop Road
P

previous trace road en route to Robinson Mountain.)

This point, 2.5 miles from the trailhead, is the turnaround for the easy hike. The climb beyond is worth it, but it certainly does not get easier. As a general note, each switchback will be shorter and steeper than the previous one.

About one-third of the way across the second switchback, the road crosses a drainage where its construction seems to defy the landslide of brick-colored lava rock. That any road at all is possible on this pile of loose cinders is a testament to U.S. Forest Service engineers. The lower peak you're trudging toward along this leg is Darton Dome. Looking behind you, though, you will catch sporadic views of the San Francisco Peaks to the west.

The second U-turn occurs smack at the 8,000-foot elevation and is marked by a vehicle gate. You have gone 3.65 miles from the trailhead by this point.

Halfway across the third switchback, look for the transition line between the red lava rock and the limestone layer. It also marks the 4-mile point. Turn around to see all the peaks, cinder cones, lava fields, and prairies to the southwest. Sharp eyes could make out Sunset Crater Visitor Center, and perhaps even where you parked your car.

At the fourth turn, the ravine on the slope beyond is festooned with huge granite hoodoos (columns of rock). On the other side, to the west, you witness postcard-quality views of the San Francisco Peaks.

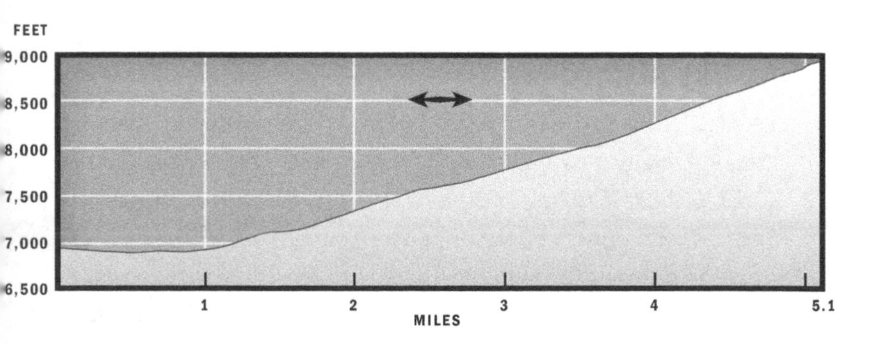

By the fourth turn, spruce and fir trees start appearing among the pines. You walk entirely along the granite cap over the basalt layer. O'Leary Mountain is a lava dome, after all, in contrast to cinder cones such as Sunset Peak.

O'Leary actually has two peaks, with the one on the north side being slightly higher. The one to the south, though, has the lookout tower, and the road that reaches it.

Just past the saddle between the two peaks—the fifth turn—you encounter a gate (and perhaps a parked vehicle). The final climb to the lookout tower is desperately steep and not always worth it in a vehicle, but enticing for hikers. However, if this gate is closed, that's the end of the hike.

Metal grating covers the steep ascent from the gate to the peak itself, which is capped with the O'Leary Lookout Tower. There are a few buildings in addition to the tower, but no public services. Remember that this U.S. Forest Service lookout tower is both a home and a workplace for whomever is stationed here. Sometimes that person will talk to visitors, perhaps even letting them climb into the tower, but sometimes he or she is working and needs to be left alone. So don't just climb up the stairs without being invited.

You've climbed to 8,900 feet, gaining more than 2,000 feet in 5.1 miles. You have plenty to gawk at from the peak with or without the tower. Return the way you came.

Nearby Attractions

People frequently visit Sunset Crater and Wupatki national monuments as a pair, and the $5 entrance fee covers both parks. It takes about 2 hours to explore either monument in any depth. Sunset Crater centers on the huge, rust-colored cinder cone that rose from the plateau a thousand years ago. (It's one of the more recent of the many eruptions that formed all of the mountains that surround you.) There is a visitor center, along with a few short walking trails around the lava flow, and a smaller crater. Due to erosion, Sunset

Crater itself has been closed to hiking since the 1970s. Sunset Crater Visitor Center: (928) 526-0502; **nps.gov/sucr.**

The loop road continues through the park to Wupatki National Monument, centered on several large pueblos built and occupied more than 700 years ago. You may follow several small interpretive trails. Wupatki National Monument Visitor Center: (928) 679-2365; **nps.gov/wupa.**

Bonito Campground, one of the few near Flagstaff, borders the park. Spaces start at $18 per night and are first come, first served. The campground is operated by the U.S. Forest Service: Flagstaff Ranger District, 5075 N. AZ 89, Flagstaff, AZ 86004; (928) 526-0866; **www.fs.fed.us/r3/coconino/recreation/peaks/bonito-camp.shtml.**

Directions

From Flagstaff, take US 89 north for 12 miles. Turn right on the Sunset Crater–Wupatki Loop Road and continue 2 miles toward the park entrance. Just before you get there (almost within throwing distance), take the left turn into the O'Leary Group Campground (on FR 545A). Off to the side of this campground is the small parking lot that serves as the trailhead. While both the campground and Sunset Crater require fees, the trailhead does not. There are no services: You'd need to pay your fee to use the visitor center's restrooms.

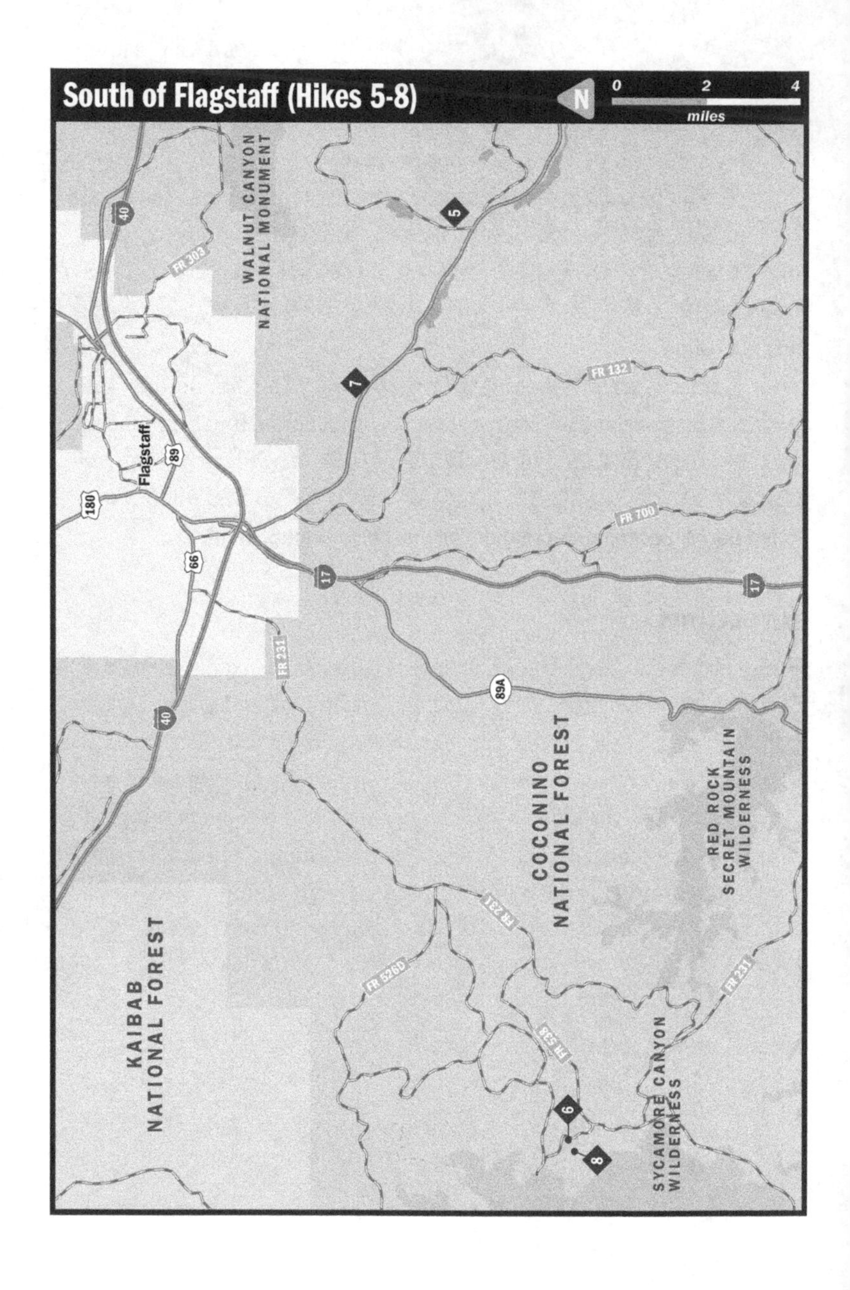

South of Flagstaff (Hikes 5-8)
N
0
2
4
miles
WALNUT CANYON NATIONAL MONUMENT
FR 303
40
Flagstaff
89
180
66
17
FR 231
FR 132
FR 700
89A
5
6
7
8
COCONINO NATIONAL FOREST
RED ROCK SECRET MOUNTAIN WILDERNESS
KAIBAB NATIONAL FOREST
FR 526D
FR 538
SYCAMORE CANYON WILDERNESS

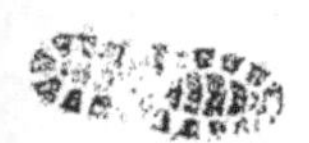

South of Flagstaff

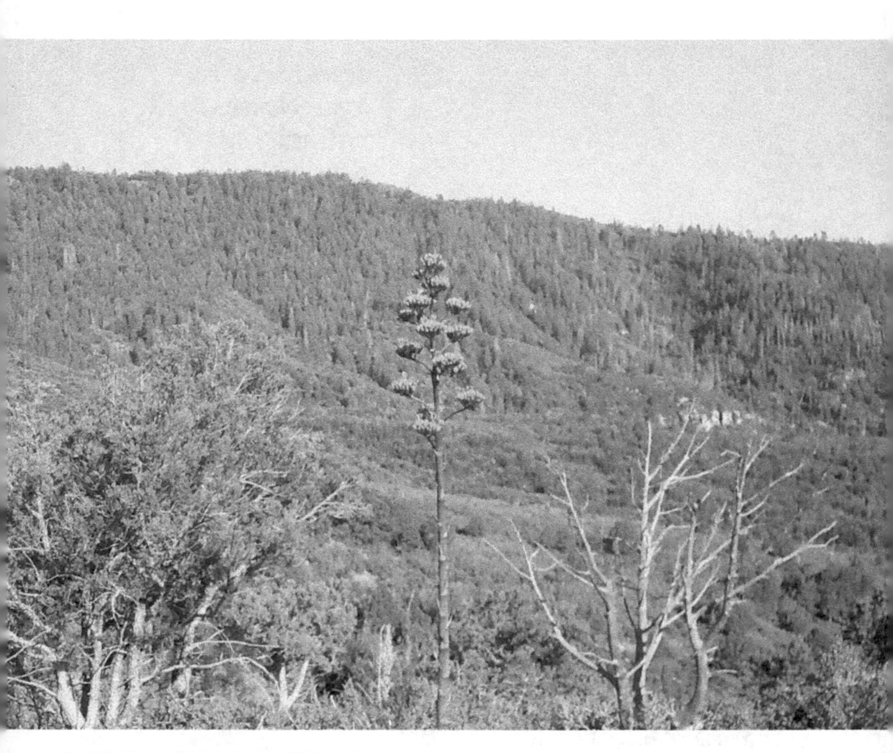

CENTURY BLOOM ON WINTER CABIN LOOP

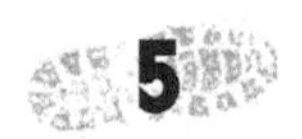

5 Anderson Mesa

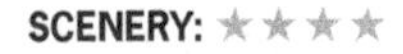

SCENERY: ★★★★
TRAIL CONDITION: ★★★★
CHILDREN: ★★★★
DIFFICULTY: ★
SOLITUDE: ★★★★

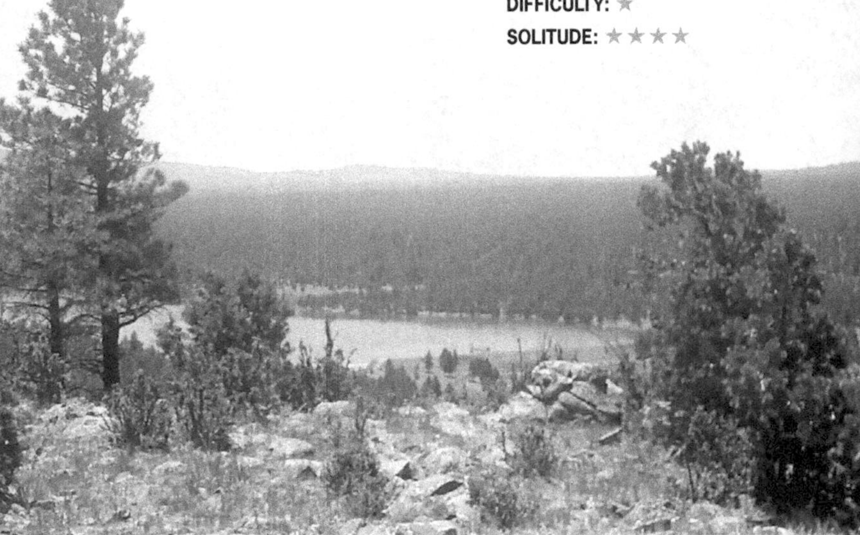

LOWER LAKE MARY FROM ANDERSON MESA

GPS TRAILHEAD COORDINATES: N35° 06.024' W111° 32.185'

DISTANCE & CONFIGURATION: 5.5-mile loop

HIKING TIME: 3 hours

HIGHLIGHTS: Two ponds, wide meadow, and scenic vistas

ELEVATION: 7,200–7,300 feet throughout

ACCESS: No fees or restrictions

MAPS: USGS Anderson Mesa

FACILITIES: None

WHEELCHAIR ACCESS: None

COMMENTS: Ponds are seasonal according to recent precipitation. Parts of the hike pass through open cattle range.

CONTACTS: Flagstaff Ranger District, 5075 N. AZ 89, Flagstaff, AZ 86004; (928) 526-0866

Overview

This easy and unpublicized hike goes around two small ponds on top of Anderson Mesa and is great for small children. The flat mesa top offers views of Lake Mary to the south and the San Francisco Peaks to the north. Part of the route follows the Arizona National Scenic Trail (AZT), a route stretching lengthwise more than 800 miles through the state from Utah to Mexico.

Route Details

From the trailhead take the singletrack, which is actually the AZT, southeast as it follows the low picket-fence line. A few forest roads in various stages of abandonment seem to go the same direction, but the singletrack was blazed precisely so that you would not have to follow these roads. You soon come to a gate allowing passage through the barbed-wire fence surrounding the extended bowl of Prime Lake.

Prime Lake and nearby Vail Lake (which you will get to) were formed 5 million years ago as air pockets in the magma pile that became Anderson Mesa collapsed. Gradually, these depressions were filled and thereby capped with clay, allowing them to trap rainwater and snowmelt. (Before hopes become too elevated, what Arizonans call lakes, folks from wetter climes might call shallow ponds.)

The trail skirts the west side of Prime Lake, passing through the bear grass, pines, and junipers that dominate the mesa. In the spring, the area can erupt in wildflowers. On a clear day, the San Francisco Peaks are visible far beyond the pond. Beyond the lake to the southeast, just shy of a mile into the hike, a second gate lets you out onto the mesa.

At the Y just past the gate, take the more obvious path, which bends sharply west (right) across the mesa. Within 0.5 mile, it reaches the edge of the mesa. A steep bank descends roughly 1,000 feet down to Lake Mary Road and, beyond it, Lower Lake Mary.

Turning left (south), the trail follows the edge of the mesa for a short bit before turning back southeast into the interior. At just

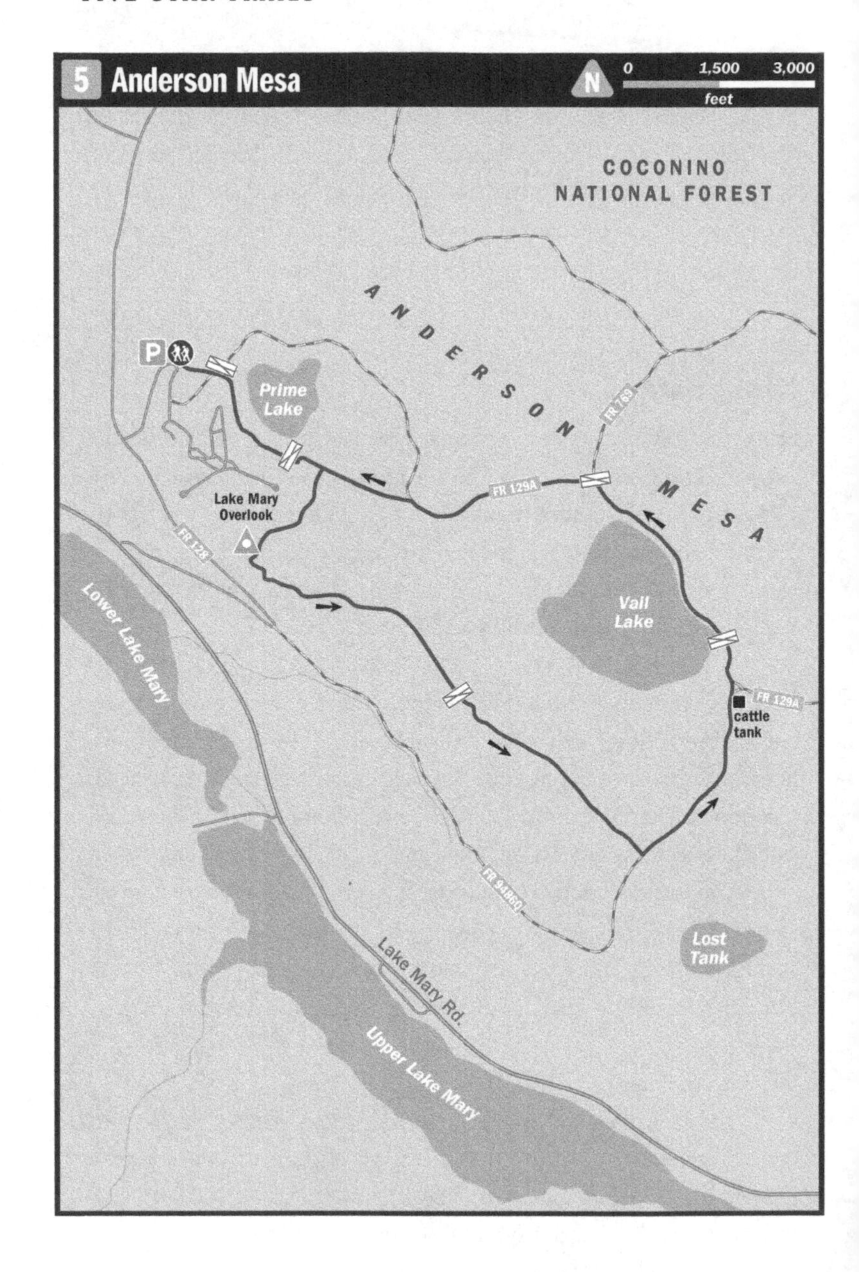
5 Anderson Mesa
N
0
1,500
3,000
feet
COCONINO
NATIONAL FOREST
ANDERSON MESA
Prime Lake
Lake Mary Overlook
FR 128
FR 129A
FR 769
Vail Lake
FR 129A
cattle tank
Lower Lake Mary
FR 9486Q
Lost Tank
Lake Mary Rd.
Upper Lake Mary

past 2 miles, you come to a gate in the barbed-wire fence, which is tightly wired and may prove difficult to open. There is no shame or consequence in conceding defeat and just climbing the fence.

All this barbed wire has nothing to do with hikers. This is an open grazing allotment, and if you haven't encountered cattle yet, it remains likely that you will, even though the hike is nearly half over. You are just as likely to encounter deer or elk, and in good weather eagles and hawks might soar overhead.

The interior of the mesa is either a meadow crowded with trees or a wide open forest, depending on how you wish to phrase it. Despite how open it looks, you can easily get lost within the sameness of it all, so stay on the trail.

At 3.25 miles, you come to a forest road (FR 129A). Beyond it the AZT continues to the south, toward Mormon Lake, and, eventually, Mexico. Turn left (northeast) on the road, though, to continue this hike. In 0.5 mile you will pass a cattle tank about a hundred feet distant to the southeast (right). At 0.25 mile past that tank, at about the 4-mile mark, you come across a decaying spur road leading to the gate into Vail Lake.

The path around the east shore of Vail Lake shows as a road on many maps, but it has been closed to motor vehicles for years. The lakes are being preserved for creatures that actually live here. For example, the cattle must drink from the tank, but the abundance of

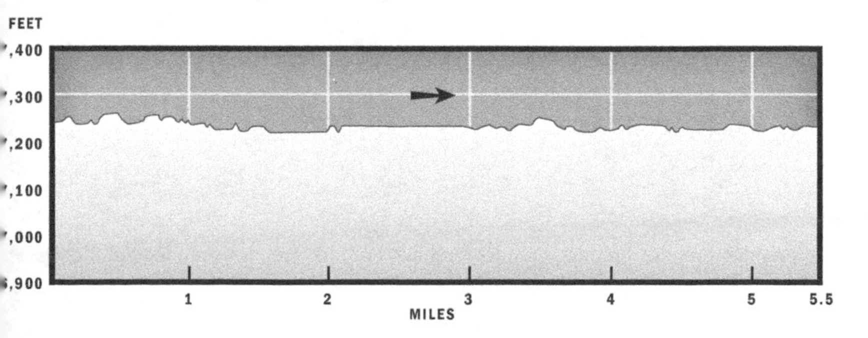

prints below your feet shows how the fence line does not impede deer or even elk. Further, the pond is a crucial habitat for ducks and frogs and all manner of little scurrying things that you might find in the weeds and mud surrounding the pond.

On the northern side of the lake, you find another gate, beyond which two dirt roads go off across the mesa. Take the one heading left (due west). In less than 0.5 mile, it will curve to the northwest; before it curves again to the north, you will see a path following what used to be a road farther northwest. (So if you find yourself going due north, you've missed it.) This track leads directly to the southern gate of Prime Lake. From there, return the way you came.

Directions

Take Lake Mary Road south from Flagstaff for about 9 miles to FR 128. The sign will say USGS OBSERVATORY AND MARSHALL LAKE. FR 128 is also the only left (north) turn for a mile in either direction. Follow the paved road up the side of the mesa, where, just past the top, the road branches in a Y. Stay right (east) toward the observatory, away from Marshall Lake. The trailhead parking lot is across the road from the observatory.

The observatory is not open to the public and is likely locked tight during daylight hours.

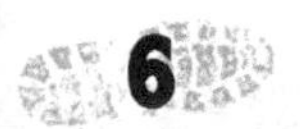

6 Kelsey Springs Loop

SCENERY: ★★★★
TRAIL CONDITION: ★★★
CHILDREN: ★★
DIFFICULTY: ★★★
SOLITUDE: ★★

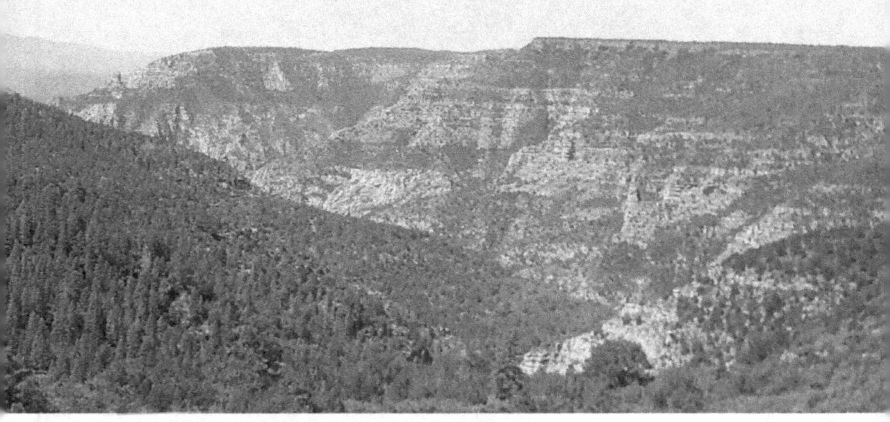

VIEW OF SYCAMORE CANYON FROM THE KELSEY TRAIL

GPS TRAILHEAD COORDINATES: *Dorsey Trailhead:* N35° 3.551' W111° 55.045'

DISTANCE & CONFIGURATION: 10-mile loop

HIKING TIME: 5 hours

HIGHLIGHTS: Scenic vistas and flowing springs

ELEVATION: 6,916 feet at trailhead to 5,239 feet at the bottom of the canyon

ACCESS: No fees; requires a high-clearance vehicle, and roads may be impassable during wet conditions.

MAPS: USFS Sycamore Canyon Wilderness

FACILITIES: None

WHEELCHAIR ACCESS: None

COMMENTS: Sycamore Canyon drains through cattle country, so water here is not safe to drink without treatment. Most of the hike is within the wilderness area, so no bikes are allowed. See note at the end about route options.

CONTACTS: Flagstaff Ranger District, 5075 N. AZ 89, Flagstaff, AZ 86004; (928) 526-0866; **www.fs.fed.us/r3/coconino/recreation/peaks/sycamore-canyon-wild.shtml**

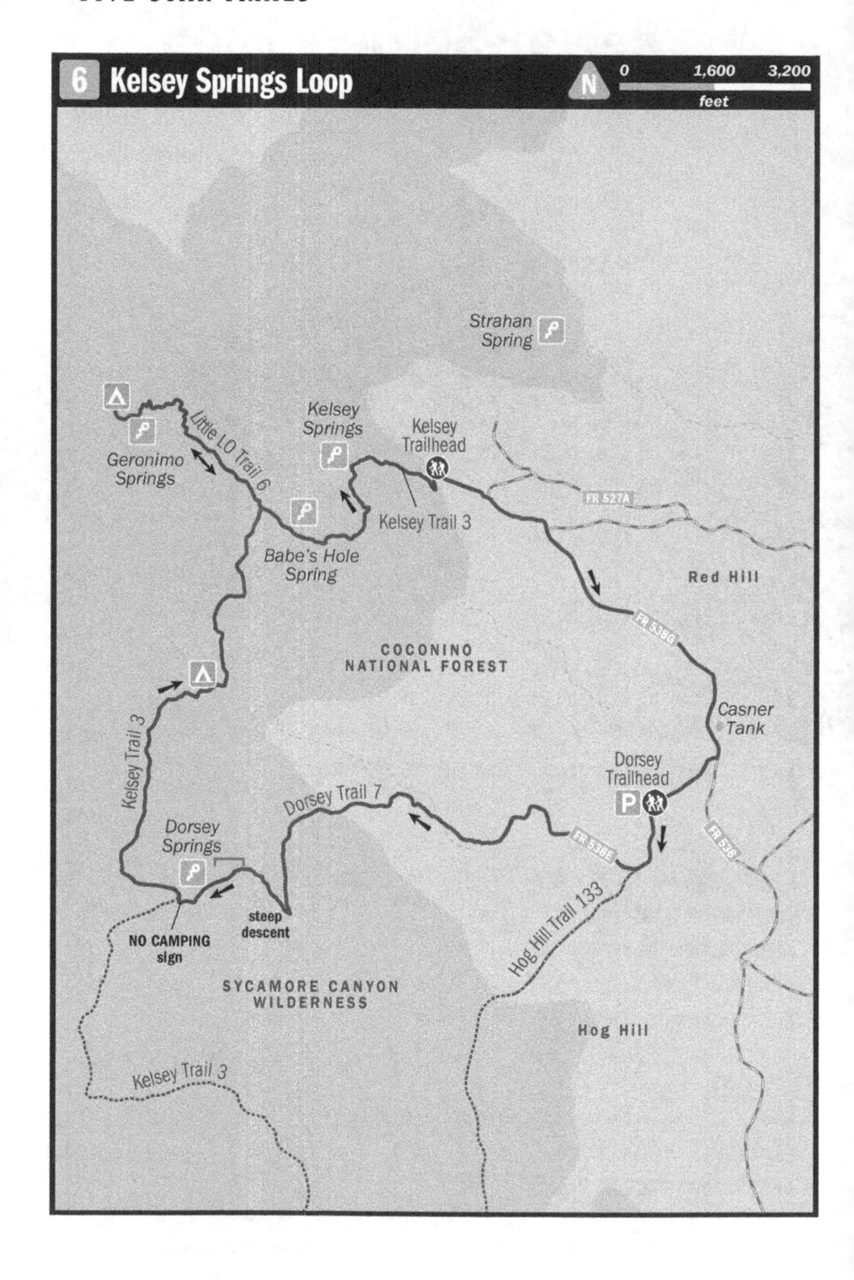
6 Kelsey Springs Loop
N
0
1,600
3,200
feet
Strahan Spring
Kelsey Springs
Kelsey Trailhead
Little LO Trail 6
Geronimo Springs
Kelsey Trail 3
FR 527A
Babe's Hole Spring
Red Hill
FR 538G
COCONINO NATIONAL FOREST
Casner Tank
Kelsey Trail 3
Dorsey Trailhead
Dorsey Trail 7
FR 538E
FR 538
Dorsey Springs
Hog Hill Trail 133
NO CAMPING sign
steep descent
SYCAMORE CANYON WILDERNESS
Hog Hill
Kelsey Trail 3

Overview

This loop follows the Dorsey Trail 7 down to Dorsey Springs, and then continues north along the edge of the canyon via Kelsey Trail 3. A short but steep spur leads to Geronimo Springs near the canyon floor. Kelsey then climbs back to its own trailhead, and forest roads lead back to the Dorsey Trailhead. This hike is near the Winter Cabin hike (see page 69).

Route Details

From the trailhead, follow the remnant road past the wilderness boundary sign (the actual legal boundary is about a mile farther in) a few hundred yards from the parking area, and into as fine a forest of pines and oaks as you are likely to experience and still get cell phone coverage. Keep an eye out for any of the several enormous examples of alligator junipers, along with the rust-colored towers of the ponderosa pines.

Within 0.25 mile, you come to the signed Y-intersection with Hog Hill Trail 133. Dorsey Trail 7 goes to the right (roughly west). The remnant road drops gently, crossing a wide shelf covered with pines and oaks, and it continues thus for the better part of a mile until the fence and deer maze mark the actual wilderness area boundary.

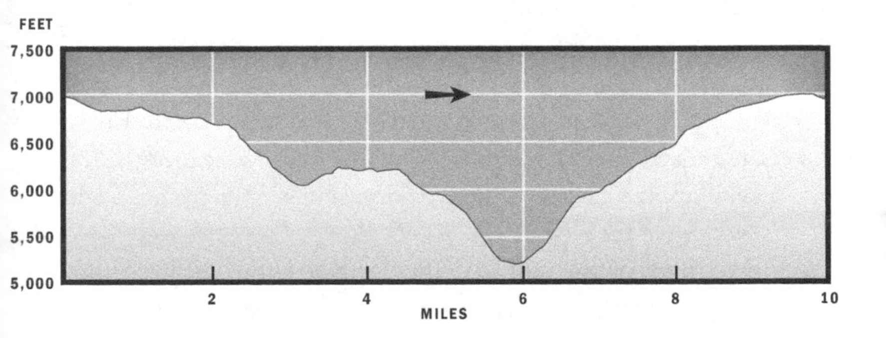

Past that, the trail becomes an easy singletrack, drifting south through thick stands of piñon pines. You pass through a small burned area and through a clearing with widely spaced junipers. But mostly you roll gently through the pines for nearly a mile.

At 2.1 miles in, the trail will enter a ravine, turning sharply north as it does so, and this marks the start of two steep and prolonged downward grades. Halfway through this first plunge, just past where one dry drainage joins another, the trail will seem to split. One trail levels off across the side of the ravine, while the other continues down along the bottom of the wash. Take the lower trail, which soon levels out across a bench sheltered by a thick stand of pines. Enjoy this quick breather before the second descent plunges down the hill toward Dorsey Springs.

Dorsey Springs is the most reliable of the several springs in the area, yet the water is not safe to drink without treating. A plastic pipe leads from the spring, but most of the time more water gurgles through the thin streambed around it, saturating a thin line of grass that goes several hundred yards down the canyon.

The sign says NO CAMPING WITHIN 200 FEET, and, predictably, about 200 feet farther south on the trail, you cross a large, well-established campsite. A few hundred yards south of that, you come to the intersection with Kelsey Trail 3, the main north–south trail in this part of the wilderness. This junction is about 1.7 miles from the trailhead.

From the junction with the Dorsey Trail 7, the Kelsey Trail 3 dips westward, heading farther into the canyon before turning north. At about 0.33 mile in, you start a substantial climb, as the thick pines thin out and transition scrub, mostly live oaks, takes over the trail side. While the bushes do not block the sun, neither do they hinder your views of the canyon.

On top of the ridge you return to pine forest. The track traces the top of the ridge, at about 6,200 feet, until a sharp turn (watch for cairns) twists to the east, following the drainage up the canyon.

At 3.2 miles, you encounter a campsite. The trail drops to

the northeast, winding along the slope until you reach the signed junction with Little LO Trail 6. You are just under 5 miles from the Dorsey Trailhead at this point.

Assuming you are not at a loss for time or energy, stay to the left, going northeast down the Little LO, which begins scrambling along the top and then the side of a finger ridge. Two distinct sets of switchbacks follow. The first is gravelly and fairly exposed. Across from you, the sheer white sandstone cliffs remind you that this is, in fact, the easy way down. The second switchback is shaded by Gambel oaks, curving over the trail like a series of archways. So, instead of slipping on loose rocks, you are slipping on loose leaves.

Toward the bottom of the switchbacks lies Geronimo Springs (it flows from the hillside roughly even with the last turn). On a good day, it gurgles into an inlet that eventually drains into Sycamore Creek. On a bad day, only the plastic pipe and wooden trough might indicate its location. Happily, this spring has more good days than bad.

The trail crosses the little creek just downstream from the springs, and on the other side you'll find a campsite beneath a rock overhang. The trail continues beyond, past another couple of well-worn campsites and eventually to the normally dry Sycamore Creek, but this overhang campsite is your turnaround spot. You've gone about 1 mile from the junction with the Kelsey Trail 3, and you climb a hard mile back up.

Back on Kelsey, continue northeast (when you regain your breath). You will soon come to Babe's Hole Spring, gushing or seeping from a stone enclosure in the streambed. From here, the trail starts to climb.

At the 8-mile mark (counting the LO spur), you skirt a sizable clearing. A little farther north, you find Kelsey Springs, marked by a high trough. These springs are a seep at best.

Past the springs, the trail turns east and climbs gradually over a shelf before the final ascent, switching back up the canyon the last 0.25 mile until you reach the Kelsey Trailhead.

From this dirt lot, follow the trailhead "driveway" to FR 538G and turn south (right). Walk on this road up the west slope of Red Hill for about 1.7 miles. Just past Casner Tank, you reach the driveway to Dorsey Trailhead.

Routing options: The Winter Cabin Loop (see page 69) also begins at the Dorsey Trailhead, and you may combine it with the Kelsey Springs Loop for a super-loop (skipping the Dorsey Trail 7). Such a loop would be 9 miles without the spurs to either Geronimo Springs or (on the Winter Cabin side) Ott Lake, both of which would add 2 and 3 miles, respectively.

Directions

From Flagstaff, follow US 66 southwest out of town until its intersection with Woody Mountain Road (FR 231). Turn left (south) on Woody Mountain past the Flagstaff Arboretum, and drive for 16 miles toward its intersection with FR 538. Turn right (north) onto FR 538. This area is open cattle range, and you may find yourself sitting in the road waiting for the cows to mosey out of your way. Continue another 6 miles over the hill until you reach FR 538E, where you turn right again. A sign marks the driveway to the trailhead.

You may reliably reach the Dorsey Trailhead with any reasonably high-clearance vehicle, while the Kelsey Trailhead requires a four-wheel-drive vehicle. If you have suitable vehicles, though, a car shuttle can save you a few miles.

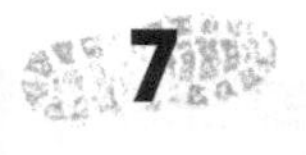

7 Sandys & Walnut Canyons

SCENERY: ★★★★
TRAIL CONDITION: ★★★★
CHILDREN: ★★★★
DIFFICULTY: ★★/★★★
SOLITUDE: ★★

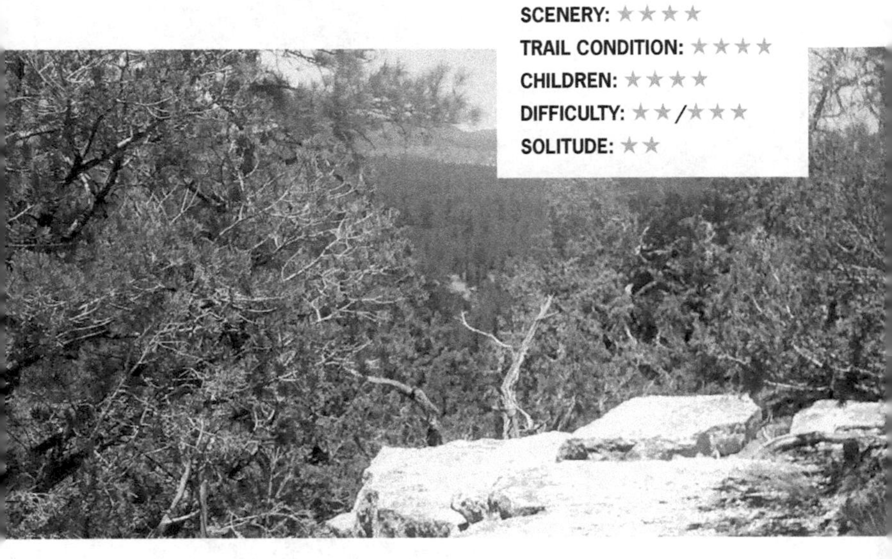

TOP OF FISHER POINT

GPS TRAILHEAD COORDINATES: N35° 07.885' W111° 36.342'

DISTANCE & CONFIGURATION: Easy hike (just Sandys Canyon): 4 miles out-and-back. Fisher Point option adds 2 miles out-and-back. Walnut Canyon option adds 1 mile to the caves, 3 miles to the stand of pines, and 4 miles to the end of the trail (all out-and-back). All options (Sandys Canyon plus Fisher Point and entirety of Walnut Canyon): 10.2 miles out-and-back.

HIKING TIME: 2–7 hours

HIGHLIGHTS: Flora and fauna, bird-watching, scenic overlook, and caves

ELEVATION: 6,825 feet at trailhead to 7,019 feet at Fisher Point

ACCESS: No fees or restrictions

MAPS: USGS Lower Lake Mary and Flagstaff East

FACILITIES: None

WHEELCHAIR ACCESS: None

COMMENTS: This hike has two optional spurs, Fisher Point and Walnut Canyon, which add to time and mileage. Not to be confused with Sandy Seep Trail 129 northwest of Flagstaff or Fisher Point Trail, a section of trail to the north of this hike. Sandys Canyon has no apostrophe—it's a last name.

CONTACTS: Flagstaff Ranger District, 5075 N. AZ 89, Flagstaff, AZ 86004; (928) 526-0866; **www.fs.fed.us/r3/coconino/recreation/mormon_lake/aztrail-fisher-point-tr.shtml**

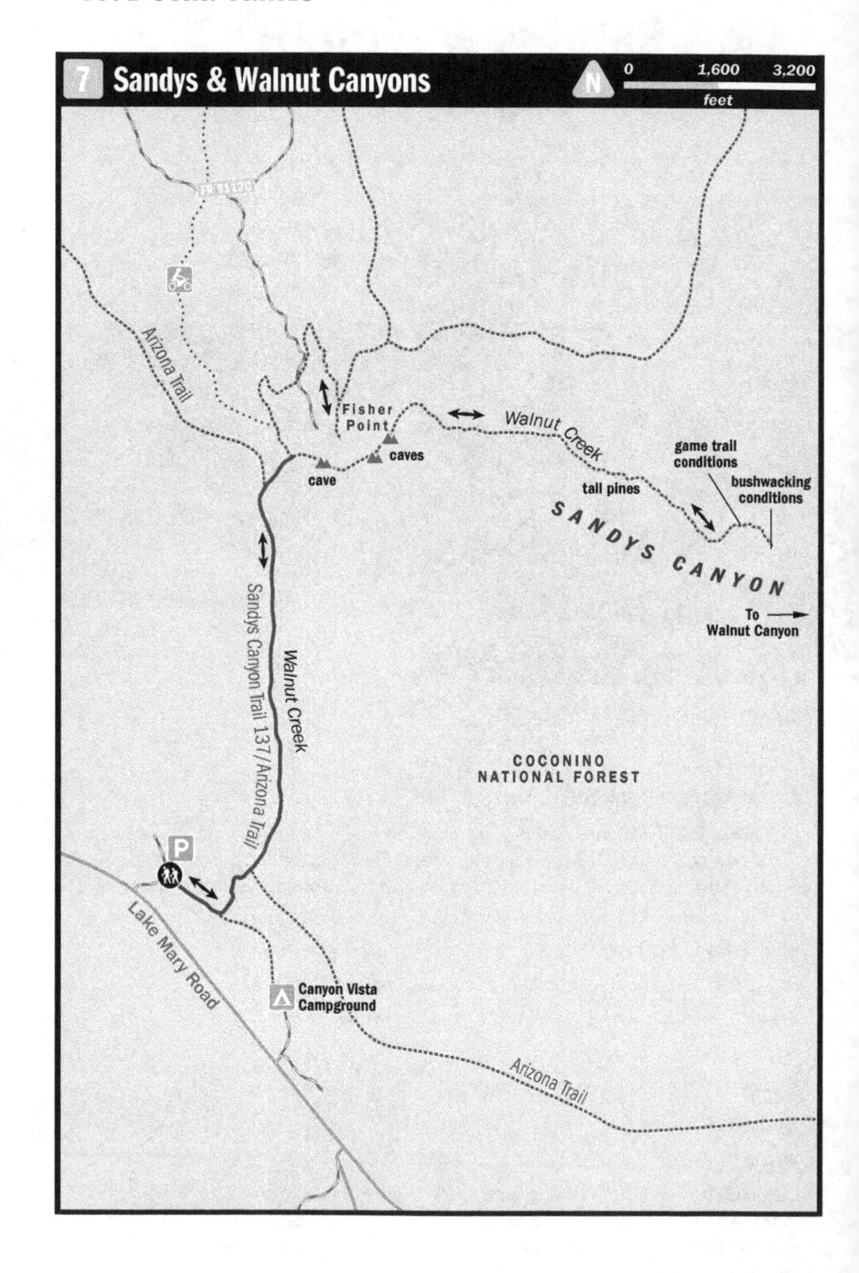
7 Sandys & Walnut Canyons
0
1,600
3,200
feet
Arizona Trail
Fisher Point
Walnut Creek
caves
cave
game trail conditions
bushwacking conditions
tall pines
SANDYS CANYON
To Walnut Canyon
Sandys Canyon Trail 137/Arizona Trail
Walnut Creek
COCONINO NATIONAL FOREST
Lake Mary Road
Canyon Vista Campground
Arizona Trail

Overview

This hike follows Sandys Canyon Trail 137 to the mouth of Walnut Canyon, where you can climb to the Fisher Point overlook and/or follow the trail deeper into scenic Walnut Canyon, which contains a few small caves. The Sandys Canyon segment is part of the Arizona National Scenic Trail (AZT), which runs north–south through the state for 800 miles, from Mexico to Utah.

Route Details

From the dirt lot, follow the well-labeled sandy track south (at first) through the pine forest. Within 0.25 mile you pass a junction with a spur trail that goes down into the ravine, past a popular climbing area known as The Pit, and then up to Canyon Vista Campground. The main trail, which you want to stay on, turns east before a short but steep descent (about 200 feet) into the ravine.

Limestone and basalt boulders of all shapes and sizes clutter the path as it follows the drainage through Sandys Canyon, crossing the wash a few times before climbing out to become a remnant jeep trail through the flat grass.

Just under 1 mile in, you pass the junction with the AZT, which joins the Sandys Canyon Trail 137 at this point. To your right, the AZT goes west 4.5 miles to the Marshall Lake Trailhead, and then

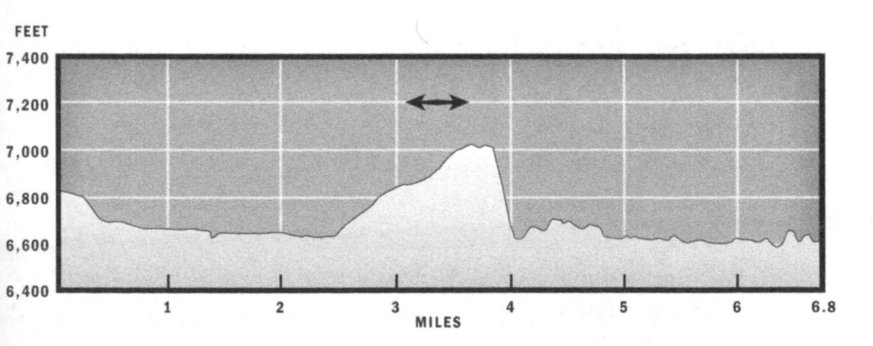

continues on roughly south all the way to Mexico. Stay straight (north) through Sandys Canyon.

Just over 1 mile later (at 2.08 miles), the trail splits at the first corner of a wide triangular intersection stretched across the meadow that fills the confluence of Sandys and Walnut canyons. As the sign will indicate, the regular AZT continues northwest from this point, going another 3.25 miles until it reaches Flagstaff on its way to the Grand Canyon and then Utah. The equestrian bypass continues northeast, going another 10.8 miles until the underpass beneath I-40. Take the equestrian bypass to your right (northeast). Within 100 yards you come to a second Y where the spur into Walnut Canyon separates from the equestrian bypass. (A third spur connects to the third Y of the triangle.) Hawks and ravens (and sometimes eagles) love this meadow and frequently soar overhead.

Within sight of the second intersection, you can see a shallow cave set in the bottom of the conical pile of limestone that supports the prominence called Fisher Point. That sensible rest stop is the turnaround for the easy hike.

To extend the hike, you face a choice: Take the AZT up to Fisher Point or follow the Walnut Canyon Trail into its namesake. Both are out-and-backs that return to this very spot, and there is no particular advantage to doing either one first. Alphabetically, though, Fisher Point precedes Walnut Canyon.

FISHER POINT: The equestrian AZT huffs up the ravine to the north. Midway up there is an apparent Y, but it is really just a detour for dirt bikes, leading to an easier means to cross the drainage farther uphill. At the top of the ravine, the trail switchbacks south across the ridge, and then follows an easy but extended series of switchbacks up the hill.

Along the way you cross a dirt road, which is a spur to FR 9112C. Just beyond that will be another big U-turn bending south. Soon, the AZT will switchback north again, but before that point you encounter the signed spur leading to Fisher Point.

Through the pines and junipers on top of Fisher Point, you

can see the triangle crossing the meadow below, as well as hawks and ravens circling about. You can also see other landmarks, such as Mount Elden, Flagstaff, and even the San Francisco Peaks if you hunt a bit for a vantage point.

Fisher Point is just over a mile from the triangle, and 3.45 miles from the trailhead. Return the way you came back to the triangle.

WALNUT CANYON: From the triangle, follow the thin track across the grass to the cave, and keep going. You soon encounter a sign extolling Walnut Canyon. According to that sign, the hike goes on about another mile, but it actually goes farther than that.

Rocks and shrubs choke the trail just past the sign, but it soon opens back up to a wide track across the grass. As you follow the winding path up the canyon, closely following the normally dry creek, you may notice that just about every tree and shrub that grows in northern Arizona has found root somewhere in Walnut Canyon. Among these leaves dart all manner of birds, lizards, and bugs.

The primary attractions, though, are the caves, both of which can be easily sighted from the trail. The mouth of the shallow cave (though deeper than the one at the mouth of the canyon) is about 0.25 mile beyond the sign, and the entrance to the deep cave about 0.1 mile past that. This last cave is deep enough to require a flashlight to explore fully, but not so deep that you could get seriously lost. But watch your head.

The deep cave is the turnaround for most hikers, yet the trail clearly continues beyond it and can be rewarding if you have the time and energy remaining. It goes up and down the north slope of the canyon, and then drops back into the drainage as the canyon bends south. The path tramples across the drainage, occasionally pushing through thick brush as it passes below towering white cliffs and everything from prickly pear cacti to spruce trees.

About 1 mile past the deep cave, or 1.5 miles past the triangle, the trail crosses through a stand of old-growth ponderosa pines. This is another fine turnaround spot, for past here it will become clear that the trail receives more traffic from deer than people. Indeed, within 0.5 mile, it degenerates into little more than a game trail, frequently blocked with deadfall, and within 0.75 mile you would be clearly bushwhacking.

If you push on to that last point, you have gone 6.8 miles from the original trailhead (assuming you also hiked up and down Fisher Point). Regardless of how far you went, return the way you came.

Directions

From Flagstaff, follow Lake Mary Road for about 6 miles from the interstates. As you leave Flagstaff city limits, look for FR 94784 to you left (east). Follow this dirt road a few hundred yards to the unofficial parking area that serves as a trailhead.

If you reach Canyon Vista Campground, you've gone too far. While the trail can be accessed from the campground, there are no day-use facilities there.

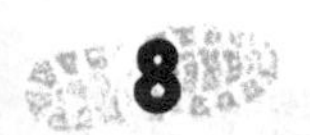

8 Winter Cabin Loop

SCENERY: ★★★★
TRAIL CONDITION: ★★★
CHILDREN: ★★
DIFFICULTY: ★★★
SOLITUDE: ★★

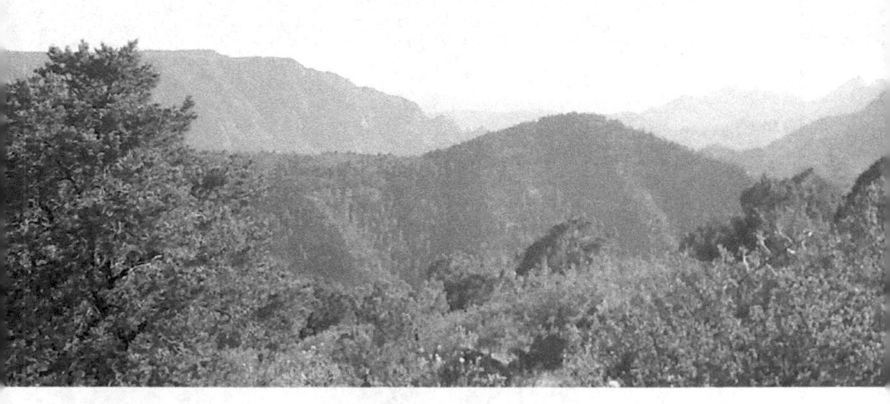

LOOKING SOUTHWARD INTO SYCAMORE CANYON FROM THE TOP OF HOG HILL

GPS TRAILHEAD COORDINATES: N35° 03.547' W111° 55.044'

DISTANCE & CONFIGURATION: 10.5-mile loop

HIKING TIME: 5 hours

HIGHLIGHTS: Scenic vistas, flowing springs, and an old cabin

ELEVATION: 6,916 feet at trailhead to 5,987 feet at Ott Lake

ACCESS: No fees; requires a high-clearance vehicle, and roads may be impassable during wet conditions.

MAPS: USFS Sycamore Canyon Wilderness

FACILITIES: None

WHEELCHAIR ACCESS: None

COMMENTS: Sycamore Canyon drains through cattle country, so water here is not safe to drink without treatment. Most of the hike is within the wilderness area, so no bikes are allowed. See note at the end about route options.

CONTACTS: Flagstaff Ranger District, 5075 N. AZ 89, Flagstaff, AZ 86004; (928) 526-0866; **www.fs.fed.us/r3/coconino/recreation/peaks/sycamore-canyon-wild.shtml**

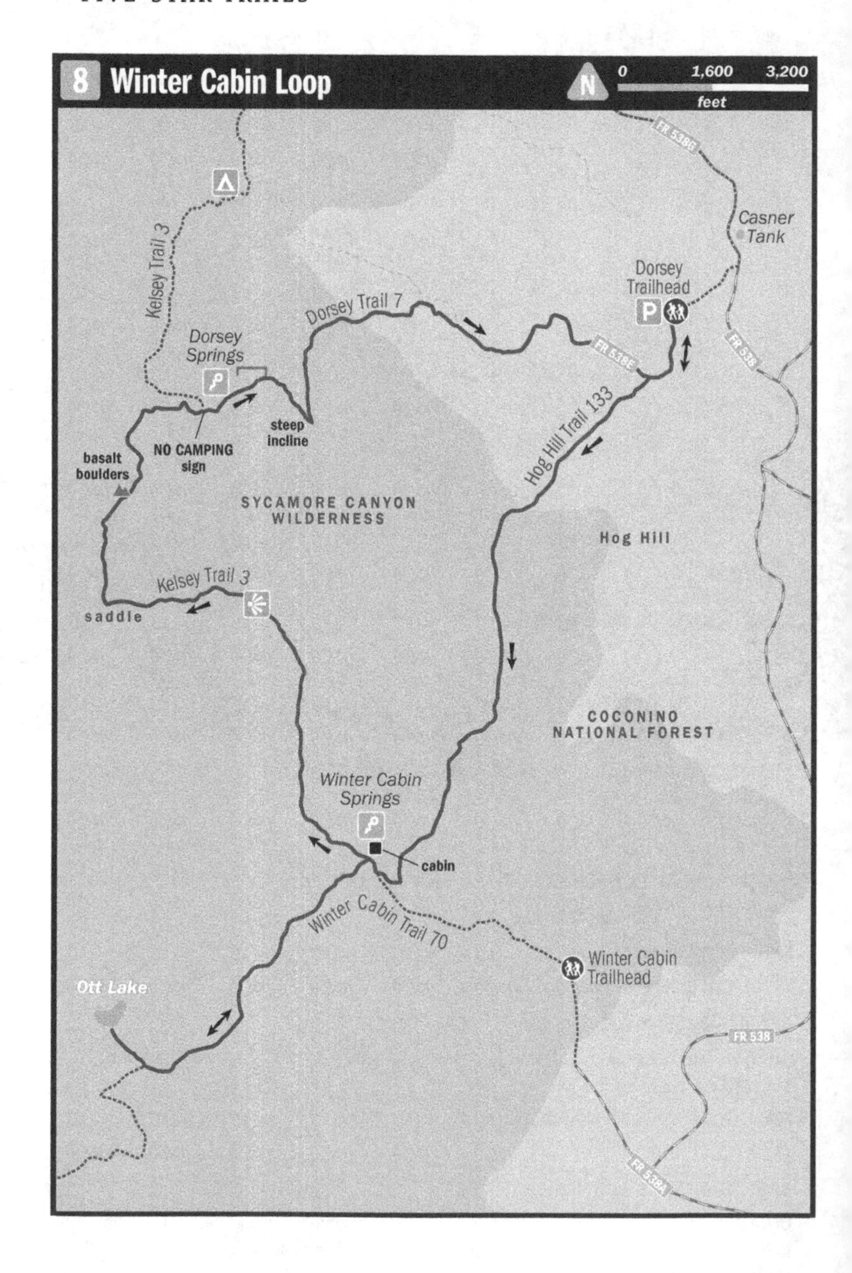
8 Winter Cabin Loop
N
0
1,600
3,200
feet
FR 538G
Casner Tank
Dorsey Trailhead
P
FR 538
FR 538E
Kelsey Trail 3
Dorsey Trail 7
Dorsey Springs
steep incline
NO CAMPING sign
basalt boulders
Hog Hill Trail 133
SYCAMORE CANYON WILDERNESS
Hog Hill
Kelsey Trail 3
saddle
COCONINO NATIONAL FOREST
Winter Cabin Springs
cabin
Winter Cabin Trail 70
Winter Cabin Trailhead
Ott Lake
FR 538
FR 538A

Overview

This loop takes the Hog Hill Trail 133 down to Winter Cabin and its nearby spring. Then, after an optional detour to Ott Lake, it follows the Kelsey Trail 3 back north along the edge of Sycamore Canyon to the Dorsey Trail 7, which leads east, up the canyon wall and back to the trailhead.

Route Details

From the Dorsey Trailhead, follow the remnant road past the wilderness boundary sign a few hundred yards from the parking area (the actual legal boundary is about a mile farther in), into a forest populated with piñon and ponderosa pines along with some enormous alligator junipers.

Within 0.25 mile, you come to the signed Y-intersection with Hog Hill Trail 133. Dorsey Trail 7 continues almost due west, as Hog Hill splits to the southwest. Take the left onto Hog Hill as it begins climbing up its namesake.

The path levels off at 6,900 feet before it approaches the actual wilderness boundary. Past here the trail becomes singletrack, and the forest deepens. Deer and elk signs abound.

A mile in, a basalt slide marks a boundary into transition scrub, where the pines clear aside for scattered junipers and manzanitas. But

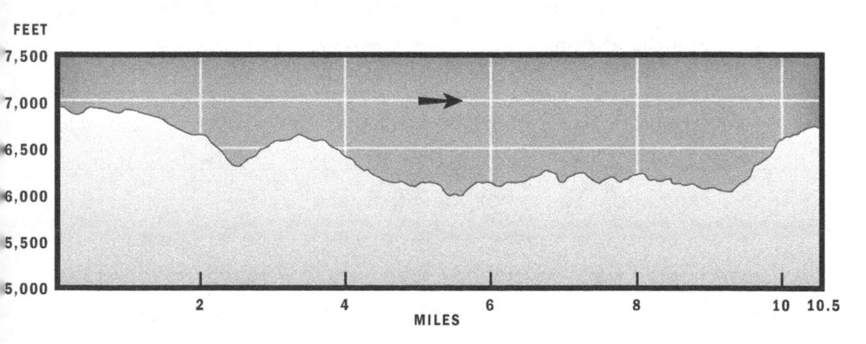

after 0.25 mile, you return to the relative shade of pines and oaks as the trail winds down the ridge to a broad shelf.

On top of this shelf, you'll see glimpses of Sycamore Canyon through the trees, but what you really need to look for are cairns marking a sudden left (essentially south) across a clearing trampled with game trails. From the shelf, the trail makes one more steep descent, switching back into a ravine. The trail climbs out of that ravine to the signed junction with Winter Cabin Trail 70. Look to your right, and you will see the cabin itself about a hundred yards down the hill. To your left, Winter Cabin Trail 70 climbs steadily southeast for just over 1 mile to the Winter Cabin Trailhead.

The cabin itself is not much: wood and mortar walls barely supporting a crumbling tin roof. Rusting remains of a woodstove and bedsprings lie behind the cabin. A frequently used campsite spreads out in front. At the corner of this campsite is the junction with Kelsey Trail 3. Immediately northeast of the cabin, a spur trail leads to Winter Cabin Springs seeping into the ravine.

OTT LAKE: The short side trip to Ott Lake is worthwhile, assuming you aren't pressed for time or energy. Continue on Winter Cabin Trail 70 to the southwest as it winds through the pines along the ridge. It continues gently up and down the canyon wall for most of a mile until it climbs to the top of a finger ridge. The pines part as manzanitas and scrub oaks take over the gravelly soil. As you turn the corner heading more westerly, the whole southern canyon comes into view.

You'll be able to see where the trail drops into the drainage and winds around Buck Ridge, where it will join the Sycamore Basin Trail, the historical cattle route connecting Flagstaff and Jerome. That's a major expedition. You're not going that far.

In fact, a few hundred yards farther you'll see the sign for Ott Lake. The spur trail cuts northwest, across a small saddle, reaching the lake within 0.1 mile. At best, Ott Lake is a marshy pond. Most of the time, it is a shallow crater where weeds sprout from dry, cracked clay.

Return the way you came to Winter Cabin. The entire side trip covers 3 miles out-and-back, making your total mileage just under 5 miles. The route now continues northwest along the Kelsey Trail 3.

UP THE KELSEY TRAIL: From Winter Cabin, the Kelsey drops quickly into, then out of, a ravine and keeps climbing at a more gradual pace for some time. After 1 mile, the trail climbs onto a scrub-covered ridge. As the trail winds to the west, brown cliffs of Coconino limestone tower to the north, while canyon vistas open to the south. The trail winds through thickets of live oaks and manzanitas, with infrequent shade from the junipers. Ahead, a rock knob stands alone like a battlement.

As you approach that landmark, the trail will turn north, climbing across the saddle that separates the knob from the rest of the canyon. Past that saddle, the pines and oaks return to shade a softer trail.

The trail continues like this, nearly due north, for a mile or so. A slide of basalt boulders signals tougher times. The trail climbs steeply northeast up the canyon. Boulders and deadfall provide regular obstacles. While the climb continues for most of a mile, the last half is easier. A green ditch full of grass leads to Dorsey Springs, but stay on the trail to reach the signed intersection with Dorsey Trail 7. At this point you have traveled 7.75 miles, including the Ott Lake spur.

Dorsey Trail 7 goes roughly east from the junction (an obvious right), crossing a well-worn campsite before bending south near the spring for which it was named. A plastic pipe leads from the spring, but most of the time more water gurgles through the thin streambed around it, watering a thin line of grass that goes several hundred yards down the canyon.

At this point, the trail climbs steeply up the canyon wall, leveling out across a shelf populated with tall piñon pines before beginning an even steeper climb.

The next climb huffs east up the ravine and then bends to go southeast up a second ravine, finally turning nearly north as you near the end of the brutality. From the springs, you have gained just under 500 feet in elevation in about 0.75 mile.

The trail climbs gently now as a singletrack rolling up through the pines until you come to the wilderness boundary. Beyond this deer maze, the Dorsey is a remnant road, crossing a wide shelf covered with pines and oaks until it reaches that familiar junction with the Hog Hill Trail 133.

Return the way you came.

Routing options: The Kelsey Springs Loop (see page 57) also begins at the Dorsey Trailhead (for similar reasons), and it can be combined with the Winter Cabin Loop for a super-loop (skipping the Dorsey Trail 7). Such a loop would be 9 miles without the spurs to either Geronimo Springs (on the Kelsey Springs side) or Ott Lake, both of which would add 2 and 3 miles, respectively.

Directions

From Flagstaff, follow US 66 southwest out of town until its intersection with Woody Mountain Road (FR 231). Turn left (south) on Woody Mountain past the Flagstaff Arboretum. Drive for 16 miles until its intersection with FR 538. Take the right (north) onto FR 538. This area is open cattle range, and you may find yourself sitting in the road waiting for the cows to mosey out of your way. Continue another 6 miles over the hill until you reach FR 538E, where you turn right again. The driveway to the trailhead is marked with a sign.

Alternate access: If you wish to bounce down to the Winter Cabin Trailhead, continue on FR 538 south, past Turkey Butte, beyond which it will degenerate into a jeep trail as it winds down the hill. FR 538H will spur off to the right (west) to terminate at the trailhead.

While the hike could be done from either the Winter Cabin or Dorsey trailheads, the latter trailhead can be reliably reached with any reasonably high-clearance vehicle, while the Winter Cabin Trailhead requires a four-wheel-drive vehicle. Starting from the Winter Cabin Trailhead adds 2.4 miles to the total trip.

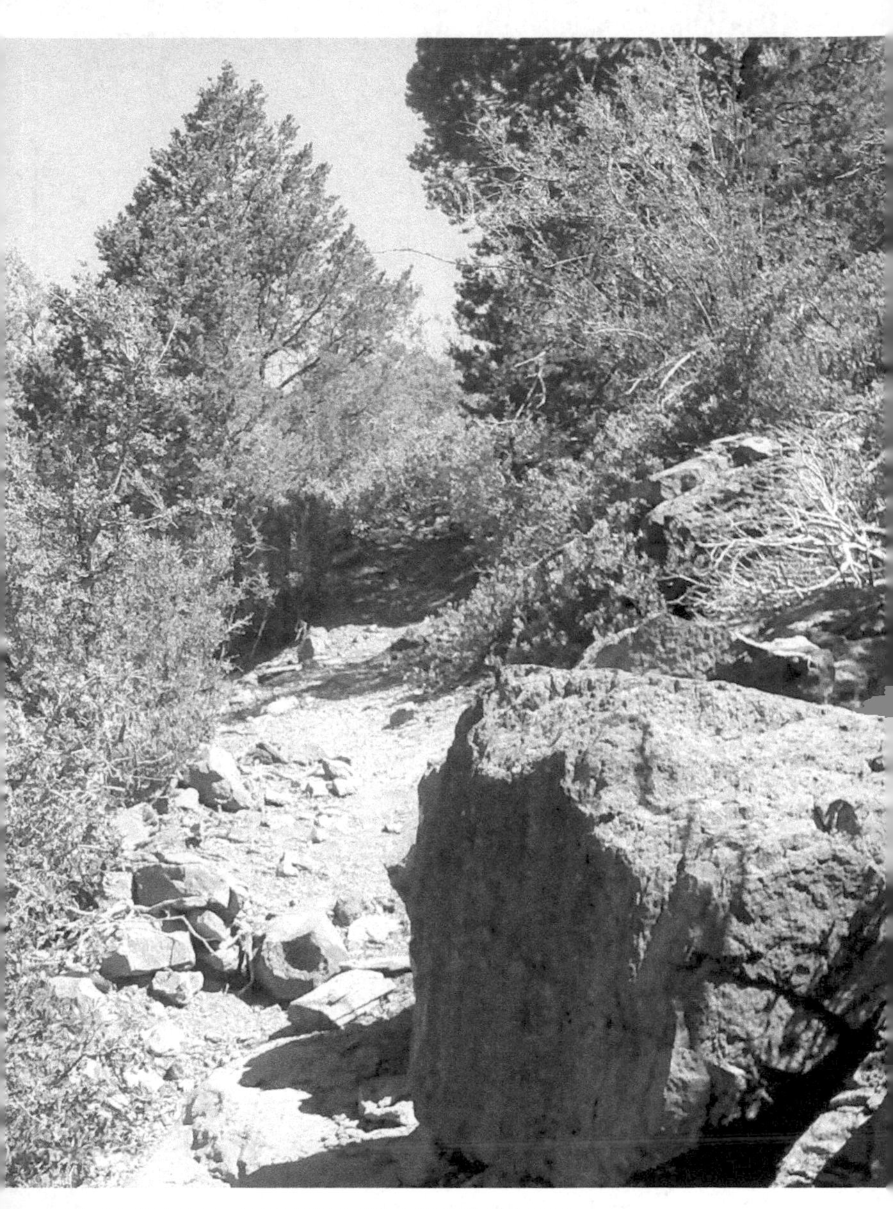

THE KELSEY TRAIL CLIMBS THROUGH TRANSITION SCRUB.

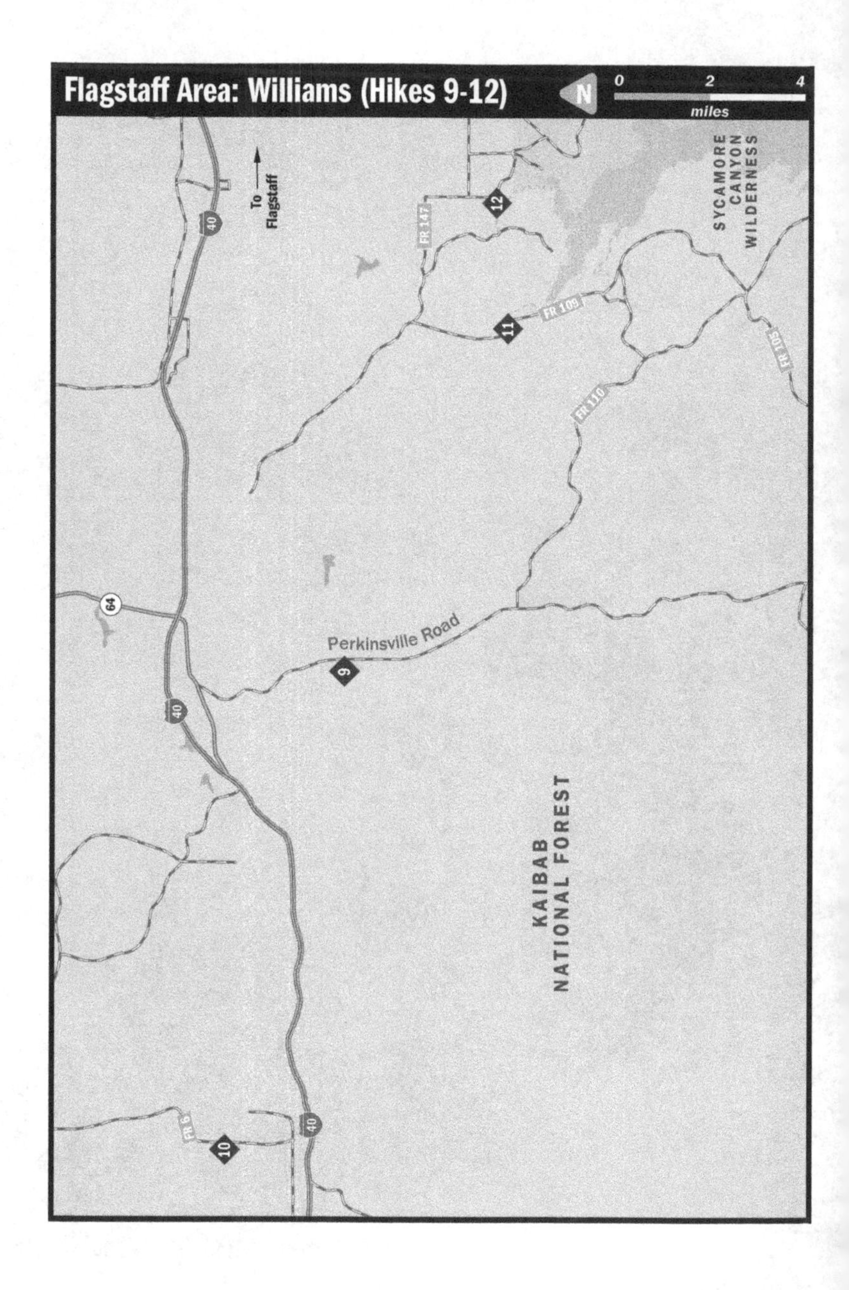
Flagstaff Area: Williams (Hikes 9-12)
N
0
2
4
miles
SYCAMORE CANYON WILDERNESS
To Flagstaff
40
12
11
FR 147
FR 109
FR 105
FR 110
64
Perkinsville Road
9
KAIBAB NATIONAL FOREST
FR 6
10

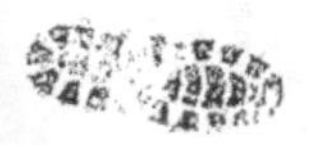

Flagstaff Area: Williams

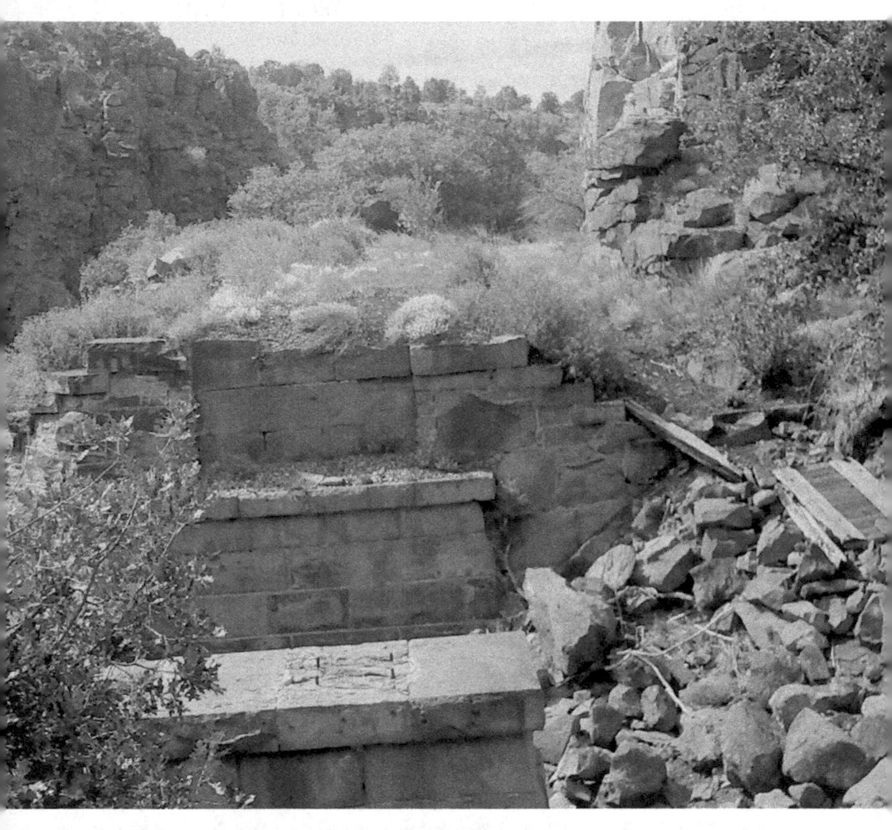

ABANDONED RAILROAD BRIDGE IN JOHNSON CANYON

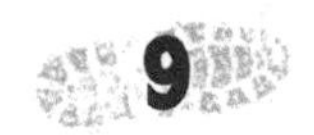

Bill Williams Mountain

SCENERY: ★★★★
TRAIL CONDITION: ★★★★
CHILDREN: ★★
DIFFICULTY: ★★★★
SOLITUDE: ★★★★
(★★ at the peak)

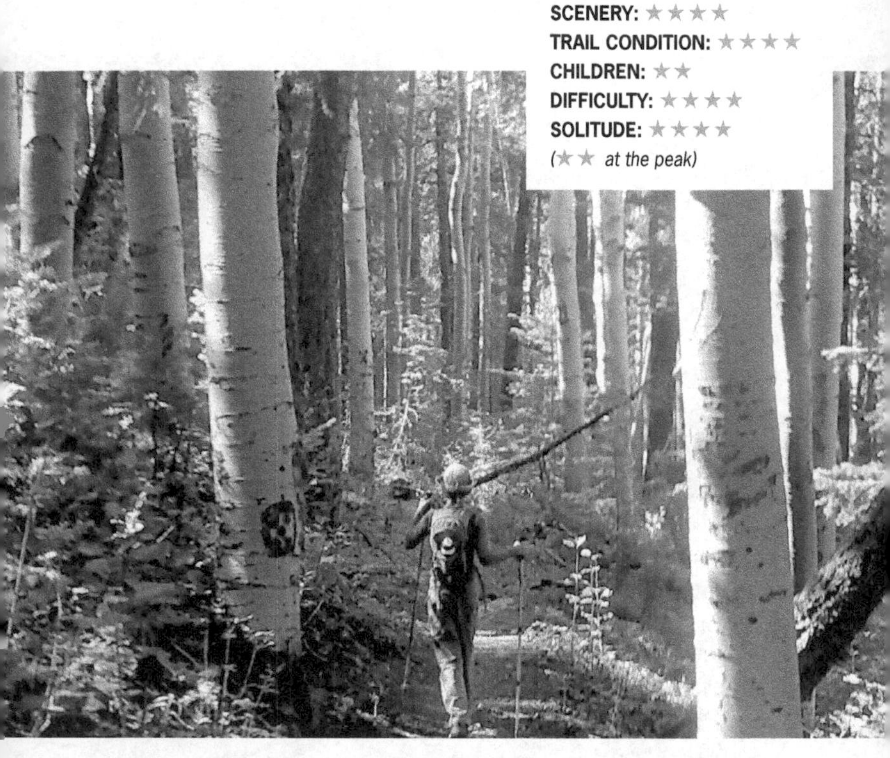

ASPENS ON BILL WILLIAMS MOUNTAIN

GPS COORDINATES: *Benham Trailhead:* N35° 12.228' W112° 10.387'
Bill Williams Mountain Trailhead: N35° 14.254' W112° 12.886'

DISTANCE & CONFIGURATION: 8.25-mile car shuttle. Benham Trail alone is 8.6 miles; Bill Williams Mountain Trail alone is 7.8 miles (both out-and-back). For an easier car shuttle, you can also drive to the top of the mountain; see "Directions."

HIKING TIME: 5 hours

HIGHLIGHTS: Panoramic vistas, wildlife, deep forests, and lookout tower

ELEVATION: 7,265 feet at Benham Trailhead and 6,947 feet at Bill Williams Mountain Trailhead to 9,256 feet at the peak

ACCESS: No fees or restrictions

MAPS: USGS Williams

FACILITIES: Restrooms and picnic tables at both trailheads; ranger station at Bill Williams

WHEELCHAIR ACCESS: None

COMMENTS: It is possible to drive to the peak, so expect company. This description is written as a car shuttle, but if that can't be arranged, either hike can be done as an out-and-back. Benham alone is 4.3 miles one-way to the peak, while Bill Williams is 3.9 miles one-way. While arguably equal in scenic value, Benham is a slightly easier climb.

CONTACTS: Williams Ranger District, 742 S. Clover Rd., Williams, AZ 86046; (928) 635-5600; **www.fs.usda.gov/kaibab**

Overview

This car-shuttle hike winds up and down Bill Williams Mountain, named for the mountain man who also lent his name to the nearby town. The hike starts up the Benham Trail to the peak, which has a working fire watchtower, and then down the Bill Williams Mountain Trail to end near the ranger station at the edge of town.

Route Details

Take the wide dirt path west from the Benham Trailhead. Keep an eye out for deer through here, especially in the morning. The trail quickly climbs a ridge. The clearing to your left (south) surrounds a private campground.

In 0.5 mile, you cross a drainage and climb a second ridge. A small burned area opens to a view of Bill Williams Mountain looming in the distance. After a full mile (wooden posts will mark the mileage), the path takes a U-turn to climb a third ridge. Shortly thereafter, you pass beneath some power lines. You can see the cut for the power lines going up the slope like an alleyway through the forest.

After another 0.5 mile, the trail winds through a lovely stand of Gambel oaks mixed in with some spruce and fir saplings and a multitude of ferns. All manner of birds may be carrying on overhead. On the far side of this stand, the switchbacks start.

Benham Trail 38 was constructed in the 1920s as an alternative to the toll road (now Bill Williams Mountain Trail 21) but abandoned in the 1950s as the modern road was completed. In the 1970s it was reopened as this recreational trail and named for H. L. Benham, a ranger who helped establish the Williams Ranger District in 1910.

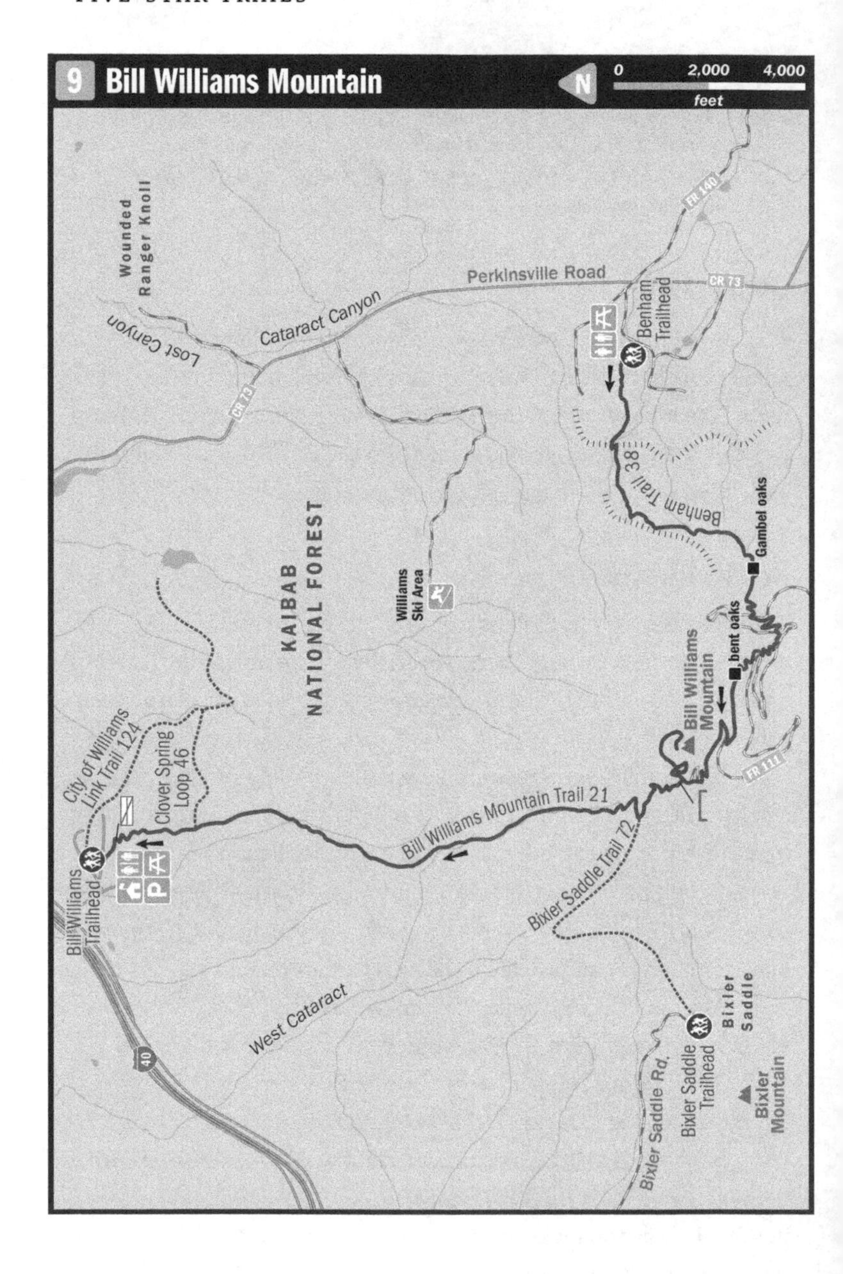
9 Bill Williams Mountain
N
0 2,000 4,000
feet
Wounded Ranger Knoll
Lost Canyon
Cataract Canyon
Perkinsville Road
CR 73
FR 140
Benham Trailhead
Benham Trail 38
Gambel oaks
KAIBAB NATIONAL FOREST
Williams Ski Area
bent oaks
Bill Williams Mountain
FR 111
City of Williams Link Trail 124
Clover Spring Loop 46
Bill Williams Trailhead
Bill Williams Mountain Trail 21
Bixler Saddle Trail 72
West Cataract
40
Bixler Saddle Rd.
Bixler Saddle Trailhead
Bixler Saddle
Bixler Mountain

The Benham marches back and forth through mixed conifers until the first road crossing, at Forest Road 111, which goes all the way to the top, at about the 2-mile mark. This juncture is about halfway in distance but less than a fourth in effort. Look to your left for the old pack trail to continue up the mountain across the road. Turn around to the east for a view of the San Francisco Peaks.

You cross this same road a second time within 0.5 mile. At the 3-mile mark, you'll find some good views to the south, and then look for the Gambel oaks bending south across the trail toward the sunshine. In season, this slope explodes with wildflowers. The trail begins a long western traverse (about 0.33 mile) before the switchbacks begin again, steeper than ever, as they march you through a third road crossing at 3.5 miles.

Before you reach the 4-mile mark, you cross the road a fourth time, clearly close to the peak now. Aspens interrupt the spruces and firs. A short segment of footpath continues to a fifth crossing, but you lose nothing by staying on the road, for only the road takes you to the peak in the end.

As you wind your way around toward the peak, though, take note of where the Bill Williams Mountain Trail 21 leaves the road to charge down the north slope. You'll be back for that. Meanwhile, stay on the road.

The road spirals around the mountain until it reaches the

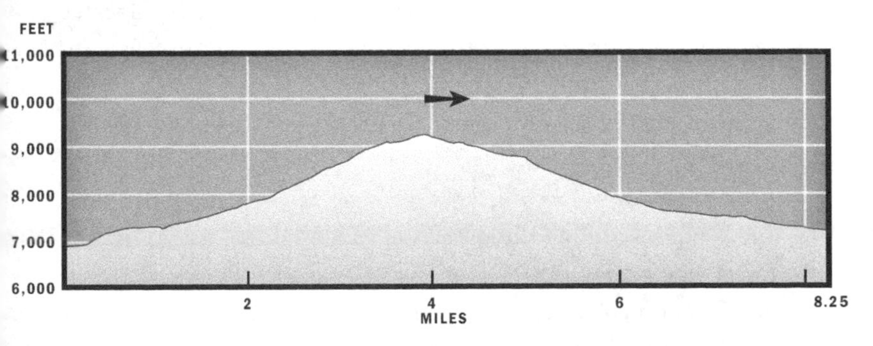

peak, crowned with antennae and transmitters of all sorts, and a fire lookout tower manned throughout the summer. Sometimes the tower ranger has time to talk, but other times he has work to do. This is the ranger's office (though he doesn't have to sleep here as is often the case at other towers). Don't just barge in uninvited.

From the peak, with or without being on the tower, you can see as far south as Mingus Mountain and as far north as the Grand Canyon. Ladybugs cover the bushes. Because this area can be reached by car, you may have plenty of nonhiker company.

Take FR 111 back down to the Bill Williams Mountain Trail 21, the path you will have noted on your way up. There is no sign, but it is the only other trail. A bench sits where the footpath meets the road. Technically, the junction is up the slope a few yards on the other side of the road, but that would lead you right to here anyway.

Switchbacks head down from the road through the old-growth mixed conifer and aspens. You can prove to yourself through here that the moss does indeed tend to grow on the north side of the tree. Looking lower, you will see mushrooms, ferns, and berries on occasion.

At 0.33 mile past the junction, you come to an intersection with the Bixler Saddle Trail 72, which leads westward to its namesake. Stay straight on Bill Williams.

At 5.5 total miles, the switchbacks straighten and the trail follows a brush-choked ravine down the slope. A great many boulders and deadfall lie strewn between the tall trees. Then, 0.75 mile later, chokecherry trees appear as the trail pulls to the right to follow the ridgeline east of the drainage. Soon you pass mile marker 2 (numbered from the Bill Williams Mountain Trailhead) posted within a field of boulders.

The path plunges down the ridge, as the deep pines open into juniper scrub and brighter sunshine. At 7.6 total miles, you pass a junction with the Clover Spring Trail 46, part of a municipal trail system in Williams. Soon after, the trail starts winding down the ridge. Not only does the grade increase, but the trail itself also becomes as hard as concrete and full of rocks.

You pass through a gate, and the trail begins switching back until it reaches a junction with City of Williams Link Trail 124. Stay straight—not right. Past this, the trail softens to an easy stroll across the meadow less than 0.5 mile to the Bill Williams Mountain Trailhead.

Directions

To Benham Trailhead: From Flagstaff, take I-40 west about 30 miles to Williams. Take Williams Exit 165, going left (south) into town on Railroad Avenue. In town, turn left (south) on Fourth Street. After a few blocks this becomes County Road 73 (Perkinsville Road). Continue 3.5 miles, past the reservoir, to FR 140, where you turn right (west). Park at the trailhead, less than 0.5 mile down the road. The trailhead has vault toilets, a few picnic tables, and some horse facilities.

To Williams Ranger Station: From downtown Williams (see above), continue west on Railroad Avenue for 1 mile, and then turn left (essentially west) at the I-40 frontage road. There will be a sign here for the ranger station as well. Continue west along the frontage road, past the motels, to the turnoff to the Williams Ranger District office. The Bill Williams Mountain Trailhead is at the south end of the parking lot. There are vault toilets and picnic tables at the trailhead; water is available at the ranger station, but it closes by 4:30 p.m. year-round.

To the peak: FR 111, which leads to the peak, can be reached from CR 73 about a mile south of the Benham Trailhead turnoff. This graded dirt road is passable in passenger cars in good weather, but it is full of steep grades and sharp turns. While there is no formal parking at the peak, there is room between the buildings for three or four vehicles.

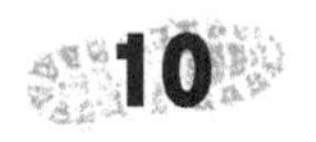

10 Johnson Canyon Railroad

SCENERY: ★★★★

TRAIL CONDITION: ★★★★★/★★★

(before the tunnel/beyond the tunnel)

CHILDREN: ★★★★/★★★

(before the tunnel/beyond the tunnel)

DIFFICULTY: ★★

SOLITUDE: ★★★★

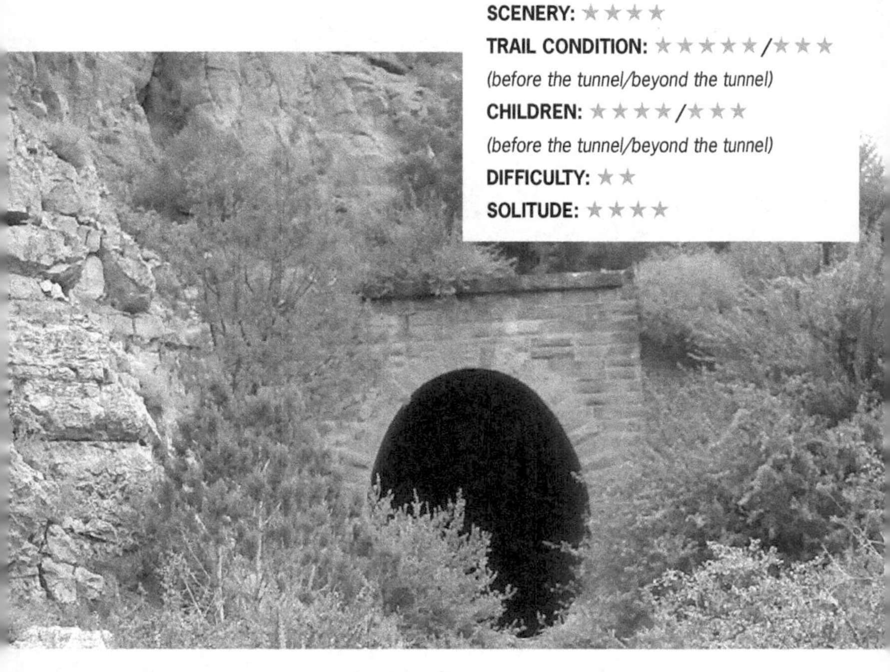

JOHNSON CANYON RAILROAD TUNNEL

GPS TRAILHEAD COORDINATES: N35° 14.679' W112° 21.705'

DISTANCE & CONFIGURATION: 6 miles for the easy hike to the waterfall; 8.25 miles for the total hike out-and-back

HIKING TIME: 4 hours for the out-and-back; 3 hours for the easy hike

HIGHLIGHTS: Bridges, railroad tunnel, and seasonal waterfall

ELEVATION: 5,926 feet at trailhead to 6,363 feet at end of hike

ACCESS: No fees or restrictions

MAPS: USGS Ashfork and McLellan Reservoir

FACILITIES: None

WHEELCHAIR ACCESS: None

COMMENTS: Easy and longer versions of this hike are described. No reliable water sources on the trail.

CONTACTS: Williams Ranger District, 742 S. Clover Rd., Williams, AZ 86046; (928) 635-5600; **www.fs.usda.gov/kaibab**

Overview

This hike follows the old railroad grade from the ruins of Welch Station, up Johnson Canyon, and through an abandoned railroad tunnel to the site of an occasional waterfall. The grade continues another couple miles up the canyon, passing the ruins of bridges and other railroad infrastructure. The easy version of this hike turns around at the waterfall.

Route Details

The trailhead is at the site of Welch Station, never much in its heyday and even less now. To the northwest of the intersection, find a large concrete pad among the brush and sunflowers: the foundation of the railroad station, and the largest remaining remnant of the settlement. Other, smaller traces remain among the brush if you wish to hunt for them. Be wary, though, when poking around here because the tall grass hides gopher holes, stumble rocks, prickly pear cactus—even the rare rattlesnake.

FR 9183Y northbound is the trail. (The southbound segment goes 0.25 mile to dead-end at the modern tracks.) The smooth lava-gravel road can be navigated by vehicle, but you must understand that it was built for trains and is maintained by no one. It is a narrow path for a full-size vehicle. Most of the tire tracks you see were made by all-terrain vehicles (ATVs).

The thin road climbs slightly up the west side of Johnson Canyon. Scrub oaks and junipers grow over the profusion of tall prairie weeds in the lower canyon, but keep an eye out for an occasional patch of wild squash.

Soon both the canyon and the road bend a little east, and a bridge carries you across a deep side channel. Immediately past the ridge you pass through a cut rock, and then around a bend before crossing beneath the angry buzz of high-voltage lines.

Below you in the canyon, now a couple hundred feet lower, you can see a wide field covered with cattle tracks. The ribbon of rock that

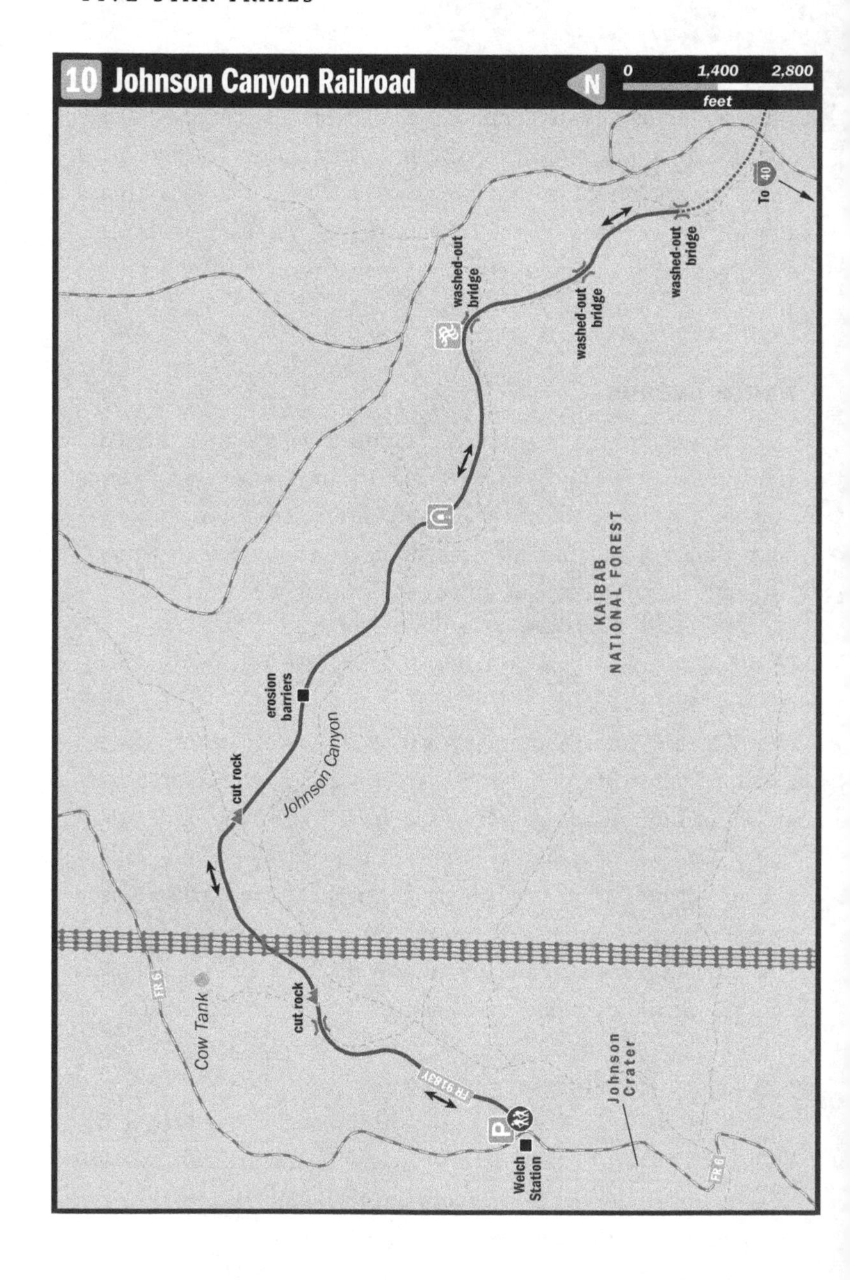
10 Johnson Canyon Railroad
N
0
1,400
2,800
feet
To 40
washed-out bridge
washed-out bridge
washed-out bridge
KAIBAB
NATIONAL FOREST
erosion barriers
Johnson Canyon
cut rock
cut rock
Cow Tank
FR 6
FR 9183Y
Johnson Crater
Welch Station
FR 6

represents the normally dry Johnson Creek passes just to the east of that clearing. Beyond the canyon, to the south, the bustle of I-40 can be made out in the distance. Ahead of you, the gravel road continues to bend toward the east.

A towering berm takes you across the next side channel, completing the turn to the east. On the far side, the grade passes through a second cut rock.

After 1.7 miles, the first of several metal-and-concrete erosion barriers lines the downslope side of the grade. In the canyon below, pines, including some small stands of ponderosa, displace the junipers. Above are short sandstone cliffs dotted with small erosion caves. As you crunch along through here, the trail bends to the south, and soon you will see the highlight: the tunnel.

The brick-lined tunnel entrance becomes clearly visible as you cross over the final, short berm. Here the graveled track stops and the trail becomes rougher dirt. During World War II, this passage, one of the few rail lines into California, stayed under 24-hour guard.

The tunnel itself extends 328 feet, and while its curve prevents sunlight from passing clean through, it can be easily navigated without a flashlight.

The Atlantic and Pacific Railroad started blasting this hole in 1881 and didn't finish until 1882. At its peak, 3,000 men worked on the project, many losing their lives to explosives or drunken

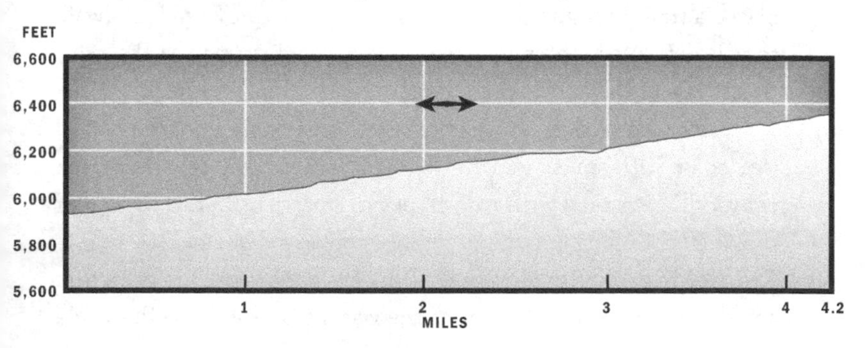

antics. The original shoring was destroyed early on through fire in 1898, a year after the Santa Fe Railroad acquired the line, and the existing masonry-and-steel boilerplate replaced it.

This railroad tunnel, the only one west of Albuquerque, had a notorious reputation. The steep grade coming into the canyon from Williams forced engineers to brake hard, which, over time, deformed the tracks and led to derailments—frequently off the trestle bridge that once spanned the chasm you just crossed. Remnants of those old wrecks reportedly still lie scattered inside the canyon.

In 1911 the railroad built a second, less steep route bypassing Johnson Canyon; eastbound (and upward bound) trains used this route. As steam trains were phased out, the 1911 route was doubletracked, and the Johnson Canyon section was abandoned entirely by 1962.

Beyond the tunnel, a rougher path hugs the cliff of what is now the north side of the narrowing canyon. Arizona walnut trees crowd the trail along with reeds and weeds. Within 0.25 mile, the trail passes a falls (when water flows) and, shortly beyond, the first washed-out bridge. At 3 miles, this is the turnaround for the easy hike.

A footpath, reinforced by ATV traffic, leads in and out of the side ravine the bridge once crossed, and the remnant grade continues, now turning clearly south. At 3.66 miles you come to your second washed-out bridge: a beautiful piece of orange masonry that once crossed the ravine, about 40 feet deep here. Once again, ATVers have blazed a trail through the ravine. Look for the improvised boardwalk to your left, cross the ravine, and follow the dirt track to the right (west) side of the opposite buttress.

Past the second bridge, you'll see occasional remnant railroad ties, some with spikes and plates still attached. You pass through a cut rock half-choked with wild grapes to emerge nearer to the top of the canyon. Rolling grasslands line the top on either side.

At the 4-mile mark, and at an elevation of 6,363 feet, you come to the third and largest of the washed-out bridges. The grade continues beyond the bridge, of course, but soon passes through private property. Return the way you came.

Directions

From Flagstaff, head west on I-40 for 44.5 miles, past the town of Williams, to Welch Exit 151. Head north on FR 6, taking care not to be misled by the many spur roads near the exit. This area is popular with RVers. Follow the graded dirt FR 6 down through the wash (lower Johnson Canyon) and then uphill. At about 14.5 miles from the exit, you will pass Johnson Crater (on the left), which is worth checking out. Another 0.25 mile past the crater, you will come to a clearing with a cattle gate on the far side of a little intersection where FR 9183Y crosses FR 6. This is it. There is no official parking area, but several pullout spots are large enough for a car.

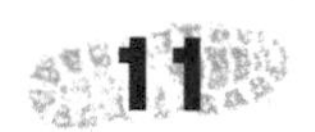

11 The Overland Trail

SCENERY: ★★★
TRAIL CONDITION: ★★
CHILDREN: ★★
DIFFICULTY: ★★★
SOLITUDE: ★★★★★

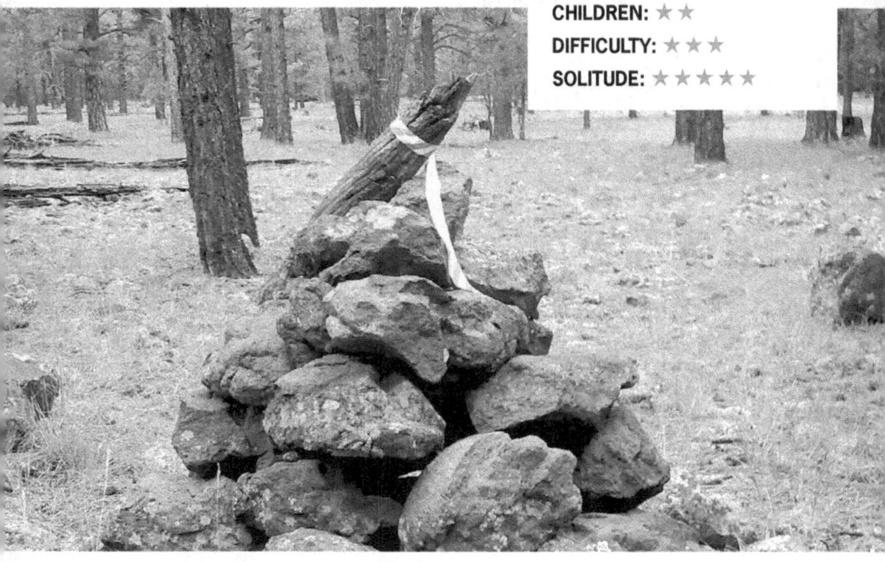

CAIRN MARKING THE OVERLAND ROAD

GPS TRAILHEAD COORDINATES: *Pomeroy Tanks Trailhead:* N35° 09.085' W112° 01.783'
Dow Springs Trailhead: N35° 15.503' W111° 98.284'

DISTANCE & CONFIGURATION: 6.4 miles out-and-back; 3.2-mile car shuttle

HIKING TIME: 4 hours; 2-hour car shuttle

HIGHLIGHTS: Old railroad route, homestead ruins, and isolated prairies

ELEVATION: Within 100 feet of 6,700 feet throughout

ACCESS: No fees or restrictions

MAPS: USGS Davenport Hill and Garland Prairie

FACILITIES: None

WHEELCHAIR ACCESS: None

COMMENTS: You will reach the start of this hike via the Sycamore Rim Loop, page 96.

CONTACTS: Williams Ranger District, 742 S. Clover Rd., Williams, AZ 86046;
(928) 635-5600; **www.fs.usda.gov/kaibab**

Overview

This hike traces a segment of the historical Overland Trail just north of Sycamore Canyon. The route, marked with cairns and ribbons, follows the historical wagon road and railroad grade across the pine-covered mesa to end at the edge of Garland Prairie. You may do it as an out-and-back, combined with the Sycamore Rim Trail to form a loop, or as an easy car shuttle from Pomeroy Tanks to Dow Springs.

Route Details

The Overland Trail originated as a wagon and pack-mule route connecting the bustling mining town of Jerome with the bustling railroad hub of Flagstaff. This short section bisects the Sycamore Rim Trail.

From the Pomeroy Tanks Trailhead, follow the short spur to the main trail. Soon you reach the first of the Pomeroy Tanks: natural water holes sunk into basins of wrinkled granite and garnished with reeds and lily pads. Many spur trails wander around these tanks, so watch for the cairns that mark the main trail. Take that trail left (north).

Just past the last of these tanks, you will encounter a large, double-trunked ponderosa tree and the signed intersection with the Overland Trail. The Overland Trail is not an actual footpath but a route marked with cairns, white ribbons, and occasional wooden posts with a mule blazed upon them.

A wide variety of ribbons of various colors decorate the surrounding pine forest. Ignore all of them except for the white ribbons.

The trick to a cairn hunt is to have the next cairn in sight before leaving sight of the last cairn. By following this discipline, your route might wobble on occasion, but you will not become lost.

The first one you look for is to the east, well within sight of the signed junction. Keep following the cairns across the ridge.

At 0.3 mile past the junction, the cairn can be hard to spot where the route jogs a little north to climb higher upon the ridge. An

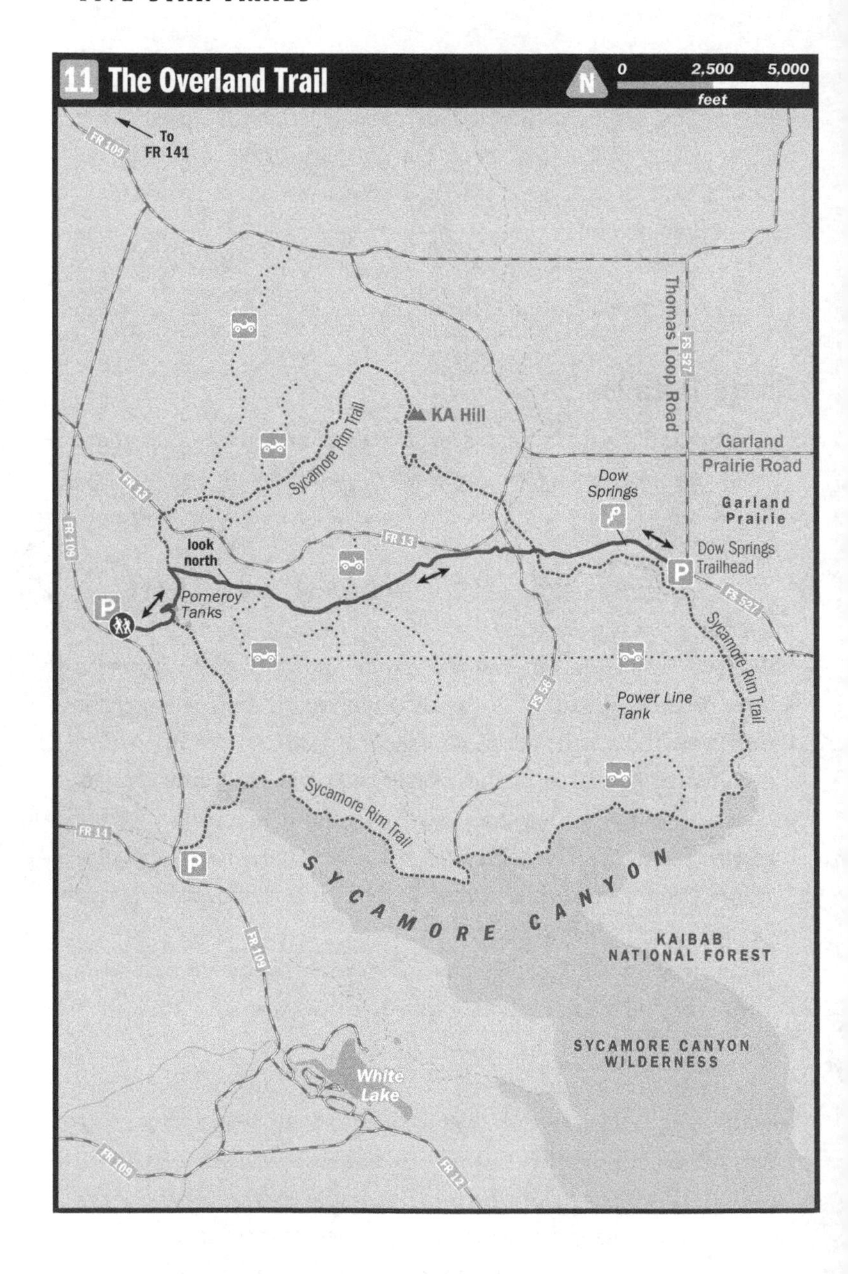

11 The Overland Trail
N
0
2,500
5,000
feet
To
FR 141
FR 109
FR 13
FR 13
FR 109
Thomas Loop Road
FS 527
KA Hill
Sycamore Rim Trail
Garland
Prairie Road
Dow
Springs
Garland
Prairie
Dow Springs
Trailhead
look
north
Pomeroy
Tanks
FS 527
Sycamore Rim Trail
FS 56
Power Line
Tank
Sycamore Rim Trail
FR 14
SYCAMORE CANYON
KAIBAB
NATIONAL FOREST
SYCAMORE CANYON
WILDERNESS
FR 109
White
Lake
FR 109
FR 12

obvious yellow sign, nailed to a tree to the left (north), will alert you to a grazing boundary. If you approach this sign, your next cairn should become more visible within a few dozen paces.

At 0.2 mile farther, the route crosses a jeep trail. This intersection is near a popular car-camping site. You may have already noticed, but it is obvious here how the route follows an old railroad grade (more correctly, the railroad grade was laid on top of the old pack route). A roadway of basalt boulders that once supported the tracks now slowly crumbles beneath the pine needles. The tracks were removed and reused long ago. Here and there, you will come across the remains of the original wooden trestles, though right through here most of them have been used in campfires.

However, in just under 1 mile farther, you will cross a second jeep trail, and past that you will come to the wooden planks and other rusting artifacts from the cowboy civilization that once inhabited the region a hundred years ago.

Shortly beyond that, you cross a third, more developed jeep trail. Look for the post when you cross. Do not be confused by ribbons on the branches over the road—they lead somewhere else. The railroad grade bends south, roughly paralleling the jeep trail, but the route continues more or less east.

The cairns lead you across the pine-studded mesa for another 0.3 mile until you approach FR 13. The Overland runs roughly parallel

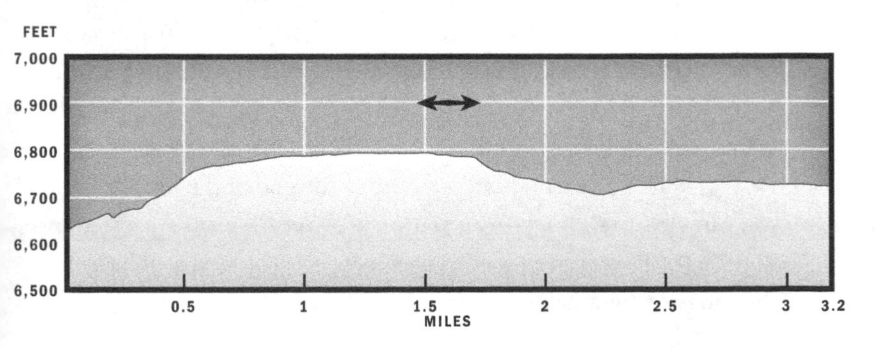

to this road, following the shallow, grassy drainage. You could walk the road and lose nothing—but what fun is that?

Shortly, you cross FR 56, about 0.1 mile south of the Midway Trailhead (see Sycamore Rim Loop profile following). Your next cairn is down the road a few yards to the south (right), in the grass. More obvious is the two-headed ponderosa pine with the white stripe painted across it. Head toward that landmark, passing two cairns in the tall grass along your way. Past the tree, the trail climbs up the ridge a bit, and about a hundred yards later you come to a second intersection with the Sycamore Rim Trail. There's a sign.

Past that intersection, the cairns can be tough to find in the thicket of saplings and Indian paintbrush starting to cover the maze of deadfall left from a forest fire. Two helpful hints: The route goes nearly due east through here, and ribbons on branches can guide you when rock piles are buried in brush.

Once you've pushed through that, you emerge at the edge of Garland Prairie, where the Overland Trail intersects with the old railroad grade just above Dow Springs. You'll have to rock-hop up onto the boulder highway that forms the old grade before you see that the route parallels the grade, bending south, to join it in skirting the edge of the prairie.

The route becomes a sporadic foot trail as you approach the end of the segment, an intersection with the Dow Springs Trailhead spur. Informational signs explain some history to your left, while to your right a few hundred feet, the crumbling remnants of an old cabin stand at the junction with the main rim trail. To your left, as well, almost within sight, is the Dow Springs Trailhead, the end of the segment.

If you left a second car here, this is the end of the hike. If not, you can either return the way you came or return via the Sycamore Rim Trail (the southern half of this loop is easier and more scenic than the northern half).

Directions

From Flagstaff, take I-40 west to Exit 167, just east of Williams. Go left (south) on FR 141. Before FR 141 bends to the east, look for FR 109 continuing south (now to your right). Follow that road to the Pomeroy Tanks Trailhead.

For directions to the Dow Springs Trailhead, see the Sycamore Rim Loop profile following.

12 Sycamore Rim Loop

SCENERY: ★★★★
TRAIL CONDITION: ★★★★★
CHILDREN: ★★★
DIFFICULTY: ★★★
SOLITUDE: ★★

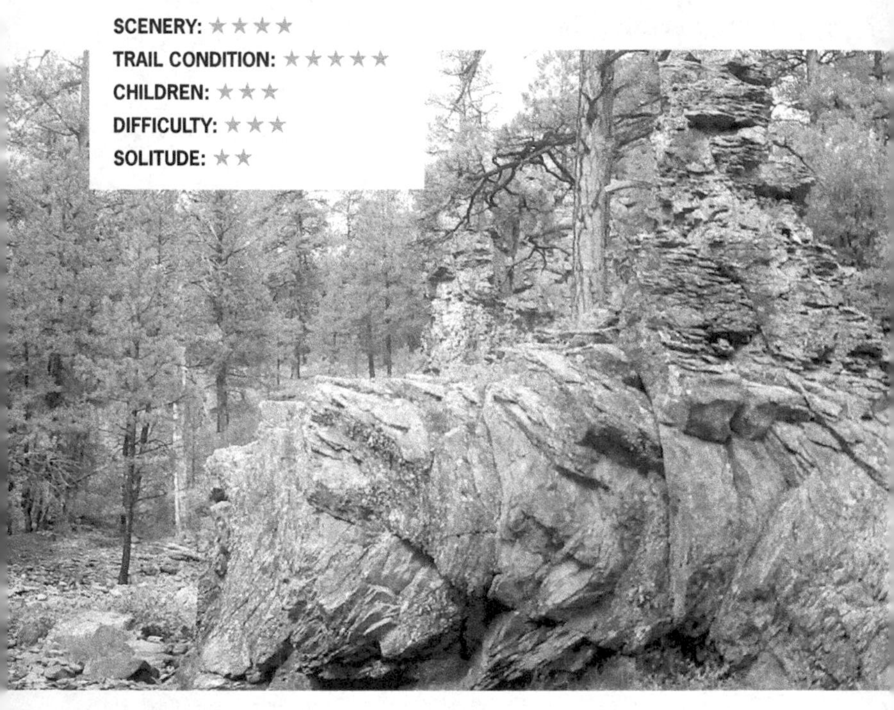

JABBA THE ROCK NEAR THE POMEROY TANKS

GPS TRAILHEAD COORDINATES: N35° 9.301' W111° 58.970'

DISTANCE & CONFIGURATION: 11.8-mile loop; easier option is 8 miles out-and-back

HIKING TIME: 6 hours; easy hike is 4 hours

HIGHLIGHTS: Flowing springs, scenic vistas, cowboy ruins, lily ponds, and a seasonal waterfall

ELEVATION: 6,778 feet at trailhead to 7,267 feet atop KA Hill

ACCESS: No fees or restrictions

MAPS: USGS Davenport Hill and Garland Prairie

FACILITIES: None

WHEELCHAIR ACCESS: None

COMMENTS: With several access points, various route combinations are possible.

CONTACTS: Williams Ranger District, 742 S. Clover Rd., Williams, AZ 86046; (928) 635-5600; **www.fs.usda.gov/kaibab**

Overview

This well-constructed loop travels past Dow Springs and the remains of the settlement there before circumnavigating the stunning north rim of Sycamore Canyon. It then turns north, past a seasonal waterfall and year-round lily ponds, before turning east to climb up and over KA Hill, then south along the edge of Garland Prairie. There are several access points, so this can be hiked in segments if desired. This hike description covers the entire loop, going clockwise from Dow Springs Trailhead.

Route Details

From the Dow Springs Trailhead, follow the short spur to the main trail. You pass several interpretive signs describing the old settlement of Dow Springs and the historical Overland Trail (see previous profile), remnants of which can be seen from this spur. When you reach the main trail, you'll find the crumbling remains of an old cabin to your right (north). After examining that, head left (south) along the trail.

In a few hundred yards, the trail winds down through boulders into a ravine leading to lily ponds. Follow the singletrack back out of the west side of the ravine. Do not take the road east across the ravine.

In about 0.25 mile, follow a spur trail east about 100 feet from the trail to a rocky outcrop on top of the ravine. This affords a view of some small rapids feeding a wading hole.

This east fork of what will become Sycamore Canyon begins to deepen and narrow as you head south along the rim. The trail angles southwest through thicker pine forest, turning more westward as it drops slightly into the canyon. You soon climb back up onto the rim, now heading essentially west through the tall pines.

At 2.3 miles, you come to a jeep trail, an unnumbered track that eventually mates with FR 56 somewhere to the north. More important, this is the first good-quality lookout point with an expansive view of the canyon. The trail slithers along the rim,

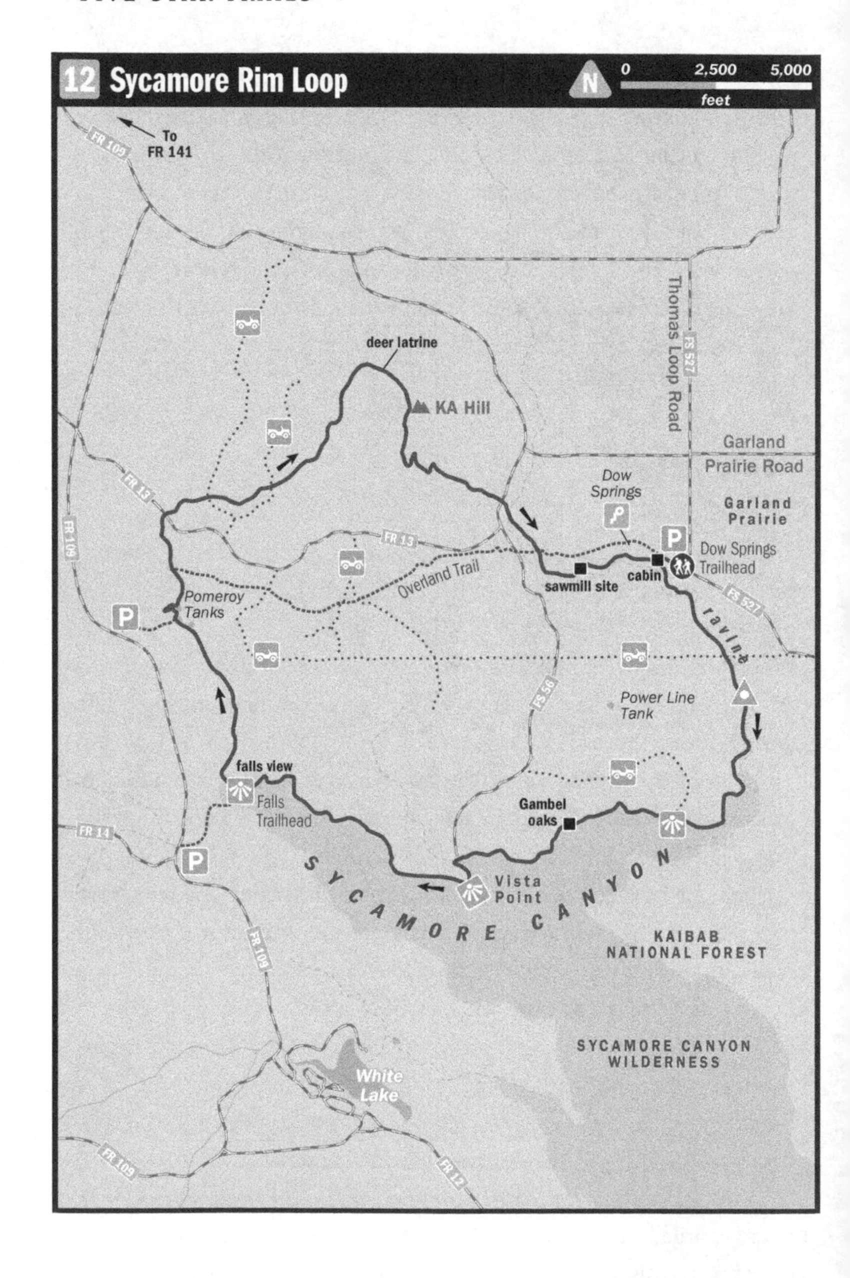
12 Sycamore Rim Loop
N
0 2,500 5,000
feet
To FR 141
FR 109
deer latrine
KA Hill
Thomas Loop Road
FS 527
Garland Prairie Road
Garland Prairie
Dow Springs
FR 13
Dow Springs Trailhead
cabin
sawmill site
Overland Trail
Pomeroy Tanks
FS 527
ravine
FS 56
Power Line Tank
falls view
Falls Trailhead
FR 14
Gambel oaks
Vista Point
SYCAMORE CANYON
KAIBAB NATIONAL FOREST
SYCAMORE CANYON WILDERNESS
White Lake
FR 12

sometimes revealing the canyon spreading out to your south but most of the time wandering through the trees. Along this way, you'll pass through a stand of mature Gambel oaks.

About 1 mile past the jeep road, 3.25 miles from your start, you come to a spur trail leading to the Sycamore Vista Trailhead, 0.25 mile north at the end of FR 56. This, of course, foreshadows Vista Point, a short climb up the ridge from the spur junction. As the name implies, you can see the whole canyon spreading south from here.

You have traveled just under 4 miles at this point. This is the turnaround for the easy out-and-back hike.

After another 0.5 mile westward, the rim and the trail bend northwest, as the ridgetop becomes more open and rocky following the west fork of the canyon. At about 5 miles it begins winding down the ridge, closing in on the canyon and soon—possibly—the falls.

Before hopes get too high, know that these falls are seasonal, only flowing in the early spring or after a recent rain. The canyon below the falls is a popular rock-climbing area. Just south of the falls, you come across a rocky outcrop with a good view of either the falling water or the dry cliffs. A few hundred yards later, at the 5.5-mile mark, the spur to the Falls Trailhead crosses the wash right above the falls, heading west to the parking area. Leaving a second vehicle here would make for an easy car shuttle.

The Sycamore Rim Trail continues, following the drainage

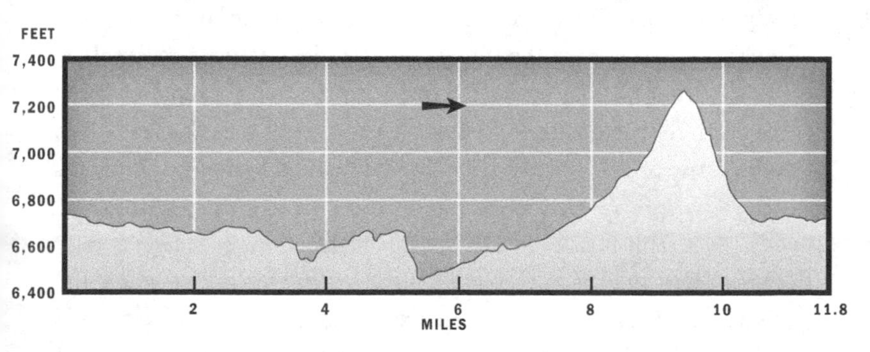

upward and northward away from the canyon. The climb levels out as you reach the first of the Pomeroy Tanks: natural water holes sunk into basins of wrinkled granite and garnished with reeds and lily pads, providing homes for small fish, frogs, and a wide variety of insects.

The spur trail to the third tank is nearly as wide as the main trail, but it is not marked by cairns and does not go up out of the canyon as the main trail does. For the main trail, look for a rock formation that resembles either a giant knotted log or Jabba the Hutt, depending on the tenor of your imagination, and go around it to the left (northeast). Or just watch for the cairns.

At nearly 6 miles you come to the intersection with the Overland Trail, a historical wagon route now marked as a recreation trail (see previous profile). This segment bisects the Sycamore Rim Loop Trail; that was the other end you passed near the Dow Springs Trailhead.

Overland Trail is not an actual footpath, but a route marked with cairns. The Sycamore Rim Loop, in contrast, continues as a trampled singletrack northwards of the wash, passing one more tank until it climbs over a rocky little ridge and crosses FR 13. The trail bends back toward the east here as it marches through the pines toward KA Hill. Along the way, it will cross two more jeep roads as it begins a gentle ascent away from the canyon.

After 1 mile the route turns north, starting the easy if steady climb up KA Hill. Along the way, alligator junipers appear among the pines and oak. Watch your step through the deer latrine. There is a small clearing near the top where deer clearly gather in numbers and hang around, as evidenced from the amount of droppings piled beneath the nibbled-to-nubs bushes. Shortly past this, the trail levels off on top of KA Hill. The peak itself is marked by a pile of boulders and a sign. This is the 8-mile mark.

KA Hill is a large lava dome piled on top of a few smaller ones. Here and there, through the trees, you will be able to see Bill Williams Mountain, the San Francisco Peaks, the grassy expanse of Garland Prairie, and the shelf north of Sycamore Canyon that you have been circumnavigating.

The trail continues almost level across the hilltop 0.1 mile before it begins a steep series of switchbacks down the eastern slopes. Within 0.25 mile, the trail levels out again deep in the pines, and within another 0.5 mile you reach FR 56 and its trailhead.

From there, the path goes across the grassy field, and then skirts the ravine as it approaches Dow Springs. Soon you reach the site of the sawmill that was once the economic heart of the historical settlement, circa 1910–1920. A few piles of rocks, scattered remains of wooden barricades, and an interpretive sign are all that remain now. The trail will dip into and climb out of the low canyon one more time before rounding the ridge to return, past the old log cabin, to the Dow Springs Trailhead spur.

Directions

From Williams, travel east on I-40 to Garland Prairie, Exit 167, and go south on FR 141 (Garland Prairie Road). The drive across the prairie is worth it all by itself. After 16 miles, FR 141 will turn sharply east, but continue straight on FR 338 (labeled in some places as FR 131). Continue due south for 1.5 miles until you see the tiny parking lot.

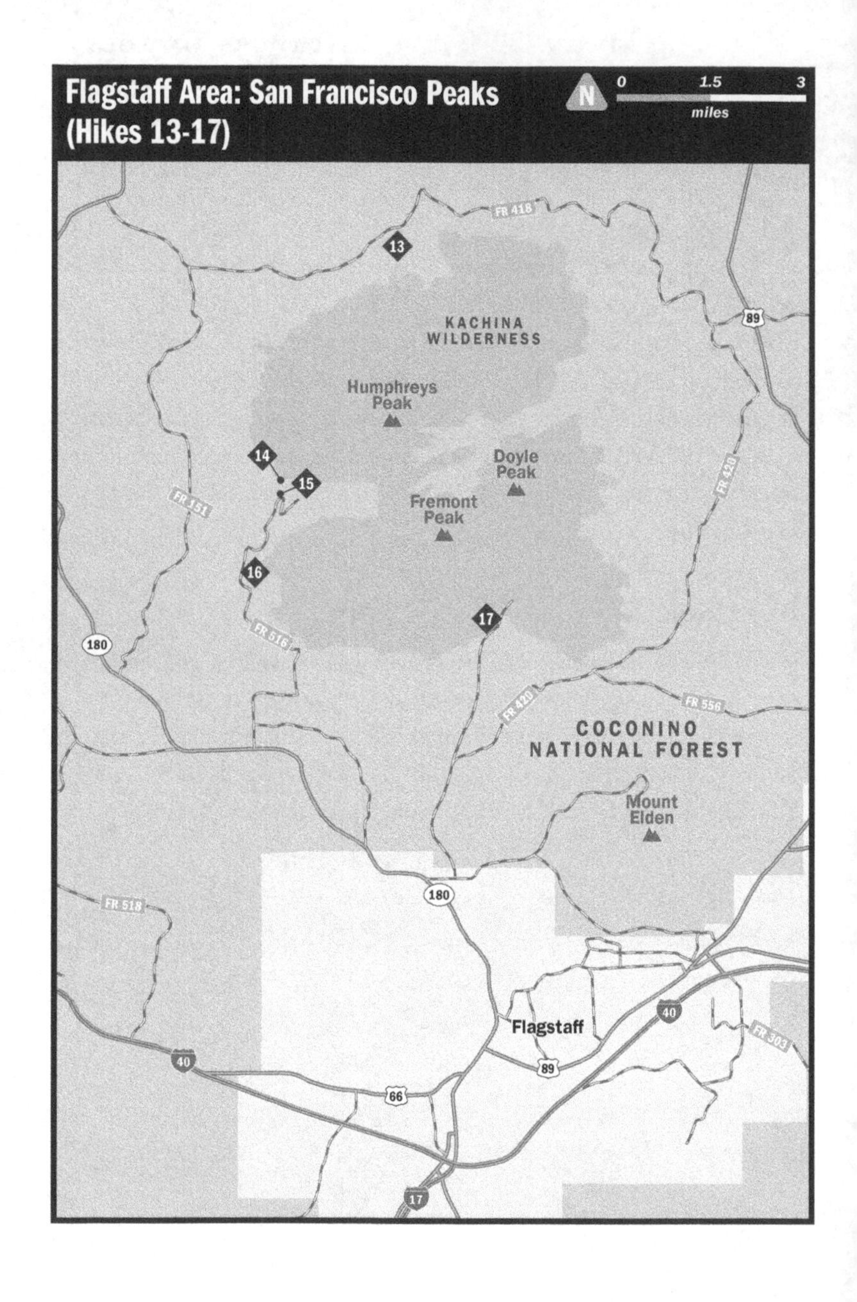
Flagstaff Area: San Francisco Peaks
(Hikes 13-17)
N
0
1.5
3
miles
FR 418
13
KACHINA
WILDERNESS
89
Humphreys
Peak
14
15
Doyle
Peak
FR 151
Fremont
Peak
FR 420
16
17
FR 516
180
FR 420
FR 556
COCONINO
NATIONAL FOREST
Mount
Elden
180
FR 518
40
Flagstaff
FR 303
40
89
66
17

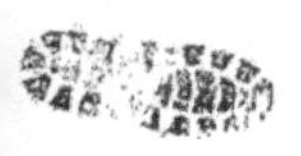

Flagstaff Area: San Francisco Peaks

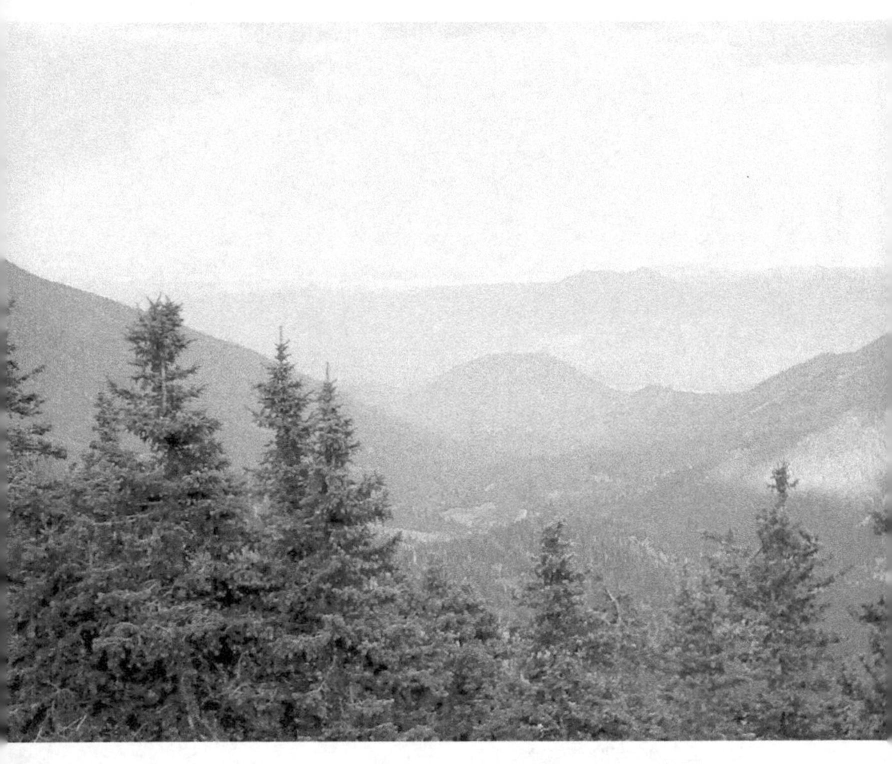

INNER BASIN OF THE SAN FRANCISCO PEAKS FROM WEATHERFORD TRAIL

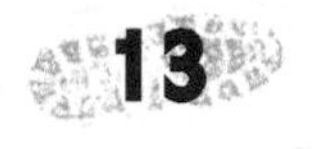

13 Abineau–Bear Jaw Loop

SCENERY: ★★★★★
TRAIL CONDITION: ★★★
CHILDREN: ★★
DIFFICULTY: ★★★★
SOLITUDE: ★★★

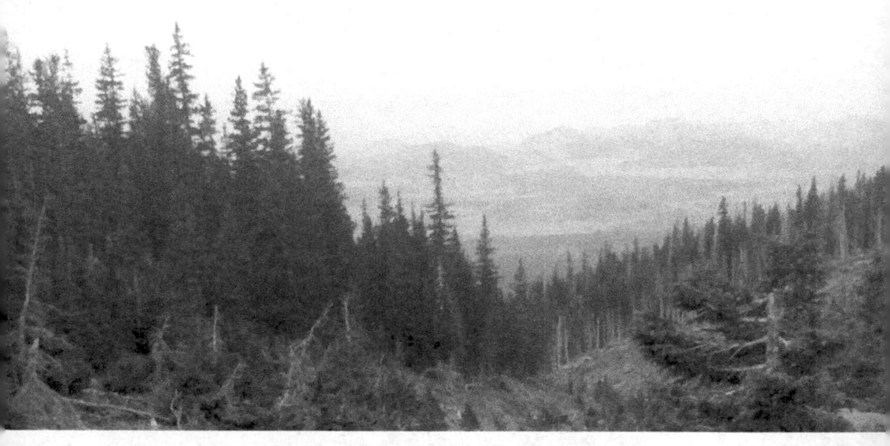

THE TOP OF ABINEAU TRAIL LOOKING NORTH

GPS TRAILHEAD COORDINATES: N35° 21.198' W111° 40.634'

DISTANCE & CONFIGURATION: 7.5-mile loop

HIKING TIME: 4 hours

HIGHLIGHTS: Vistas, deep forests, and wildlife

ELEVATION: 8,550 feet at trailhead to 10,293 feet at the junction of Waterline Road and the Abineau Trail 127

ACCESS: No fees

MAPS: USGS White Horse Hills and Humphreys Peak

FACILITIES: None

WHEELCHAIR ACCESS: None

COMMENTS: No water available. At high altitudes, weather can change quickly, particularly during the late-summer monsoons. Easier in a high-clearance vehicle. May be closed during heavy snow.

CONTACTS: Flagstaff Ranger District, 5075 N. AZ 89, Flagstaff, AZ 86004; (928) 526-0866; **www.fs.fed.us/r3/coconino/recreation/peaks/abineau-bear-jaw-tr.shtml**

Overview

This loop uses two trails and a road to go up and down the far northwestern slopes of the San Francisco Peaks. Starting on Bear Jaw Trail 26, you wind upward through mixed conifers and aspens to the Waterline Road. That utility-access road takes you to the bottom slopes of Mount Humphreys, the tallest peak in the state. From there, follow the Abineau Trail 127 down the canyon of the same name and back to the trailhead.

Route Details

BEAR JAW: A 0.5-mile spur leads from the trailhead to the Kachina Wilderness boundary, a sign-in log (sign it), and a Y-intersection. Just getting to this point is reward enough, with gravel singletrack running through mixed conifers, aspens, and tall grass. Two trails head southward up the slopes of the San Francisco Peaks: the Abineau Trail 127 to the right and the Bear Jaw Trail 26 to the left. The latter is the easier of the two climbs, so go left on Bear Jaw.

Bear Jaw skirts an open prairie for the first 0.3 mile before turning north into the aspens and pines. It dips in and out of Reese Canyon as it starts a relatively gentle ascent up the slope.

Just shy of 1.5 miles, the path climbs a little hill past two huge ponderosa pines standing guard on either side of the track. On top of the hill, the doubletrack trail seems to divide the rust-colored ponderosas from the white-and-olive aspens. On the far side of the hill, you pass a sign proclaiming the actual wilderness boundary.

The old wagon track starts a steep and rocky climb from here. By the second mile, you've cleared 9,000 feet. At 0.25 mile later the trail enters Bear Jaw Canyon. Views of the San Francisco Peaks open before you, while a ravine plunges steeply to your left. Across the ravine, aspens bend over the trail like archways, seeking the sunlight.

The trail goes down the hill and around the ravine, and then starts switchbacking steeply up the hill. In addition to gravity, you must contend with roots and stumble-rocks littering the narrow path.

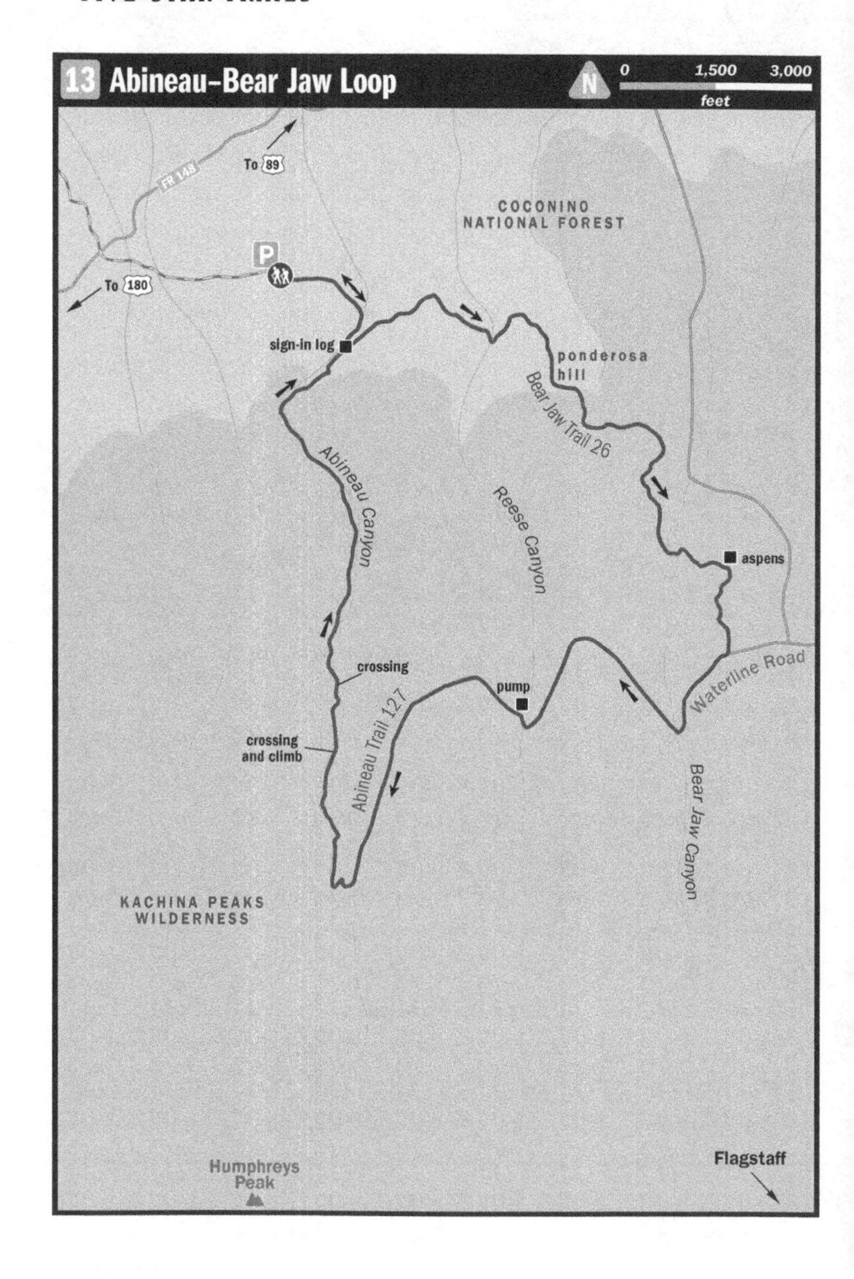
13 Abineau–Bear Jaw Loop
N
0
1,500
3,000
feet
To 89
FR 148
To 180
COCONINO
NATIONAL FOREST
sign-in log
ponderosa
hill
Bear Jaw Trail 26
Abineau Canyon
Reese Canyon
aspens
crossing
pump
Waterline Road
crossing
and climb
Abineau Trail 127
Bear Jaw Canyon
KACHINA PEAKS
WILDERNESS
Humphreys
Peak
Flagstaff

A steep 0.5 mile and 500 feet farther up, the trail goes from brown to black as you pass through a stand of aspens. These trees aren't just related: Aspens often reproduce by cloning themselves from a common root structure. All these pillarlike trees are technically the same organism, genetically identical, and joined by a common root. A stand of aspens in Utah—much like this one—contends for the title of largest single living organism.

Just shy of 3 miles, and probably surrounded by that same aspen(s), Bear Jaw intersects the Waterline Road at a brisk altitude of 9,723 feet.

WATERLINE ROAD: The Waterline Road circumnavigates much of the San Francisco Peaks, maintained as a service road for the—wait for it—municipal water line that delivers water from the high mountain springs down to Flagstaff. To the east (left), it winds around toward Lockett Meadow and the Inner Basin. To the west (right), it heads up toward Mount Humphreys and, more important, Abineau Trail 127.

Throughout, Waterline is a graded dirt road fenced in by thick stands of aspens and spruces. Here and there, a water pipe pokes through the gravel. It goes like this for a solid 2 miles. A little pump house on the upslope side of the road marks your halfway point. Beyond this, you'll notice the climb becomes a bit steeper.

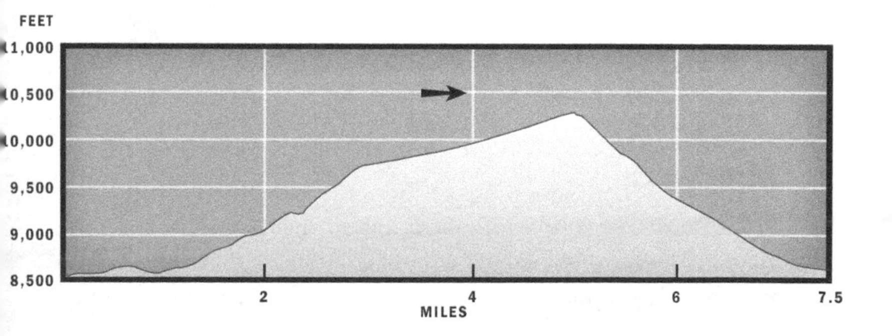

At 5 miles Waterline Road dead-ends at a pile of rubble and deadwood from a 2005 avalanche. The slopes to the west, Mount Humphreys and beyond, are closed to hikers; there are no dedicated trails except the Abineau Trail 127 charging down the canyon. Before you start on that, look to the north. This point is just over 10,000 feet in altitude. On a clear day you can see all the way to the Grand Canyon.

ABINEAU TRAIL 127: You can thank the U.S. Forest Service that any trail is here at all, for the massive slide of rocks and trees obliterated the route in 2005. Huge piles of deadwood still litter Abineau Canyon almost all the way down. Fire is not the only way to kill a lot of trees in a hurry.

The path picks its way through this wooden maze along the bottom of the drainage until it finally climbs the western bank a bit after 0.5 mile. Dwarfish, Christmas-quality spruce trees poke through the gaps in the piles of logs. As you continue down the canyon, these yield to taller trees as oxygen becomes more available.

Mule deer and elk wander these woods, and this side of the slopes offers the best hope of seeing a black bear—particularly in early mornings. That best hope, to be sure, is thin, but the trail is not overrun with traffic like those on the other side of the mountain, and sharp eyes do have a good chance of finding signs of the bear's passing.

At 5.5 miles you cross the canyon a second time. Mixed conifers, aspens, and an occasional alligator juniper now crowd the trail. At 6.5 total miles you pass another wilderness boundary sign, dropping below 9,000 feet in the process. At 0.5 mile later, you return to the Y and the spur back to the trailhead.

Directions

From Flagstaff, take US 180 north toward the Grand Canyon. After about 19 miles, and just past mile marker 235, turn right (east) on FR 151. Follow this graded dirt track for about 1.5 miles until its intersection with FR 418. Go left (staying east) on FR 418 for about 3 miles, where the road terminates at the trailhead.

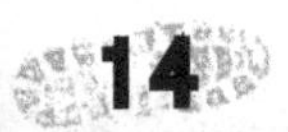

14 Humphreys Trail

SCENERY: ★★★★★
TRAIL CONDITION: ★★★★
CHILDREN: ★
DIFFICULTY: ★★★★★
SOLITUDE: ★

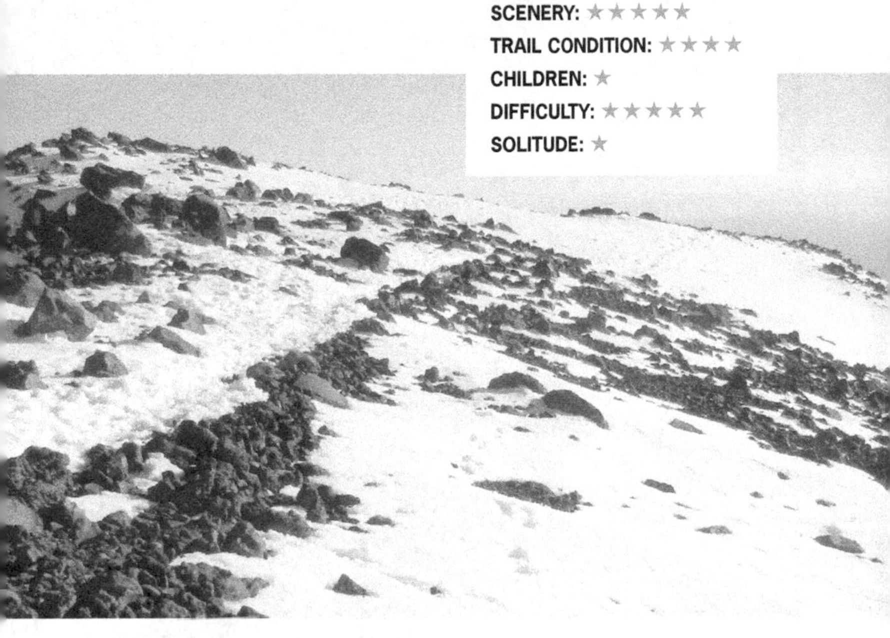

THE FIRST FALSE SUMMIT OF HUMPHREYS PEAK

GPS TRAILHEAD COORDINATES: *Humphreys Trailhead:* N35° 19.876' W111° 42.696'

DISTANCE & CONFIGURATION: 8 miles to the saddle and back; 10 miles to the peak and back

HIKING TIME: 6 hours minimum; see Comments

HIGHLIGHTS: Four layers of ecozone and the highest point in Arizona

ELEVATION: 9,294 feet at trailhead to 12,623 feet at the peak

ACCESS: No fees or restrictions; free backcountry permit required in winter months

MAPS: USGS Humphreys Peak

FACILITIES: Outhouses at trailhead; restaurant and gift shop at ski resort 0.25 mile up the road

WHEELCHAIR ACCESS: None

COMMENTS: Weather can change quickly at high elevations, especially during late summer—a very bad place to be during a thunderstorm. No hiking off-trail above the tree line. If you are not acclimated to the altitude, the last mile to the peak can be a slow, hard trudge.

CONTACTS: Flagstaff Ranger District, 5075 N. AZ 89, Flagstaff, AZ 86004; (928) 526-0866; **www.fs.fed.us/r3/coconino/recreation/peaks/humphreys-tr.shtml**

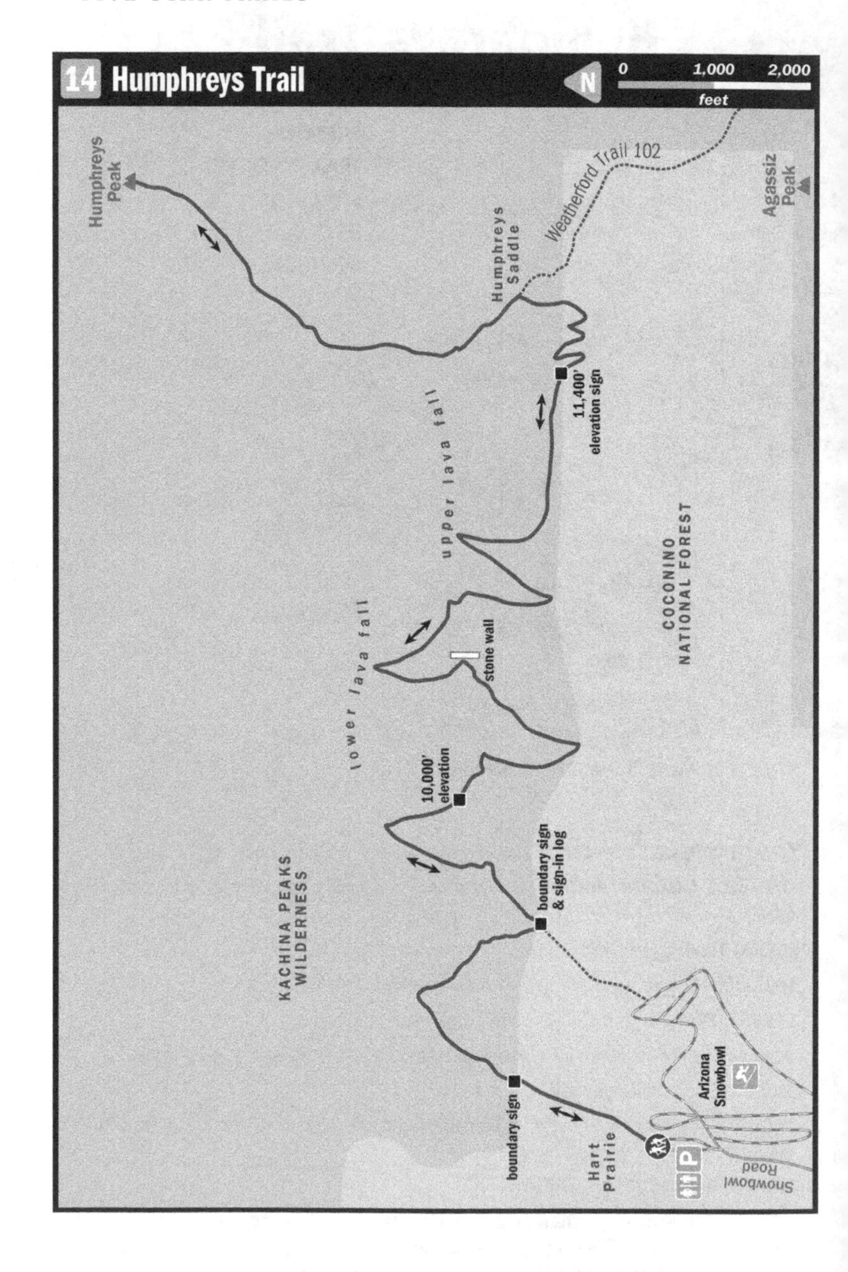
14 Humphreys Trail
N
0
1,000
2,000
feet
Humphreys Peak
Weatherford Trail 102
Agassiz Peak
Humphreys Saddle
11,400' elevation sign
upper lava fall
COCONINO NATIONAL FOREST
lower lava fall
stone wall
10,000' elevation
boundary sign & sign-in log
KACHINA PEAKS WILDERNESS
Arizona Snowbowl
boundary sign
Hart Prairie
P
Snowbowl Road

Overview

This popular trail makes the arduous march from the bottom of the Snowbowl ski resort up the slopes through different ecozones to arrive at Humphreys Saddle. The trail then climbs even farther above the tree line to the peak of Mount Humphreys, the highest point in Arizona. That status makes this trail quite popular.

Route Details

From the trailhead, take the dirt path straight across the meadow (roughly north), crossing under the chair lift and over some steel cables. The meadow is the eastern edge of Hart Prairie stretching to your left. To your right, your destination looms over you, filling most of the horizon.

In 0.3 mile, you enter the trees, passing a Kachina Wilderness boundary sign and a social trail to the lower ski lodge. Stay straight (north) on the main trail.

The trail is crisscrossed with the roots of the aspens and spruces that tower overhead. The climb is already steep, yet a mere foreshadow of climbing to come. The early part is quiet once you're away from the prairie. The only sound might be the wind, your footfalls, or your panting because you are already higher than on any hike in Sedona.

The trail bends softly around back south, and at 0.9 mile you

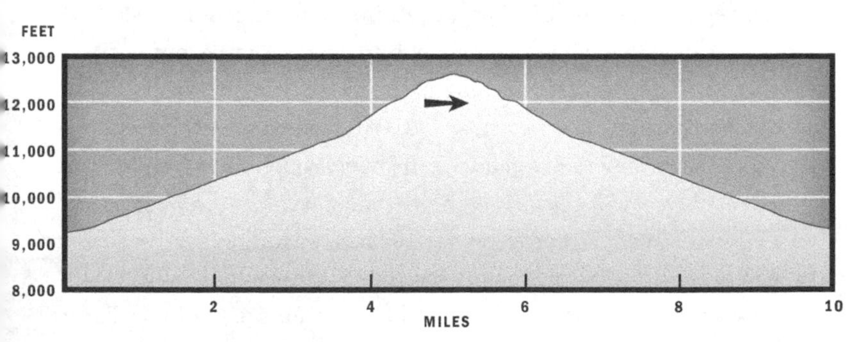

encounter the second Kachina Wilderness boundary sign, a sign-in log, and a T-intersection. To the right (south), a spur trail leads down to the upper ski-resort lodge. To the left (northeast), the main trail continues up the mountain. Go left.

At 1.5 miles you cross the 10,000-foot elevation line. At 0.3 mile later, the switchbacks begin. Most of the Us have social trails—none of which are part of the official trail—heading straight across the slope. If in doubt, make the U-turn and keep climbing.

Midway through the first switchback, a low stone wall lines a ravine crossing. At 2.1 miles you are halfway to the saddle in terms of distance, though only about a quarter of the way in terms of effort.

The next switchback touches the edge of a lava fall. A wide river of gray basalt covered with bright green-and-yellow lichen runs all the way down the slope. Climb out a few steps, and the southern horizon opens up before you with a view of Kendrick Mountain on the far side of Hart Prairie.

Two more bends in the trail bring you back to this same lava fall, only higher up. This is the 3-mile mark, and 20 feet shy of the 11,000-foot line.

Around the corner to the south, views of Snowbowl and Mount Agassiz begin to emerge from behind the increasingly smaller trees. You pass the 11,400-foot sign, which warns against off-trail hiking above this elevation. Past here the remaining switchbacks are going to be rocky and stairstep-steep. The stumpy bristlecones are all that's left growing this high—high enough to obstruct views but not high enough to provide any meaningful shade.

At nearly 4 miles even, and 10,800 feet, you reach Humphreys Saddle, a gravelly shelf straddling the midway point between Mounts Humphreys and Agassiz; it is also the junction with the Weatherford Trail (see page 124). You can't actually see Humphreys Peak from here—those are all false peaks, each one just tall enough to block the view of the taller peak behind it—but you can see the Inner Basin, the tree-lined remains of the caldera of the now-extinct volcano you have been climbing.

In its fiery prehistoric heyday, the volcano reached as high as 16,000 feet. Major eruptions some 200,000 years ago reduced it to these scattered prominences, 4,000–5,000 feet lower but still the tallest peaks in the state.

White-throated swifts soar and dive around these peaks, hunting for tiny insects. And the scrubby little yellow-and-brown flowers you see among the rocks are San Francisco Peaks groundsel, a distant relation to the sunflower. This high-altitude flower grows nowhere else and is the reason you must remain on the trail above the tree line.

The final push up from the saddle puts the *hump* in *Humphreys*. It is barren, rocky, and steep (gaining 900 feet in about 1 mile, which is a steep grade at any altitude), and for all the wind, it has chokingly little oxygen. You will climb three heartbreaking false summits before finally reaching the real one. But at this top, the highest point in Arizona, you can see southward below the Mogollon Rim, past Sedona, into the smust (dusty smog) at the horizon. Even better, turning northward offers views of the Grand Canyon and mountain peaks in Utah.

Return the way you came.

Directions

From Flagstaff, take US 180 north about 7 miles to Snowbowl Road. Turn right (north) and follow this paved but sharply winding road about 7 miles to the bottom of the ski resort and two large trailheads on either side of the road. Humphreys Trailhead is to the north, on the left side of the road opposite the Kachina Trailhead. These trailheads remain open even after the ski resort closes.

15 Kachina Trail

SCENERY: ★★★★
TRAIL CONDITION: ★★★★
CHILDREN: ★★★
DIFFICULTY: ★★
SOLITUDE: ★★

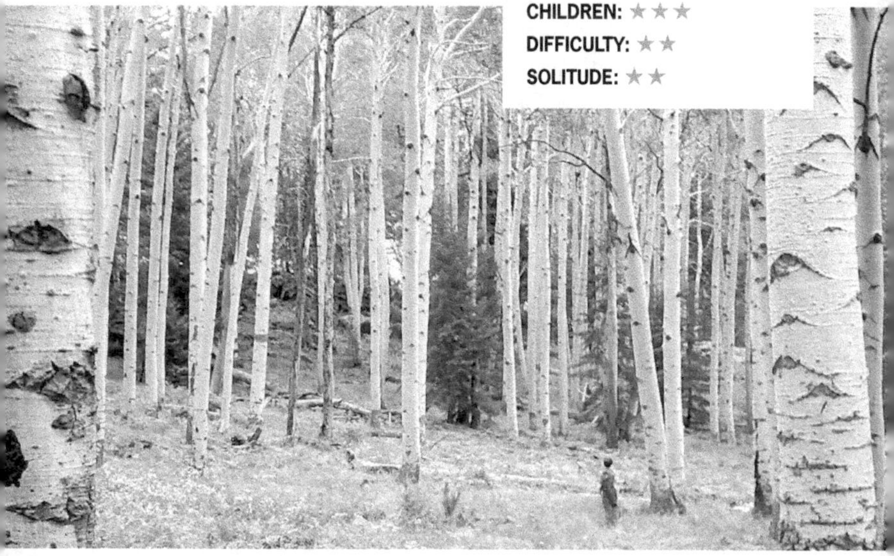

ASPENS AT THE EAST END OF THE TRAIL

GPS TRAILHEAD COORDINATES: *Kachina Trailhead:* N35° 19.624' W111° 42.684' *Freidlein Prairie Trailhead:* N35° 17.826' W111° 39.087'

DISTANCE & CONFIGURATION: 11.6 miles out-and-back; easier version is 5.4 miles out-and-back. A car shuttle would be 5.8 miles.

HIKING TIME: 6 hours; 3 hours for the easy version or car shuttle

HIGHLIGHTS: Vistas, foliage, and wildlife

ELEVATION: 9,260 feet at Kachina Trailhead to 8,576 feet at Freidlein Prairie Trailhead

ACCESS: No fees or restrictions; Freidlein Prairie Trailhead requires a high-clearance vehicle.

MAPS: USGS Sunset Peak

FACILITIES: Outhouses at Humphreys Trailhead, across the road from the Kachina Trailhead. See also "Nearby Attractions."

WHEELCHAIR ACCESS: None

COMMENTS: Excellent spot for wildflowers in the spring and colored leaves in the fall. While described as an out-and-back, this hike can also be done as a car shuttle.

CONTACTS: Flagstaff Ranger District, 5075 N. AZ 89, Flagstaff, AZ 86004; (928) 526-0866; **www.fs.fed.us/r3/coconino/recreation/peaks/kachina-tr.shtml**

Overview

The relentlessly scenic Kachina Trail 150 crosses the southern slopes of the San Francisco Peaks from the Snowbowl ski resort at the west end to the Weatherford Trail on the east. It provides a fine route to see many of these mountains' splendors without huffing into the higher altitudes.

Route Details

At the trailhead, cross the log and head toward the signs. The trail plunges east through aspens and mixed conifers rising from a bed of ferns, moss, and brush. Mixed conifers, here, means nearly all of them, as the trail passes between the high range of the pines and the low range of the spruces and firs. Here and there the dirt is broken up by roots or moss-covered boulders. Several small, grassy clearings break this canopy, the first one occurring within 0.3 mile.

At 0.6 mile, you enter the wilderness area, marked by a sign, a registry, and some overhead power lines. At 0.2 mile later, the trail passes the boulder playground: a pile of lichen-covered boulders, about the size of playground equipment and riddled with social trails blazed by children of all ages exploring them.

Squirrels scamper about on the boulders and deadwood, while birds including Clark's nutcrackers and Steller's jays carry on overhead. Just past 1 mile, the trail starts its first sustained drop, entering a ravine and then climbing quickly out of it.

At the top of the climb the trail seems to disappear into a pile of boulders, and many of the sandals crowd turn around here. The trail continues, though. Simply cross the boulders as best as you can, heading toward the double-trunked tree to the east. By the time you reach the tree, the continuing footpath will be obvious. That path quickly turns to pass below a short basalt cliff before bending back east to continue down the slope. After the trail winds around a few more boulders, the trees part a bit, revealing some views to the south.

At 1.6 miles, you cross a wash and climb out to encounter a

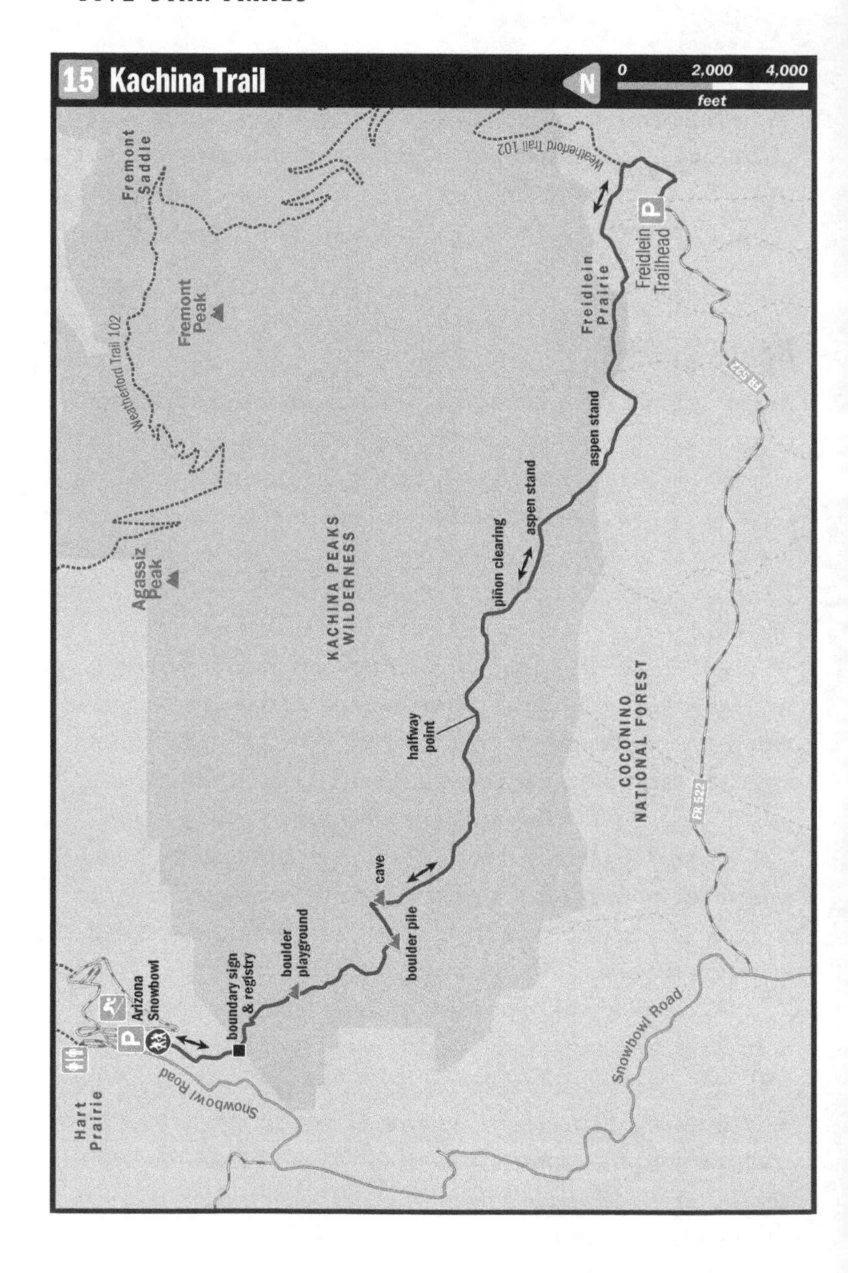
15 Kachina Trail
N
0
2,000
4,000
feet
Fremont Saddle
Fremont Peak
Weatherford Trail 102
Agassiz Peak
KACHINA PEAKS WILDERNESS
Freidlein Prairie
Freidlein Trailhead
aspen stand
aspen stand
piñon clearing
halfway point
cave
boulder pile
boulder playground
boundary sign & registry
Arizona Snowbowl
Hart Prairie
Snowbowl Road
COCONINO NATIONAL FOREST
FR 522

shallow cave beneath an overhang of basalt. At the 2-mile mark, damage from the forest fire has opened wide vistas of Hart Prairie and lands beyond. At 0.25 mile later, though, you will have returned to the boulders and the trees.

On the far side of these trees, the route climbs up the slope of a grass- and fern-covered clearing. On a clear day you can see all the way into Oak Creek Canyon. In the middle of the clearing, at 2.7 miles, a group of trees provides a fine resting spot for enjoying the view. This is the turnaround for the easy hike.

From the trees, the trail drops, soon passing back into the tall trees. It winds through the spruces and pines and aspens, across a couple of large washes, and then, at 3.2 miles, climbs a bit to a wide, grassy slope dotted sporadically with piñon pines. To the left (north), the San Francisco Peaks (specifically Agassiz and Fremont peaks) tower above, while to the right (south) can be seen Hart Prairie and beyond.

The eastern stretch of the Kachina is less traveled but popular with deer and elk. Elk are particularly active in the fall, when the bull elk bugle during breeding season.

On the far side of this prairie, at about 4 miles, the trail enters a huge stand of towering white aspens. Then it crosses a fern-filled clearing into another stand of aspens. This pattern repeats for the better part of the next mile, even as the path starts dropping more steeply down the slope.

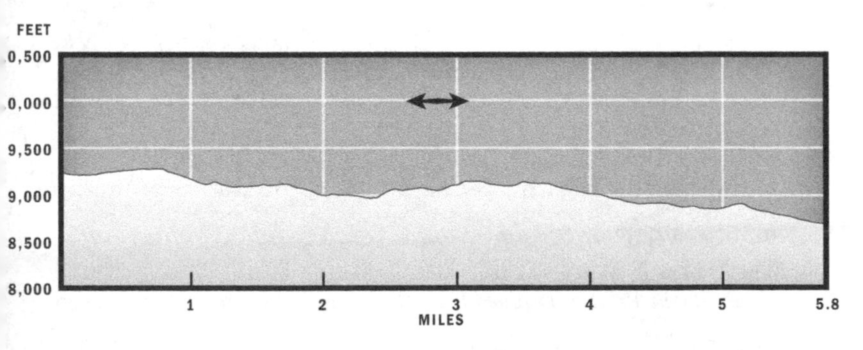

At close to 5 miles, the trail reaches the edge of Freidlein Prairie. It meanders 0.3 mile through this broad grassland before it reaches a Y-intersection. To the left, it continues east another 0.3 mile until it ends at a T-intersection with the Weatherford Trail. To the right, it drops south for 0.4 mile to the Freidlein Prairie Trailhead. If you stashed a car at that spot, take the right. If not, return the way you came.

Nearby Attractions

The Snowbowl is open during the summer, offering sky rides on its ski lift, a disc-golf course (disc golf is an obsession in Flagstaff), and the Peak Side Café at the Agassiz Lodge, where you might discover how high altitudes makes burgers taste better. The sky rides, which land you a few hundred feet shy of Agassiz Peak, run $12 for adults (free for kids 7 and under), but it's closed at the first hint of lightning. Lunch at the Peak Side runs $8–$15 a plate, not including beer. The gates to the lodge area close at 5 p.m., but the trailheads are below the gates. The Snowbowl can be reached at (928) 779-1951 or surfed at **arizonasnowbowl.com**.

Directions

To Kachina Trailhead: From Flagstaff, take US 180 north about 7 miles to Snowbowl Road. Follow this paved but sharply winding road about 7 miles to the bottom of the ski resort and two large trailheads on either side of the road. The Kachina Trail 150 is at the south end of the south trailhead.

To Freidlein Prairie Trailhead: Look for FR 552 about 2 miles up Snowbowl Road from US 180. Take FR 522 east for 3 bumpy miles, past the dispersed camping area, until it terminates at the trailhead.

16 Veit Springs Loop

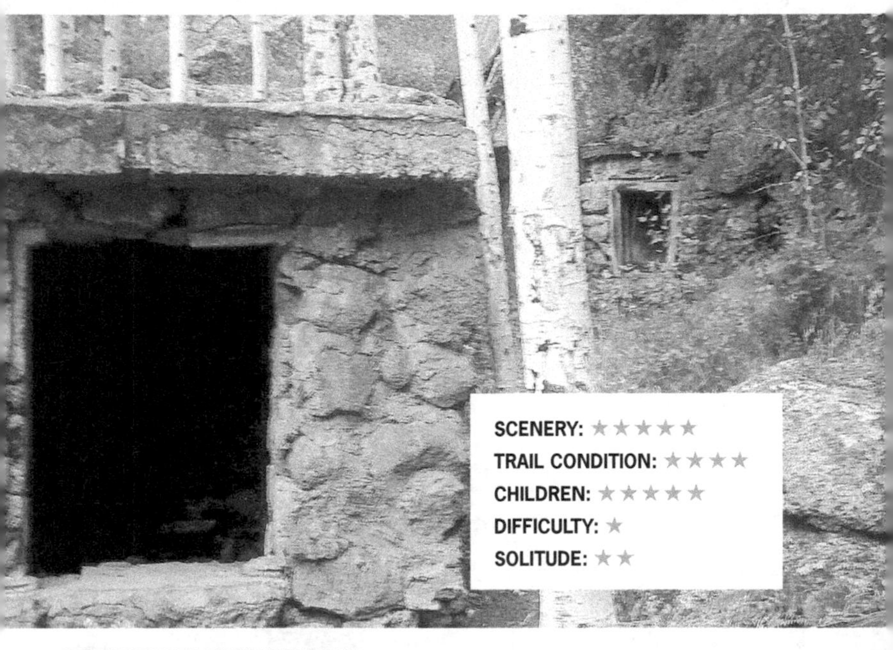

SPRINGHOUSES NEAR VEIT CABIN

GPS TRAILHEAD COORDINATES: N35° 18.580' W111° 43.141'

DISTANCE & CONFIGURATION: 2-mile loop, including all spurs

HIKING TIME: 1.5 hours

HIGHLIGHTS: Springs, petroglyphs, frontier cabins, old-growth forest, and wildlife

ELEVATION: 8,650 feet at trailhead to 8,450 feet at bottom of wash

ACCESS: No fees or restrictions

MAPS: USGS Sunset Peak

FACILITIES: None

WHEELCHAIR ACCESS: None

COMMENTS: The hike circles inside the Lamar Haines Memorial Wildlife Area and is sometimes called the Lamar Haines Trail for this reason. Treat any spring water before drinking.

CONTACTS: Flagstaff Ranger District, 5075 N. AZ 89, Flagstaff, AZ 86004; (928) 526-0866; **www.azgfd.gov/outdoor_recreation/wildlife_area_lamar_haines.shtml.** *Note:* The hike is on state land but entirely surrounded by the Coconino National Forest, so the U.S. Forest Service (see phone number above) is more likely to have useful answers about local conditions.

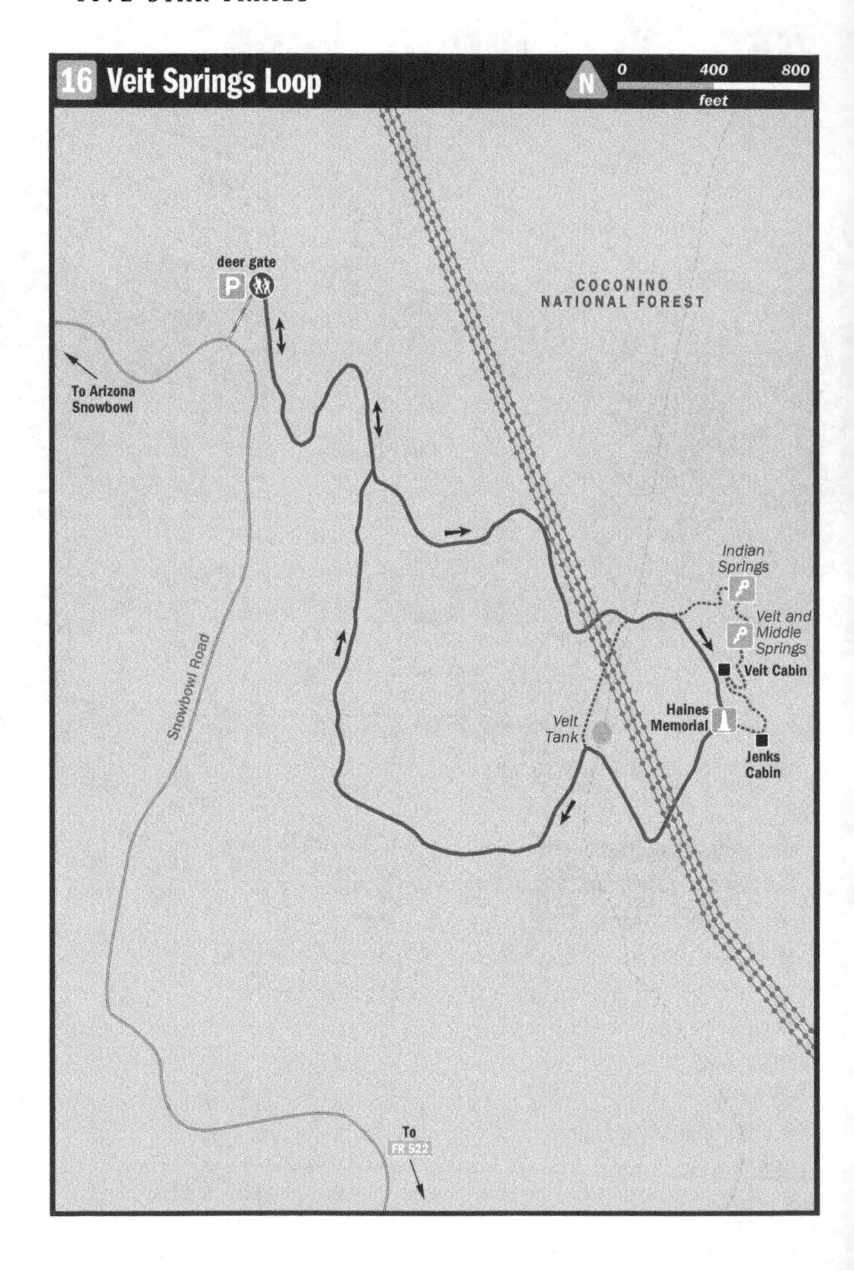
16 Veit Springs Loop
N
0
400
800
feet
deer gate
P
COCONINO
NATIONAL FOREST
To Arizona
Snowbowl
Snowbowl Road
Indian
Springs
Veit and
Middle
Springs
Veit Cabin
Haines
Memorial
Veit
Tank
Jenks
Cabin
To
FR 522

Overview

This short, easy loop passes through the old Veit homestead and associated ruins before circling through the old-growth forest and wetland meadows back to the trailhead. The Veit place was built near three springs, one of which (Indian Springs) is surrounded by petroglyphs.

Route Details

Go through the deer gate and climb the hill to the old road. This is the hardest part of the hike. The road, still usable but closed to the general public, heads south, switchbacks north around the point of the ridge, then switchbacks south into the drainage. All this happens in less than 0.3 mile.

At that 0.3-mile mark, the path splits: The wider remnant road continues due south, while a footpath heads to the east. Go east (left) on the footpath. You pass through tall aspens and spruces, and then wind into the main drainage, crossing twice beneath power lines. At the second encounter with the power lines, you find yourself at an informal intersection. An unmarked spur trail goes north, while a wider spur trail follows the power lines south. This hike reaches the other side of both spurs. Meanwhile, follow the fiberglass signs directing you down the trail straight ahead.

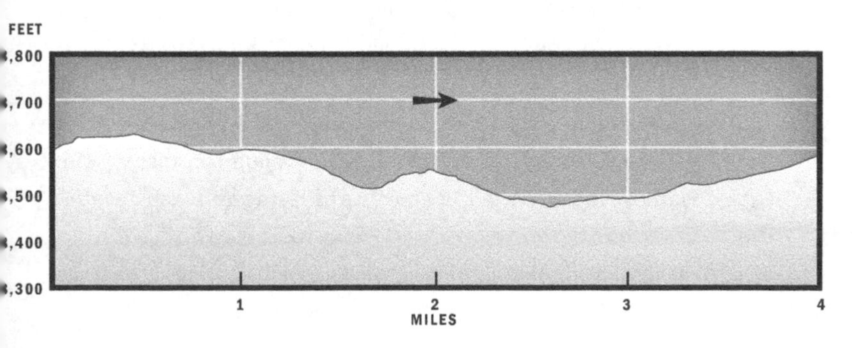

The marked trail cuts inside all the cool stuff for some reason, so if you just want to make a quick loop through some trees, that's your route. If you want to see the cowboy ruins, though, take the wide dirt path heading north from the marked trail to the Veit Cabin (within sight).

Ludwig Veit built this cabin in 1892 as part of his 160-acre homestead claim. The structure has been cut to 5 feet tall to prevent anyone from entering it. While enough doorway remains to crawl through, all you'll find inside are dirt and spiders.

A thin spur heads north, while the main path continues east. Go north to find the springhouses. A stone shed surrounds Canadian, or Veit, Spring, while a separate stone enclosure protects Middle Spring, which flows from the base of the ridge. The spur continues northwest along the base of the ridge to a limestone cliff. Indian Springs seeps up inside a small cave at the base of the cliff, while a few intact rock paintings decorate the face of the rock. A maze of trails wanders through the grass and rocks and trees, with one trail going south toward the power-line junction. But you are better off returning the way you came to the Veit Cabin.

From there a wide path runs east, parallel to the marked route. The trail passes a sometimes-pond (but mostly a weedy little depression) to arrive at a fence and a sign indicating the site of the Jenks Cabin. The Jenks family bought the homestead from Veit in 1928. All that remains of their dwelling is a rectangular depression beside the trail. The spur trail that continues east doesn't go anywhere in particular, fizzling out instead up the hill at the wilderness boundary.

From here, the social trail turns south and rejoins the marked trail at the Haines Boulder, indicated by a plaque commemorating Lamar Haines. The Arizona Department of Game and Fish acquired the parcel from the Jenks family in 1948 to preserve it as a water source for wildlife. Today the area is maintained by private donations, including donations from the Lamar Haines Foundation.

The unified trail, now the remnant road, continues south, winding down into the wash. The slopes are filled with tall pines, aspens, spruces, and firs. Abert's squirrels have the run of the place, and mule deer and elk are often seen as well. The wash itself widens into a marshy meadow, reinforced by the stone retaining wall that formed Veit Tank. On the west side of this wall, a spur trail charges straight up the ravine to the power-line junction, thereby cutting the loop in half. Unless you are somehow tired, continue straight along the road.

The road exits the wash to reenter the old-growth forest before turning north and returning to the trail split. Return the way you came.

Directions

From Flagstaff, take US 180 north about 7 miles to Snowbowl Road. Turn right (north) to follow this paved but sharply winding road about 5 miles to the turnout on the right. The gravel parking lot holds about 10 cars. If you reach a wide parking lot to the left, you've gone too far.

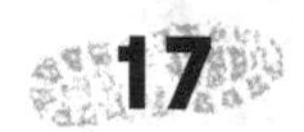

17 Weatherford Trail

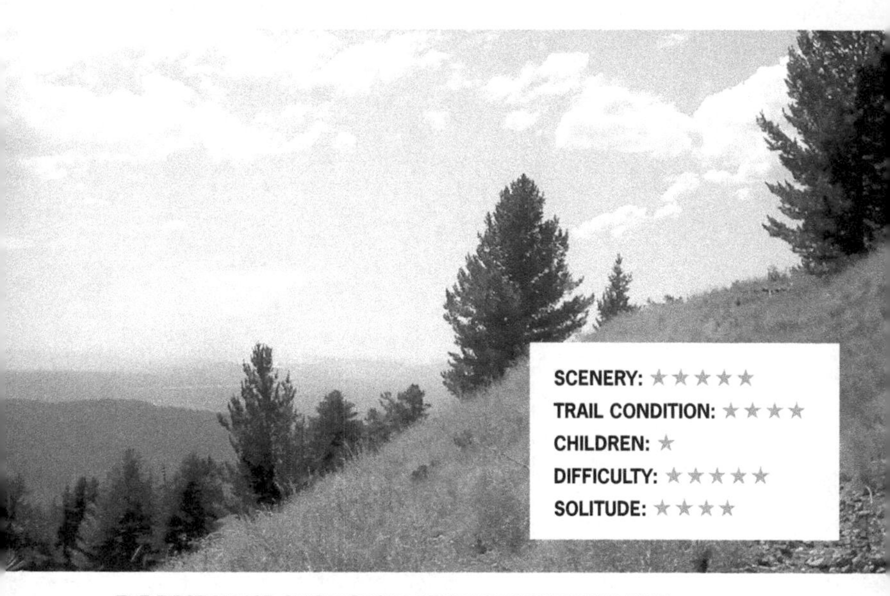

SCENERY: ★★★★★
TRAIL CONDITION: ★★★★
CHILDREN: ★
DIFFICULTY: ★★★★★
SOLITUDE: ★★★★

THE FIRST MAJOR SWITCHBACKS UP THE WEATHERFORD TRAIL

GPS TRAILHEAD COORDINATES: *Freidlein Prairie Trailhead:* N35° 17.826' W111° 39.087'
Humphreys Trailhead: N35° 19.876' W111° 42.696'

DISTANCE & CONFIGURATION: 19.4 miles total out-and-back. Easy hike to Doyle Saddle is 12 miles out-and-back. Medium hike to Fremont Saddle is 16 miles out-and-back. A car shuttle combining Weatherford Trail 102 with Humphreys Trail 151 would be 14–16 miles. A loop hike combing Weatherford, Humphreys, and Kachina trails would be 18–20 miles. See Comments.

HIKING TIME: Easy hike: 6 hours; medium hike or car shuttle with Humphreys: 8–9 hours; full hike or full multitrail loop: 10–12 hours. See Comments.

HIGHLIGHTS: Scenic vistas, wildlife, and arboreal forests

ELEVATION: 8,627 feet at trailhead to 12,000 feet at Agassiz Saddle

ACCESS: No fees; high-clearance vehicle recommended for Freidlein Prairie Trailhead.

MAPS: USGS Humphreys Peak

FACILITIES: None

WHEELCHAIR ACCESS: None

COMMENTS: No reliable water available on the trail. Weather can change quickly at high altitudes, so come prepared. Off-trail hiking prohibited at higher altitudes. Doyle and

Fremont saddles are reversed for some reason on the USGS map; look again at the mileage and the altitude gain.

An out-and-back along the entire Weatherford Trail 102 would require an early start and an aggressive pace to finish in daylight. The San Francisco Peak Suicide Loop combines the Weatherford, Humphreys (see page 109), and Kachina (see page 114) trails to loop back to Freidlein Prairie Trailhead. That's 18 miles, 20 if you go all the way to the peak. The easiest way do the entirety of the Weatherford Trail 102 is to set up a car shuttle at the Humphreys Trailhead and combine this hike with Humphreys Trail 151.

CONTACTS: Flagstaff Ranger District, 5075 N. AZ 89, Flagstaff, AZ 86004; (928) 526-0866; **www.fs.fed.us/r3/coconino/recreation/peaks/weatherford-tr.shtml**

Overview

Originally constructed as a toll road up to the San Francisco Peaks, Weatherford Trail 102 is definitely the scenic route up into and across the Kachina Wilderness. The San Francisco Peaks have four climate zones stacked on top of each other, and the Weatherford goes through all of them, in addition to providing a view of everything from the Inner Basin to Sycamore Canyon.

Route Details

UP THE SOUTHERN SLOPE: From the trailhead, a 0.4-mile spur leads through the pines and ferns to the eastern tail of the Kachina Trail 150. Go right (east) on the Kachina for another 0.3 mile until you reach the junction with the Weatherford. Looking north, the San Francisco Peaks fill the horizon. That's where you're going.

The Weatherford actually starts 1.7 miles farther south at Schultz Pass, but that was the epicenter of the 2010 Schultz Fire and may be closed for some time. Even if open, that passage will be both difficult and depressing for the next decade at least.

So head north (left) on the Weatherford, exiting the broad grasslands of Freidlein Prairie and up the slope into the pines. Soon you cross the Kachina Wilderness boundary, and 0.3 mile later you come to a register. Sign in and keep climbing.

Weatherford Road was built in the 1920s to bounce tourists up to the peaks in Model Ts. The Great Depression doomed it as a

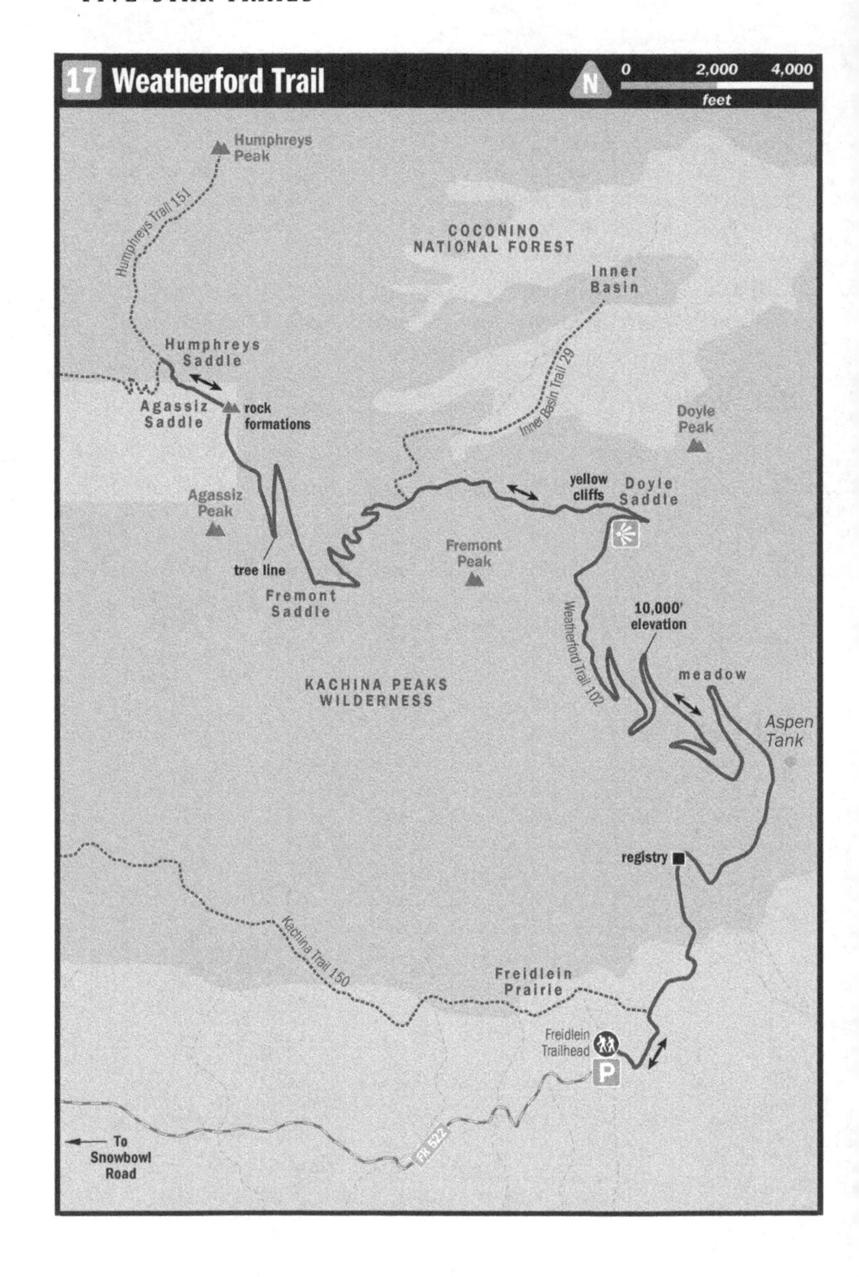
17 Weatherford Trail
N
0
2,000
4,000
feet
Humphreys Peak
Humphreys Trail 151
COCONINO NATIONAL FOREST
Inner Basin
Inner Basin Trail 29
Humphreys Saddle
Agassiz Saddle
rock formations
Doyle Peak
Agassiz Peak
yellow cliffs
Doyle Saddle
Fremont Peak
tree line
Fremont Saddle
Weatherford Trail 102
10,000' elevation
KACHINA PEAKS WILDERNESS
meadow
Aspen Tank
registry
Kachina Trail 150
Freidlein Prairie
Freidlein Trailhead
P
To Snowbowl Road
FR 522

commercial enterprise, but the route was resurrected as a recreational trail in the 1980s.

The road proceeds up Weatherford Canyon with the trail occupying the downslope half of the road, while accumulated deadfall clogs the other half. At 2 miles, you pass a thin spur trail going off through the pines to Aspen Tank—not worth it unless you need to filter water or hydrate your livestock.

After 0.3 mile, the trail switchbacks across a little meadow, foreshadowing the first set of serious switchbacks. Over the next mile, three long switchbacks will take you up 300 vertical feet of grassy slope. Stands of aspens separate wide vistas of Flagstaff and, on clear days, Oak Creek Canyon. With each turn the view gets better. After the third leg, the trail turns to cross the ridge and the views disappear behind a thicket of aspens.

At 3.8 miles, you touch upon 10,000 feet in elevation and start a second set of switchbacks. The road here climbs through a corridor of spruce trees where ravens and Clark's nutcrackers go about their noisy business. The first four legs of the switchbacks stretch another mile and bring you up 400 feet.

You cross another grassy slope with one last excellent vista of Flagstaff before one last switchback, noticeably steeper and rockier, covers the last hump to Doyle Saddle.

Doyle Saddle, at 10,850 feet and right on 6 miles, separates

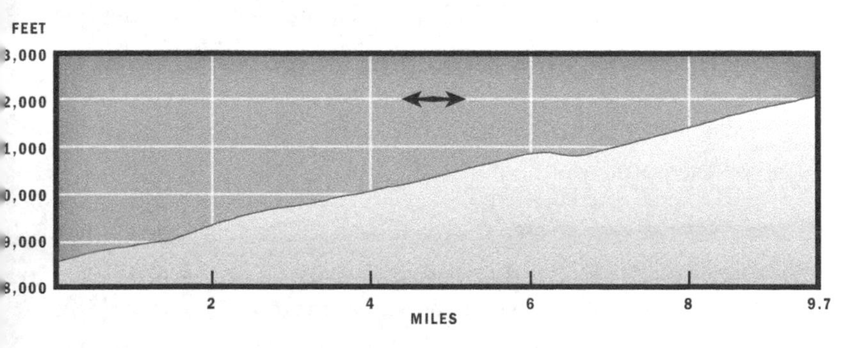

Doyle Peak to the northeast from Fremont Peak to the southwest. It is a popular campsite for thru-hikers, as evidenced by the effort put into the nearby campfire rings. This is the turnaround for the "easy" hike.

ACROSS THE INNER BASIN: The road drops now from Doyle Saddle, passing yellow cliffs and little stands of spruces to wind into the Inner Basin, the remnant caldera of a volcano that once towered 16,000 feet above prehistoric Flagstaff. Now it is a broad bowl lined with aspens and mixed conifers. The road circumnavigates the southwestern wall of this bowl, hovering around the 10,000-foot line. Following this road will likely slow your pace. Some causes may be the altitude, the climb (you'll gain 600 feet in 1 mile), or the occasional rock slides that reduce the road to a footpath, but mostly it will be because of gawking at the basin.

After 1 mile you reach the junction with the Inner Basin Trail 29, which descends tauntingly to the northwest, down into the old caldera to eventually reach Lockett Meadow (that's a different hike). Weatherford heads upward, to the southwest, in a series of short, steep switchbacks through the fir trees.

At the 8-mile mark you reach Fremont Saddle, separating Fremont and Agassiz peaks at an altitude of 11,400 feet, which is why you're panting. The saddle consists of a gravelly little meadow with some rusting junk strewn about and an established campfire site. Firewood trails head off in many directions, but the Weatherford continues roughly north, leaving the far side of the saddle to cut across the eastern slopes of Mount Agassiz. This is the turnaround for the medium-length hike. *Important:* This is the turnaround to take if you wish to be certain of finishing an out-and-back hike in daylight.

THE TREE LINE AND BEYOND: On the far side of Fremont Saddle a sign warns: 11,400 FEET—NO CAMPING ABOVE THIS ELEVATION. NO HIKING OFF-TRAIL. $500 FINE. Beyond it, the road crosses the slopes of Mount Agassiz (the second-tallest peak in Arizona) through a dwarfish thicket of bristlecone pines and cork-bark firs. Not satisfied with this height, the trail switchbacks up the mountain through this last alpine forest. By the end of these switchbacks, at 9 miles and 11,800 feet, you are hovering at the tree line.

Past the switchbacks, the road evaporates to a narrow track threading through the basalt slides that dominate the slope. Here and there, stubborn subalpine firs still push their way up through the soil, but none will ever grow taller than you. Deadwood, bleached as white as bone, is scattered among the rocks. As you come around the corner, even that disappears. There is nothing but you, the rocks, the clouds, and precious little oxygen filling the gaps in between.

As the track turns westward around Agassiz, it passes through large, jagged rock formations. At 9.4 hard miles you reach Agassiz Saddle, a rocky ridge just north of Mount Agassiz. Here, at 12,000 feet, depending on where you stand, the Weatherford Road ended. The ski lifts of Snowbowl stretch across the slopes below. As you gaze farther, the western horizon is visible, from the Mogollon Rim to the Grand Canyon if the day is clear.

Weatherford Trail 102 continues northward as a rough, scree-filled goat path bouncing you down and then across the slope. After 0.25 mile, it drops down to Humphreys Saddle and its junction with Humphreys Trail 151 (see page 109). The Weatherford Trail 102 terminates here.

It takes another 1 mile up Humphreys to reach the tallest point in Arizona, but that mile is one of the hardest you can hike in this state on an established trail. If you've set up a car shuttle at Snowbowl, Humphreys will take you there in 3 steep miles.

Directions

From Flagstaff, take US 180 north about 7 miles to Snowbowl Road. Take Snowbowl Road up about 2 miles to FR 522. Take FR 522 east for 3 bumpy miles, past the dispersed camping area, until it terminates at the trailhead. See page 113 for directions to Humphreys Trailhead if you are planning a car shuttle.

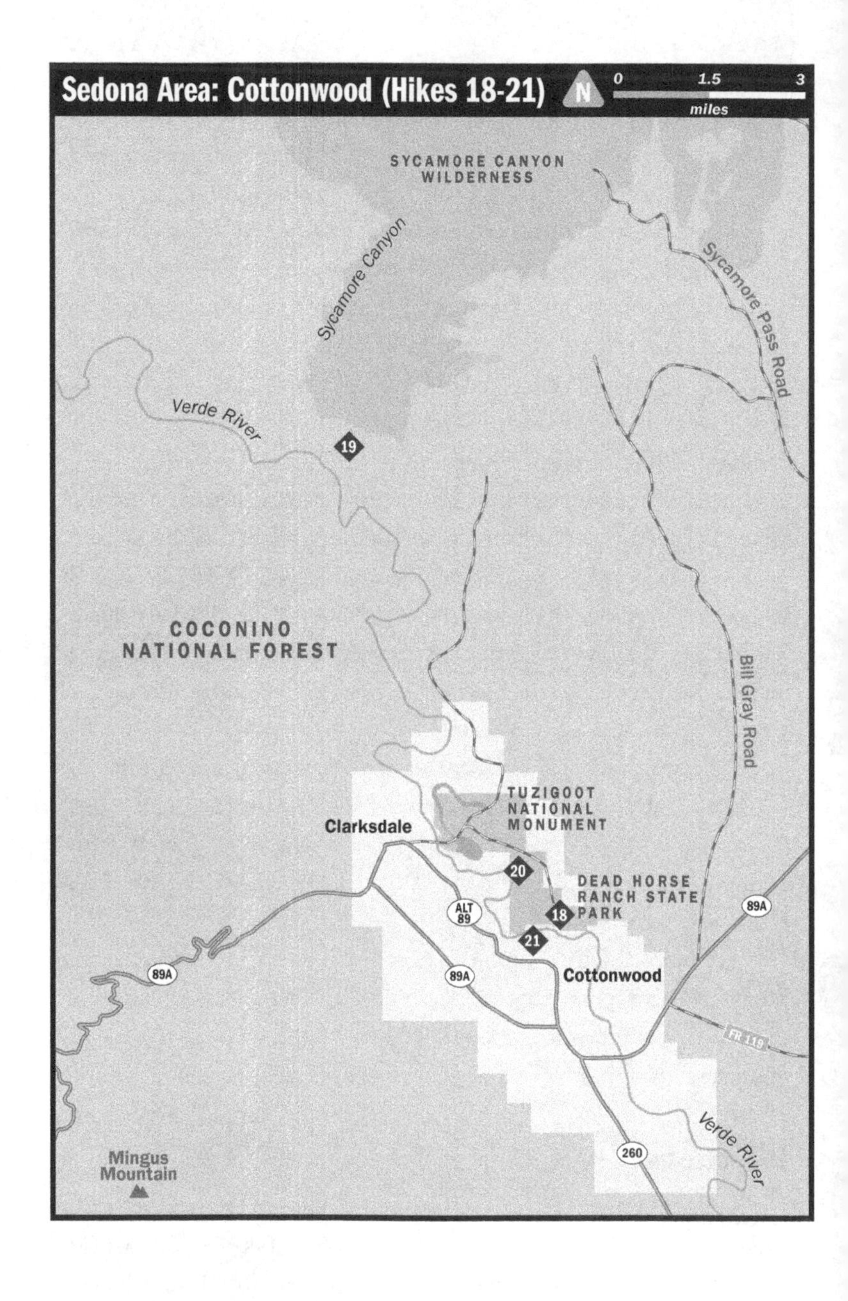
Sedona Area: Cottonwood (Hikes 18-21)
N
0
1.5
3
miles
SYCAMORE CANYON WILDERNESS
Sycamore Canyon
Sycamore Pass Road
Verde River
19
COCONINO NATIONAL FOREST
Bill Gray Road
TUZIGOOT NATIONAL MONUMENT
Clarksdale
20
DEAD HORSE RANCH STATE PARK
18
ALT 89
89A
21
89A
89A
Cottonwood
FR 119
Verde River
260
Mingus Mountain

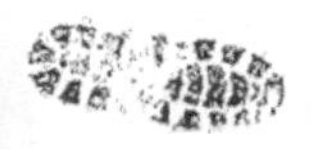

Sedona Area: Cottonwood

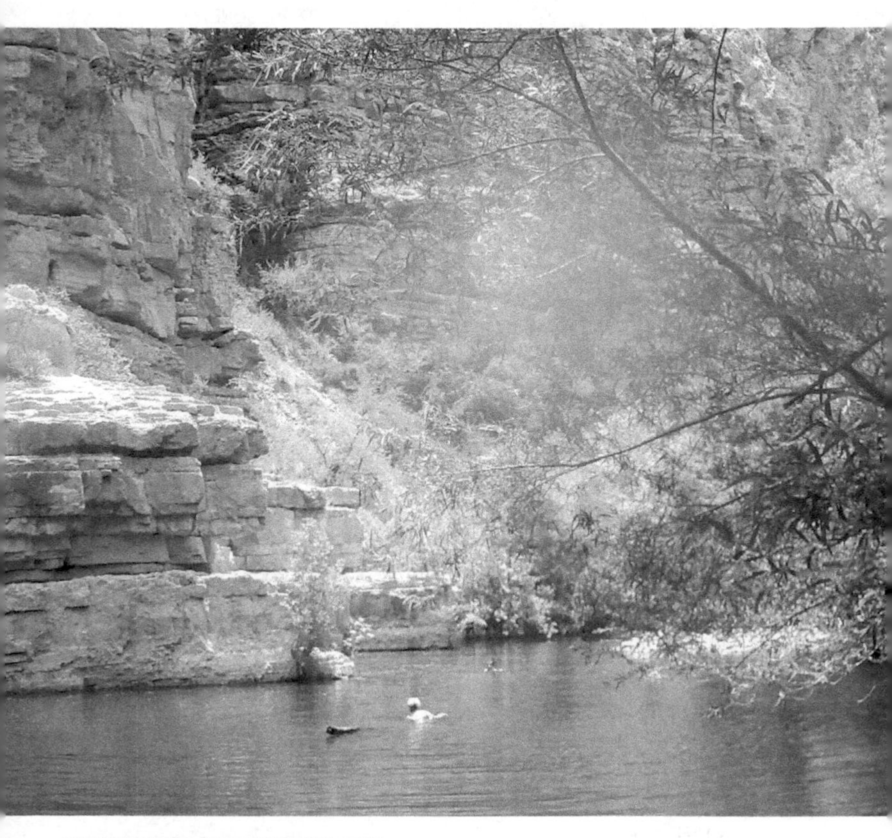

SWIMMING HOLE ON PARSONS TRAIL

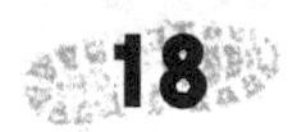

Lime Kiln Trail

SCENERY: ★★★★
TRAIL CONDITION: ★★★★
CHILDREN: ★★
DIFFICULTY: ★★
SOLITUDE: ★★★★★

OCOTILLOS ON SOUTHERN LIME KILN TRAIL

GPS TRAILHEAD COORDINATES: *Dead Horse Ranch State Park terminus, at park boundary:* N34° 45.815' W111° 59.702'
Red Rock State Park terminus: N34° 81.942' W111° 83.650'

DISTANCE & CONFIGURATION: 15-mile car shuttle

HIKING TIME: 8 hours

HIGHLIGHTS: Historical route and transition from high desert to low forest

ELEVATION: 3,471 feet at trailhead to 4,278 feet at highest point

ACCESS: Dead Horse Ranch State Park has a day-use entrance fee of $7 per vehicle; parking near Red Rock State Park or at Deer Pass Trailhead requires a Red Rock Pass. See "Directions" for more details and options.

MAPS: See the route at **azstateparks.com/Parks/DEHO/downloads/DEHO_Lime_Kiln_Trail_c.pdf.**

FACILITIES: Restrooms and water at both state parks and Deer Pass Trailhead; about two-thirds of the journey has vault toilets.

WHEELCHAIR ACCESS: For restrooms

COMMENTS: Best done as a car shuttle. A far shorter hike can be had by parking a vehicle at either Bill Grey Road near the trail crossing or at the Deer Pass Trailhead. These waypoints divide the hike roughly in thirds about 5 miles per segment.

CONTACTS: Red Rock Ranger District, P.O. Box 20429, Sedona, AZ 86341; (928) 282-4119; **www.fs.fed.us/r3/coconino/recreation/red_rock/lime-kiln-tr.shtml;** Dead Horse Ranch Trails Coalition, 2011-B Kestrel Rd., Cottonwood, AZ 86326; (928) 639-0312

Overview

This trail traces the old wagon route that connected Cottonwood and Sedona before the construction of AZ 89A. From Dead Horse Ranch State Park, it climbs out of the high desert, crosses the prairie, tunnels beneath AZ 89A, and then climbs into the hills around Scheurman Mountain before descending to the road near the entrance to Red Rock State Park.

Route Details

This description takes you southwest to northeast, yet there are compelling reasons to go the other way. For one, northeast to southwest goes generally downhill. Another consideration is that while Dead Horse Ranch, as a campground, is open all the time, it would be logistically challenging to stage a car shuttle and make the 15-mile hike in time to enjoy Red Rock before it closes at 5 p.m. In the end, though, northeast to southwest puts a hiker in the low desert, where shade is nearly nonexistent, at the height of the afternoon sun. That realization proved decisive. In cooler weather, it may not be as compelling, and you can simply follow the hike in reverse of this description.

A number of spur trails within Dead Horse Ranch State Park lead to or become the Lime Kiln Trail 82. Head for the most straightforward access—near the bridge and the intersection of the Main Park Road and the North Campground Road. The trail that crosses the North Campground Road is the one you want. It soon bends northeast, past the campground boneyard, and climbs into and out of the wash to arrive at the site of the old lime kiln, just below the trail and dug into the side of the wash. There isn't much left here, but you can definitely see where they did the work. The kiln site is the start of the mileage.

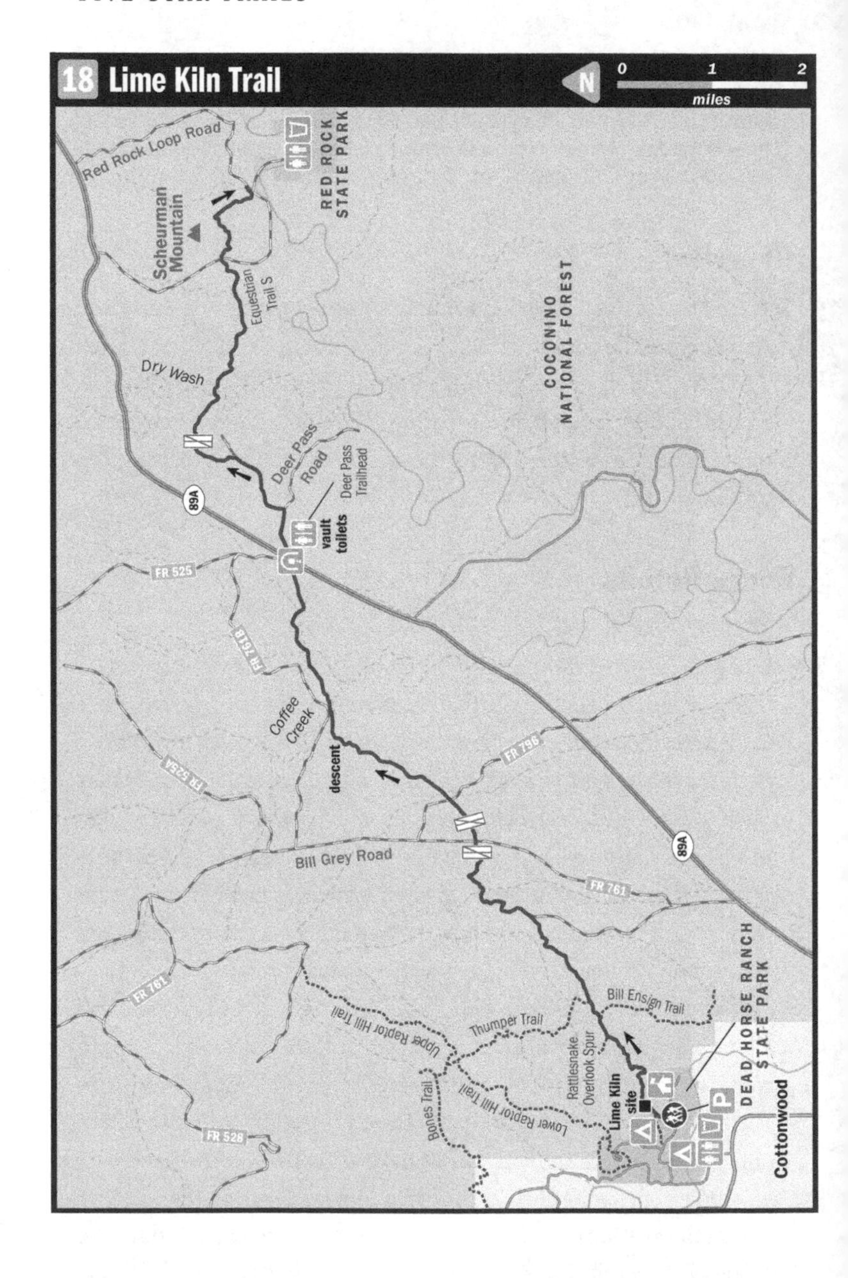
18 Lime Kiln Trail
0
1
2
miles
Red Rock Loop Road
RED ROCK STATE PARK
Scheurman Mountain
Equestrian Trail S
COCONINO NATIONAL FOREST
Dry Wash
Deer Pass Road
Deer Pass Trailhead
vault toilets
89A
FR 525
FR 761B
Coffee Creek
descent
FR 796
FR 525A
Bill Grey Road
FR 761
Bill Ensign Trail
Thumper Trail
Upper Raptor Hill Trail
Rattlesnake Overlook Spur
Bones Trail
Lower Raptor Hill Trail
Lime Kiln site
FR 528
DEAD HORSE RANCH STATE PARK
Cottonwood

The path intersects other park trails as it traverses the high desert north of Cottonwood, which spreads out behind you. You pass junctions with, in order, Rattlesnake Overlook spur, the Bill Ensign Trail, and the Thumper Trail.

The remnant road (once the principal wagon route connecting Cottonwood and a tiny ranch settlement called Sedona) winds through creosote, shrubby paloverde trees, various agave species, and pipe-stemmed ocotillos as it crosses this dry plateau. Throughout, look for the 2-foot-tall caged cairns that regularly mark the route. Those cairns lead you steadily northeast, across the hills, with junipers replacing the paloverdes as you go.

At about 1.5 miles the trail winds in, along, and across a distant spur of FR 761 (though you won't find a sign to that effect). After about 0.5 mile, cairns mark a singletrack that leaves the road to climb up and across some low hills.

Beyond those rocky hills, at about 3.5 miles, the trail joins a different spur of FR 761. The road bends here, creating an apparent Y: Go left (east), not right (south). Look for the cairn. Soon the road leads to a well-used bonfire site. A singletrack leads you due east from here, passing through a gate on its way to Bill Grey Road (FR 761), a wide, graded dirt highway across the prairie.

There is no official trailhead here, but the shoulder is wide enough to accommodate a car if you wanted to shorten the hike in

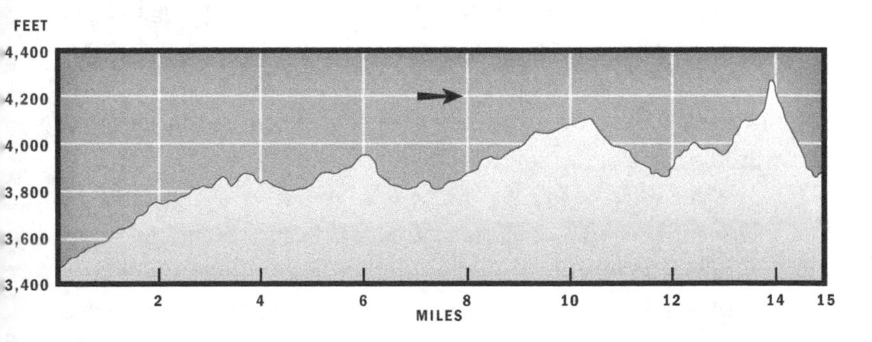

one direction or another and leave a vehicle here. Yet another spur road crosses the trail a few hundred yards east, and then you pass through a second gate.

After crossing rangeland of tall grass, wildflowers, creosote, and occasional cat's-claw, the trail climbs into some hills, paralleling a jeep trail. The latter trail, to tell the truth, presents better footing in many places than the sandy singletrack, and you could follow it instead and lose nothing. The singletrack joins the jeep trail anyway shortly before descending down the hill into a broad valley. Before starting that drop, you can see many of the rock formations that have made the little ranch village of Sedona world-famous in more modern times. The descent is the 5.5-mile mark.

Be sure, though, to stay on the singletrack as it splits from the road before crossing the first big wash, Coffee Creek. The trail represents a shortcut across the overgrazed pasture until the next wash. Past that, it rejoins the road and climbs up and around some small hills before leveling out to cross the prairie once again.

At 7.5 miles, a small wooden sign marks where the trail departs the road toward its very own underpass beneath AZ 89A. A gate guards the concrete tunnel half-filled with tumbleweeds. Beyond, the trail climbs briefly to Deer Pass Trailhead, and the vault toilets there will likely be a welcome sight. (There are, however, no other conveniences.)

The trail follows Deer Pass Road a bit before crossing it, going through a gate, and following a jeep trail past the sewage pastures. Reclaimed wastewater irrigates these fenced fields, as numerous signs will inform you. You'll have to draw your own conclusions as to why it is necessary to advertise this.

This dirt road has numerous spurs, creating some Y-intersections, so it is important to find the cairn. In one particular spot, about 11 miles in, the cairns lead you to a locked gate. The fence on either side is no longer intact, so circumventing it is no trouble, but finding the cairn afterward can prove troublesome. It's to the right (east), down the road.

Don't go uphill: That's the wrong way. Eventually, the road drops into Dry Wash (which normally lives up to its name). The route then follows the forest road (FR 9184) northeast out of the canyon, as pines and junipers become thicker and the soil redder.

Several equestrian trails cross the road, most designated with a letter. Look for Equestrian Trail S, which is also marked by a cairn, taking off to the right (northeast) and up the hill. If you cross a second wash, you've missed it.

Trail S climbs the hill and then turns left to follow the top of the ridge roughly north. From this ridgetop you can see high-income housing to your left (west) and Red Rock State Park to the right (east). After 0.25 mile, the trail descends to cross the paved Red Rock Loop Road and then, across the road, climbs again to the top of a small saddle, where the Scheurman Mountain Trail 56 meets it. Stay straight (roughly north) to start winding down the hill through basalt rubble and thickets of junipers. Just as you can see the entrance to Red Rock State Park, the trail turns left to cross a wash before climbing one last hill. The trail terminates at Red Rock Loop Road, about 100 feet north of the park entrance.

Nearby Attractions

Dead Horse Ranch State Park: With more than 400 developed acres and 100-plus campsites ranging from tent sites to rental cabins, this state park serves as the largest campground in the region. It also features fishing lagoons and access to the Verde River and numerous trails, including the south tail of Lime Kiln. Entrance to the park for day use is $7 per vehicle or $3 per pedestrian. Call (928) 639-0312 or visit **pr.state.az.us/parks/VERI.** There is also an equestrian concessionaire on-site, in the event that you don't want to travel the trail on your own feet; call (928) 634-5283 or visit **trailhorseadventures.com**.

Red Rock State Park: This park lies on the banks of Oak Creek, where it winds through the red-walled canyon 5 miles south of Sedona. A number of short, easy trails travel through the pines, junipers, and grassy fields within this 286-acre nature preserve and environmental-education center. It's day-use only—no camping available. Hours are 8 a.m.–5 p.m. daily. Entrance fee is $10 a vehicle or $3 for pedestrians. Call (928) 282-6907 or visit **pr.state.az.us/parks/RERO.**

Directions

Dead Horse Ranch State Park is on AZ 89A within Cottonwood, south of the intersection with AZ 260, near the noted historical downtown district. Day-use parking is near the fishing lagoons.

To get to Red Rock State Park, take AZ 89A 13 miles north of Cottonwood, or drive 5 miles south of Sedona to Red Rock Loop (the southern end: do not take the northern end by the high school). Proceed on Red Rock Loop another 3 miles to the park entrance. Farther east on Red Rock Loop, as it turns to graded dirt, you can find some parking spots on the side of the road, though parking here requires a Red Rock Pass.

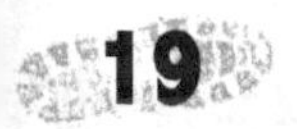

19 Parsons Spring

SCENERY: ★★★★

TRAIL CONDITION: ★★★★★

CHILDREN: ★★★★★/★★★

DIFFICULTY: ★/★★

SOLITUDE: ★

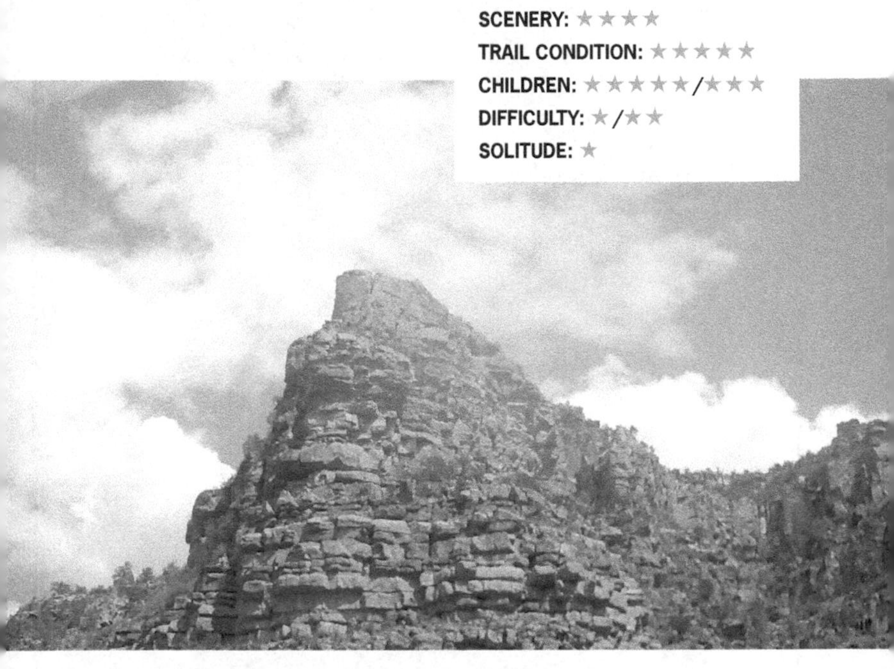

ROCK FORMATIONS NEAR THE MOUTH OF SYCAMORE CANYON

GPS TRAILHEAD COORDINATES: N34° 51.853' W112° 04.162'

DISTANCE & CONFIGURATION: 8.5 miles out-and-back; easy hike is 3.4 miles out-and-back

HIKING TIME: 4 hours plus time for swimming; 2 hours for the easy hike

HIGHLIGHTS: Swimming holes, geology, and flowing springs

ELEVATION: 3,766 feet at trailhead to 3,810 feet at end of hike

ACCESS: No fees or restrictions

MAPS: USGS Clarkdale S.E. and Sycamore Basin; the U.S. Forest Service also publishes an excellent Sycamore Canyon Wilderness map.

FACILITIES: None

WHEELCHAIR ACCESS: None

COMMENTS: This hike has an easier alternative. Despite being spring-fed, Sycamore Creek drains through cattle country, presenting a risk for giardia. There is no camping within the hike area.

CONTACTS: Red Rock Ranger District, P.O. Box 20249, Sedona, AZ 86341; (928) 282-4119; **www.fs.fed.us/r3/coconino/recreation/red_rock/parsons-tr.shtml**

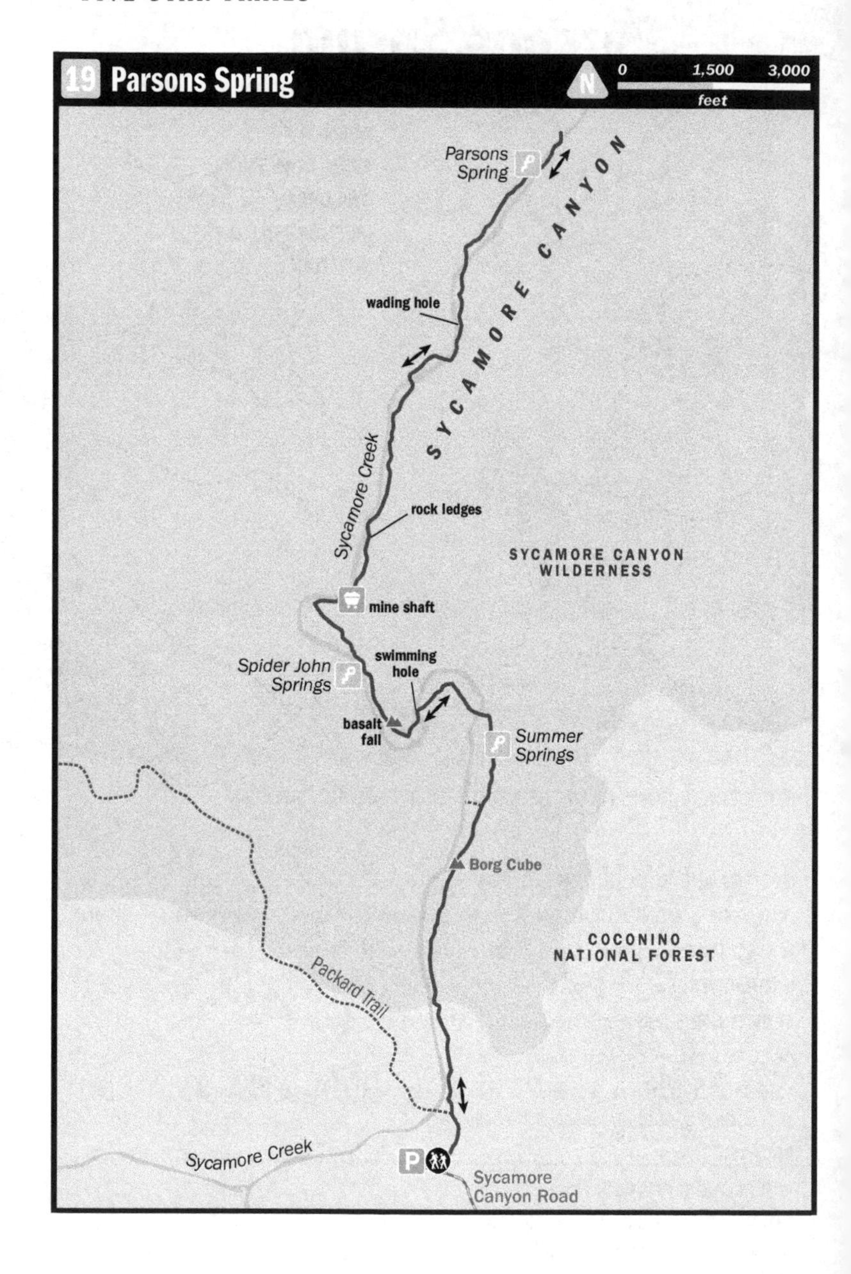

19 Parsons Spring
N
0
1,500
3,000
feet
Parsons Spring
SYCAMORE CANYON
wading hole
Sycamore Creek
rock ledges
SYCAMORE CANYON WILDERNESS
mine shaft
swimming hole
Spider John Springs
basalt fall
Summer Springs
Borg Cube
COCONINO NATIONAL FOREST
Packard Trail
Sycamore Creek
P
Sycamore Canyon Road

Overview

This easy-to-follow trail dips quickly into Sycamore Canyon, where it winds back up the canyon, crossing the spring-fed creek several times, revealing numerous riparian and geologic features. The easy version turns around at the swimming hole.

Route Details

From the barren little parking lot, the trail winds steeply but quickly down into the canyon; this is the only serious grade on the hike. As you wind down the slopes, you'll see an excellent view of your destination canyon. At the bottom, at about 0.2 mile and a drop of 180 feet from the trailhead, you enter the wilderness area at the junction with Packard Trail. Packard goes west across the canyon, and then north across Packard Mesa. Go right (north) on Parsons Trail 144.

Sycamore Creek babbles nearby as you wind through monstrous cottonwood trees. No camping is allowed here, but you will spot remnants of campsites past here and there. The trail winds away 10–20 yards from the bank to the east to bisect riparian trees (you know, the ones with leaves) and mesquite trees. Birds chirp overhead, lizards scurry through the rocks and cottonwood leaves beside your boots, and huge ants patrol the sidewalk-wide trail. Pay attention: Where there are lizards, there are snakes.

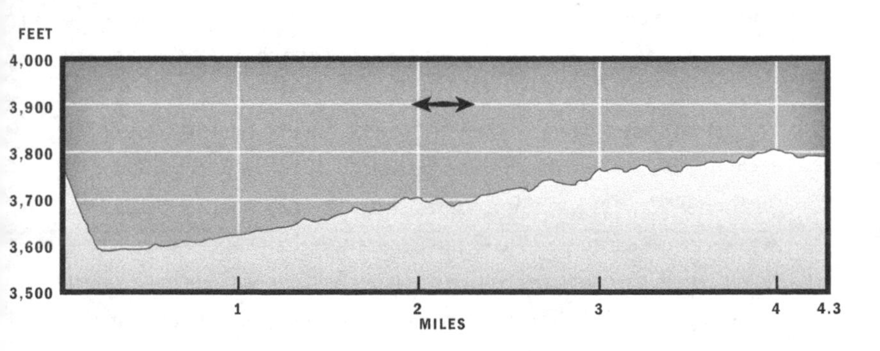

Here and there, boulders have plopped into the dry grass from the cliffs above. Keep an eye out for the Borg Cube, a house-sized basalt boulder that, from a certain angle, resembles a rough-hewn cube. At about 3.66 miles, you might see a spur trail to the left (west) that will bring you, after about 200 yards, to a lovely spot at the south end of an island in the creek.

After about 1 mile of mesquite, the trail drops, the grass greens, and the shade deepens as you return to the babbling creek. You will first pass Summer Springs, gushing from beneath rocks and roots just below the path of the trail. Just past that, you make your first crossing.

Caged cairns mark most of these crossings, though you are largely on your own in the boulder fields that can separate them by a hundred yards or more. This first one is fairly straightforward, however, and nearly due west.

You hike up and down a bluff, continuing west as the creek bends around you to the north before you rejoin it, at 1.7 miles, at the second crossing. Trot across a small rapids from a good-sized and popular swimming hole immediately upstream. You can see a sizable if shallow cave on the salmon-colored cliff opposite the trail. Most of the locals end their hike here, and this is the turnaround for the easy hike.

The trail continues steeply up the bank, across a rockfall of blue basalt, the remnants, of course, of some ancient lava flow. You lower a bit to Spider John Springs, where water gushes from the bottom of the cliffside beneath three small caves.

Just past this, at 2.5 miles, one of the many small caves you might have noticed turns out to be a mine shaft. The giveaway is the regular proportions and partially bricked-over opening. This is the only shaft that goes to any depth into the cliff, but beware: By crawling into one, you are placing more faith in the engineering acumen of whatever miner dug this 100-plus years ago than is perhaps wise.

At this point, the trail consistently follows the base of the towering red cliffs. The rectangular striations make it appear as a massive fortification of some sort. Across from you, the opposing canyon wall seems even more dramatic: Long, vertical sections have sheared off, giving it the appearance of an enormous, fossilized picket fence. Several erosion caves can be found in the side as you occasionally navigate more rock ledges or blue basalt boulders.

At about 3.25 miles, the trail drops back to the creek for the third crossing. A fourth crossing happens within 0.25 mile, and then you stroll past a series of wide, clear wading holes before the fifth crossing takes you back to the west side of the canyon.

You hike up and down a rocky bluff and cross a sandy shelf covered with scrub oaks before descending to the final crossing of the route. Immediately upstream, you'll find the series of springs and seeps collectively known as Parsons Spring. A couple of caves can be seen on the west bank. A profusion of plants lines these banks, including both wild grape and poison ivy.

This is the turnaround point. The trail continues past this mark for about 0.1 mile before disappearing in the dry boulders beyond the last, small seep. Return the way you came.

Nearby Attractions

Tuzigoot National Monument sits atop a hill overlooking what is now Cottonwood. Here, more than 1,000 years ago, the Sinaguan people built themselves an apartment complex. You can tour the remains at the national monument. Entrance fee is $5 for adults, free for children. The monument is open 8 a.m.–6 p.m. through the summer and until 5 p.m. the rest of the year. Call (928) 634-5564 or visit **nps.gov/tuzi.**

Directions

From Cottonwood, take AZ 89A south, past the city limits, to the Tuzigoot National Monument turnoff (there will be signs). Before you get to the monument, take the only left turn, which is FR 131 (Sycamore Canyon Road). Follow this graded dirt road for 10.5 miles until you reach the trailhead.

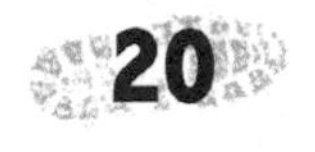

20 Verde River Greenway North

SCENERY: ★★★★
TRAIL CONDITION: ★★★★
CHILDREN: ★★★★
DIFFICULTY: ★★
SOLITUDE: ★★

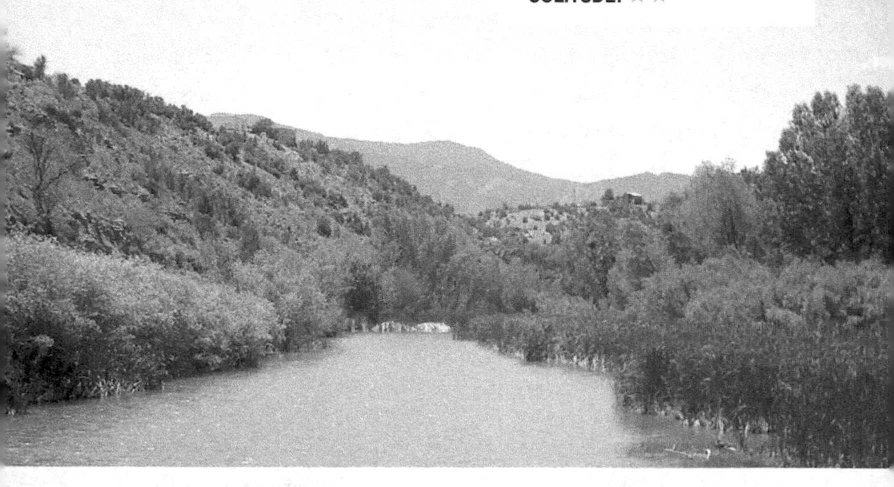

THE MIGHTY VERDE RIVER FLOWING THROUGH ITS GREENWAY

GPS TRAILHEAD COORDINATES:
Western trailhead–Verde River access: N34° 46.010' W112° 02.257'
Toppock Marsh Trailhead–Dead Horse Ranch State Park east end: N34° 45.781' W112° 01.277'

DISTANCE & CONFIGURATION: 3 miles out-and-back

HIKING TIME: 2 hours

HIGHLIGHTS: Verde River access, mesquite bosk, bird-watching, and fishing

ELEVATION: Approximately 3,300 feet throughout

ACCESS: The river access has no fee but is day-use only. Dead Horse Ranch State Park has a day-use entrance fee of $7 per vehicle.

MAPS: USGS maps are insufficiently accurate, so pick up the Cottonwood Chamber of Commerce's good street map of Cottonwood, available at either visitor center at the highway junction or at the downtown jail and from a number of local merchants. Dead Horse Ranch State Park also has a free map of the trails within that park.

FACILITIES: None

WHEELCHAIR ACCESS: None

COMMENTS: Despite what may be shown on some maps, this route does not actually cross the river. Do not confuse this Verde River Greenway with a trail of the same name within Dead Horse Ranch State Park.

CONTACTS: Dead Horse Ranch State Park, 2011-B Kestrel Rd., Cottonwood, AZ 86326; (928) 639-0312; **pr.state.az.us/parks/VERI**

Overview

The hike route follows the north bank of the Verde River between Clarkdale and Cottonwood. Starting at a popular swimming hole, the trail parallels the riverbed, and then, as the river bends south, winds through a bosk of mesquite trees and a wide field within the bounds of Tuzigoot National Monument before returning to follow the river once more. The trail terminates at an alternate trailhead within Dead Horse Ranch State Park.

Route Details

From the river access and swimming hole, proceed east along the north bank of the river; any of the social trails will do. All of these trails funnel through the tall cottonwoods and sycamores. The river corridor narrows as you go, and you are soon reduced to one path heading up the bank through the mesquite trees. Spray-painted arrows guide you along the bank for just under 0.5 mile to a break in the fence, allowing the trail to join the road.

Continue east along the road. To your left (north), the wide, fenced-off field was once filled with copper tailings from mines in the mountains behind you. Straight ahead, the adobe tower of Tuzigoot looms above.

Within 0.25 mile the road ends, but spray-painted arrows indicate a sidewalk crossing a concrete-and-stone floodwater runway. Below, to your right, the Verde flows around an irrigation-diversion embankment. The sidewalk leads to a gate marking the national park boundary. Go through the gate. There's no charge to use this trail.

The trail now winds through a beautiful bosk of Arizona mesquite, providing the first shade you've had since leaving the

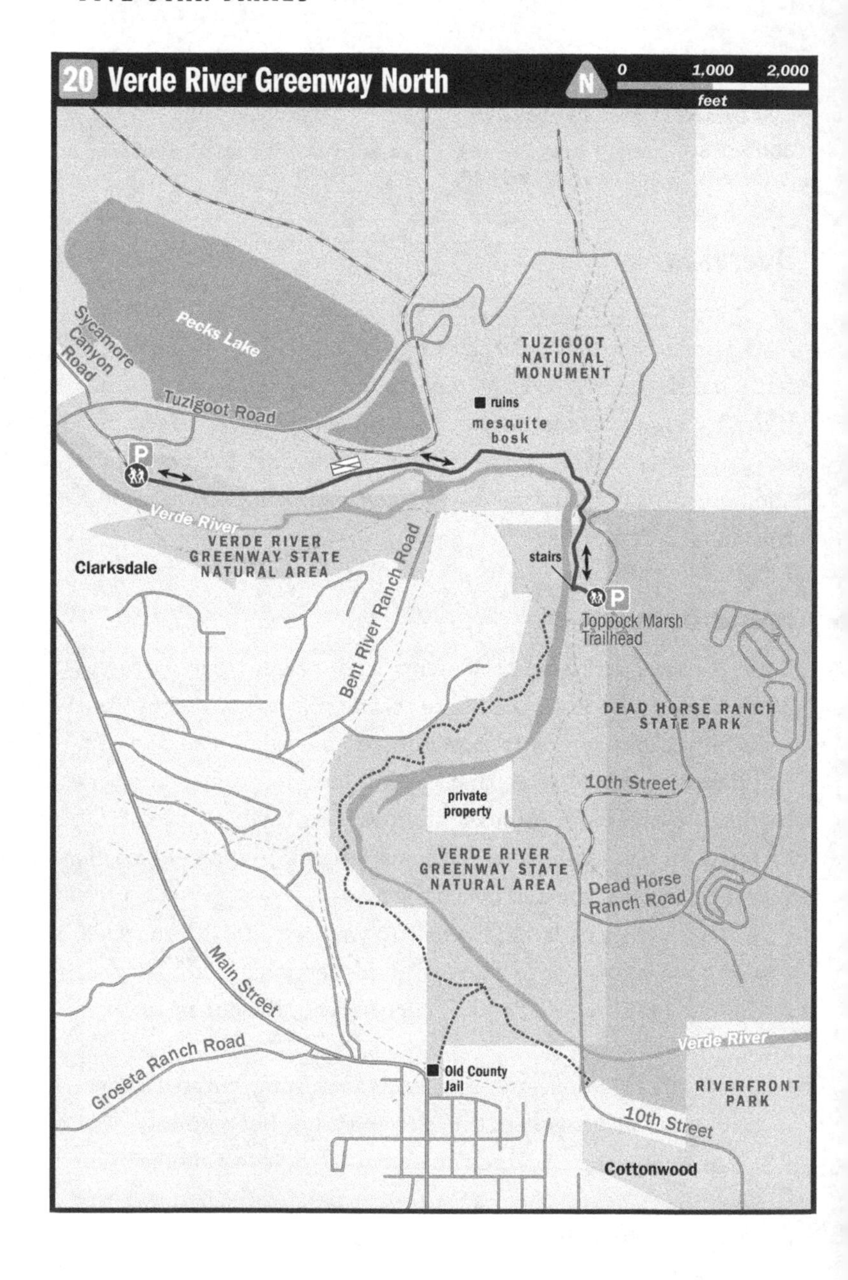
20 Verde River Greenway North
N
0
1,000
2,000
feet
Pecks Lake
Sycamore Canyon Road
Tuzigoot Road
TUZIGOOT NATIONAL MONUMENT
ruins
mesquite bosk
P
Verde River
VERDE RIVER GREENWAY STATE NATURAL AREA
Clarksdale
Bent River Ranch Road
stairs
P
Toppock Marsh Trailhead
DEAD HORSE RANCH STATE PARK
10th Street
private property
VERDE RIVER GREENWAY STATE NATURAL AREA
Dead Horse Ranch Road
Main Street
Groseta Ranch Road
Old County Jail
Verde River
RIVERFRONT PARK
10th Street
Cottonwood

river. On the far side of this bosk, the landscape opens into a weed-choked arroyo, and the trail comes to a Y. The trail to your left goes north, forming a long loop around the arroyo that is of more interest to mountain bikers. The trail to your right continues east straight across. Stay right.

Across the arroyo you come to a second Y in the path. The trail to the left is the other end of the northern loop. It also has a spur leading to a gigantic sycamore tree. That spur is worth exploring, but it's a dead end. The trail to your right leads down to the river and continues on.

The trail cuts down the sandy embankment into the marshy banks of the Verde. Colored ribbons now guide you through the willows, salt cedars (also known as tamarisks), and tall reeds. As you pick your steps through the marsh, you are also bending south, along with the river. The route emerges onto an angler trail hugging the now-steep and hard dirt banks of the river. By this point, you are definitely heading south.

Continue along this bank, popular with local anglers, for about 0.1 mile, where you encounter a stairway. This leads up to a short spur trail to the parking lot of the Toppock Marsh Trailhead. Return the way you came.

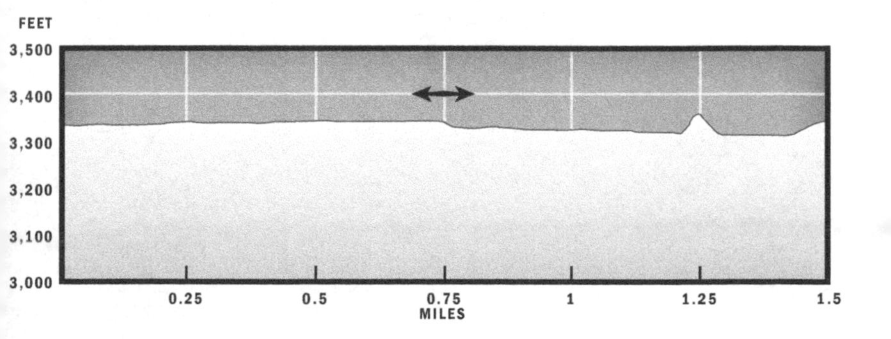

Nearby Attractions

Tuzigoot National Monument sits atop a hill overlooking what is now Cottonwood. Here, more than 1,000 years ago, the Sinaguan people built themselves an apartment complex. You can tour the remains at the national monument. Entrance fee is $5 for adults, free for children. The monument is open 8 a.m.–6 p.m. through the summer and until 5 p.m. the rest of the year. Call (928) 634-5564 or visit **nps.gov/tuzi.**

Directions

From Cottonwood, take AZ 89A south, past the city limits, to the Tuzigoot National Monument turnoff (there will be signs). Cross the bridge and look for a dirt road turning off to the right. That dirt road will wind down to a dirt lot near the river access. The final bit of the road is steep but doable in a passenger vehicle. The trailhead has no services.

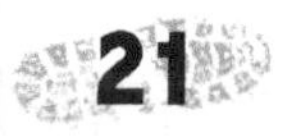

21 Verde River Greenway South

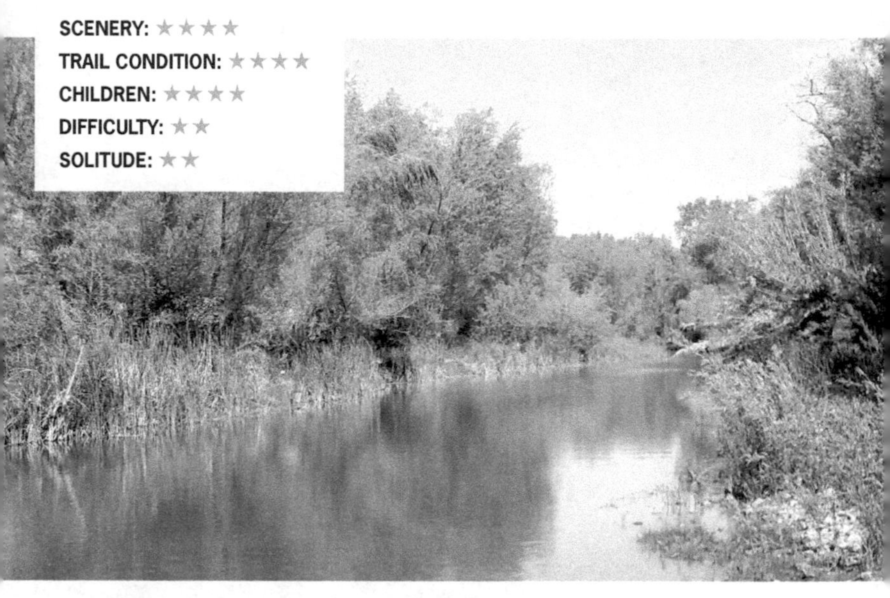

SCENERY: ★★★★

TRAIL CONDITION: ★★★★

CHILDREN: ★★★★

DIFFICULTY: ★★

SOLITUDE: ★★

THE VERDE RIVER FLOWING THROUGH RIVERFRONT PARK IN COTTONWOOD

GPS TRAILHEAD COORDINATES: *Riverfront Park:* N34° 44.964' W112° 01.309'
Jail Visitor Center: N34° 44.976' W112° 01.623'

DISTANCE & CONFIGURATION: 4 miles out-and-back

HIKING TIME: 2 hours

HIGHLIGHTS: Verde River access, riparian woodlands, and historical downtown Cottonwood

ELEVATION: Approximately 3,300 feet throughout

ACCESS: No fees or restrictions

MAPS: The USGS maps are insufficiently accurate, so pick up the Cottonwood Chamber of Commerce's good street map of Cottonwood, available at either visitor center at the highway junction or the downtown jail and from a number of local merchants.

FACILITIES: Restrooms and drinking fountains at Riverfront Park

WHEELCHAIR ACCESS: Possible on the Jail spur

COMMENTS: Much of the trail runs right up against private property, so be cool. The section of the Verde covered here is not recommended for swimming or wading. See Verde Greenway North (previous profile) for a good swimming hole. Despite what may be shown on some maps, this route does not actually cross the river. Do not confuse this Verde River

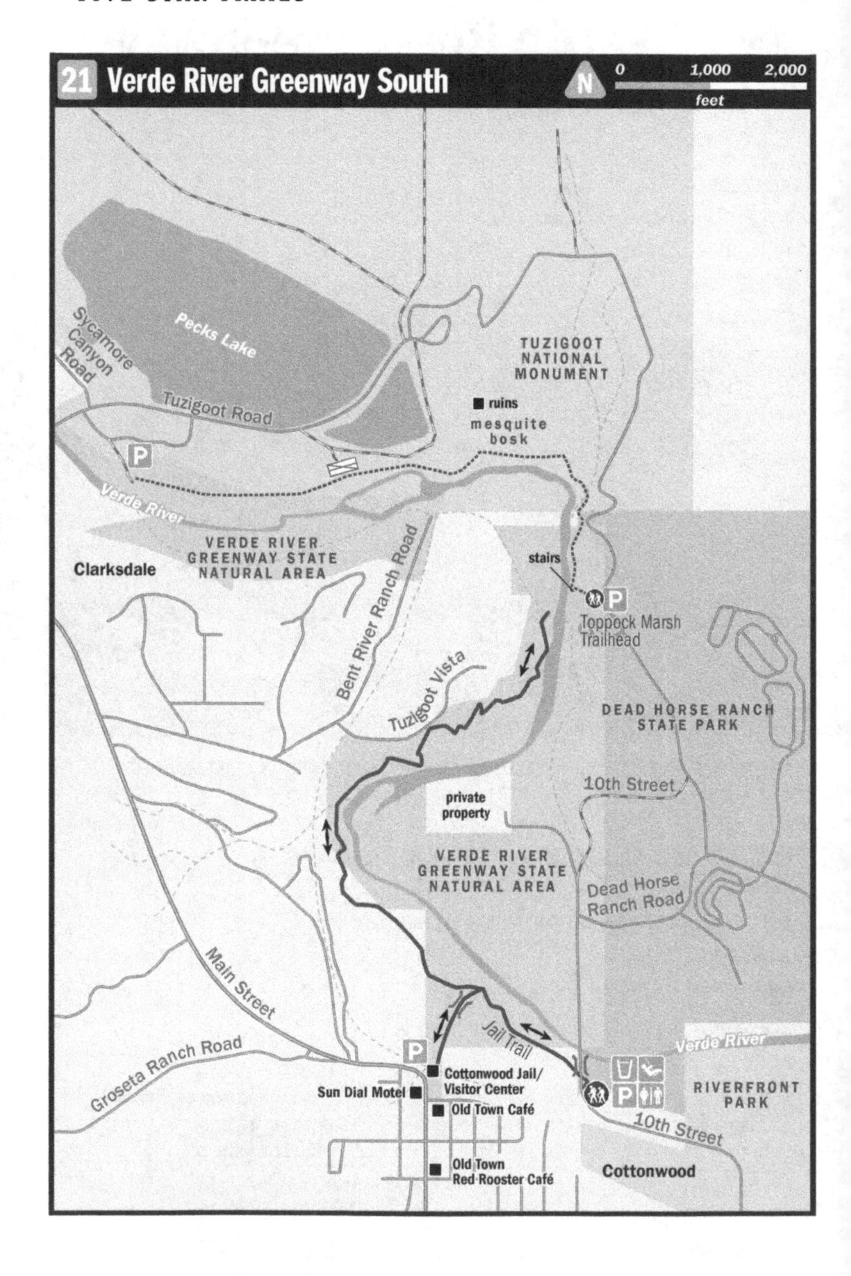
21 Verde River Greenway South
N
0
1,000
2,000
feet
Pecks Lake
Sycamore Canyon Road
Tuzigoot Road
TUZIGOOT NATIONAL MONUMENT
ruins
mesquite bosk
Verde River
VERDE RIVER GREENWAY STATE NATURAL AREA
Clarksdale
Bent River Ranch Road
stairs
Toppock Marsh Trailhead
Tuzigoot Vista
DEAD HORSE RANCH STATE PARK
10th Street
private property
VERDE RIVER GREENWAY STATE NATURAL AREA
Dead Horse Ranch Road
Main Street
Jail Trail
Verde River
Groseta Ranch Road
Cottonwood Jail/ Visitor Center
Sun Dial Motel
Old Town Café
RIVERFRONT PARK
10th Street
Old Town Red Rooster Café
Cottonwood

Greenway with a trail of the same name within Dead Horse Ranch State Park.

CONTACTS: Dead Horse Ranch State Park, 2011-B Kestrel Rd., Cottonwood, AZ 86326; (928) 639-0312; **pr.state.az.us/parks/VERI**

Overview

This obscure little trail goes from Riverfront Park (across the river from Dead Horse Ranch State Park) along the riverbed. A spur goes to the visitor center in downtown Cottonwood. The remaining trail passes through astounding riparian woods until it terminates at the riverside.

Route Details

Trails riddle Cottonwood's Riverfront Park. From the parking area (by the ball fields and playground), take any of them west and continue as they all funnel toward the 10th Street Bridge at the west end of the park. Once there, find the signs for the Jail Trail, and follow this trail under the bridge.

The Jail Trail starts out as a rock-lined path across the sandy wash south of the river, far away from any shade. The Verde River flows somewhere beyond the tangle of reeds to your right. The traffic of Cottonwood flows beyond the buildings to your left.

In just over 0.25 mile, you come across a side trail heading

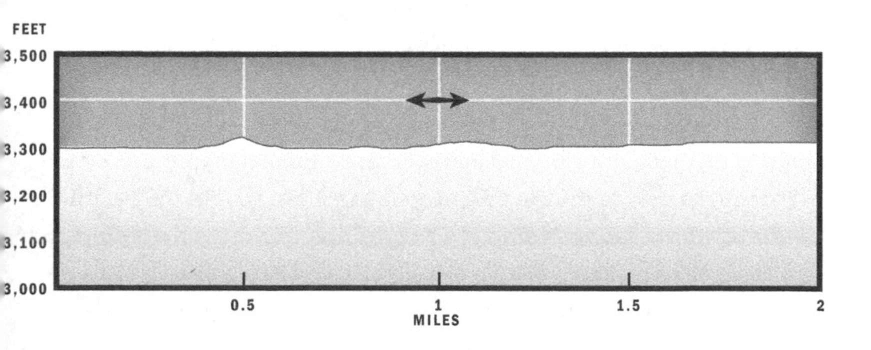

left (south) even as the main trail continues across the barren sand. Actually, should you go straight, you'd find that the path inexplicably dead-ends a couple hundred yards later, still in the middle of the wash. Take the left.

In a few hundred feet, you'll see a dirt path continuing west through the trees that line the wash. Remember that. The Jail Trail continues south, though, across a bridge, past some interpretive signs, to the Cottonwood Jail, a tiny stone building that now serves as a visitor center. It stands in historical downtown Cottonwood, which is mostly motels, bars, bookstores, and antiques shops (see "Nearby Attractions").

The jail can also be used as an alternate trailhead. It has parking for about six cars and more parking along the street.

When you have satisfied your curiosity, return to the dirt path going west through the trees. This undesignated trail is the heart of the hike, as it passes beneath the shade of cottonwoods and sycamores or across grassy, sandy glades. This area provides outstanding bird-watching, with sightings of species from hummingbirds to herons.

This route hugs the edge of the Verde River Greenway State Natural Area boundary, passing frequently within sight of private backyards. Huge cairns bound in cages mark the actual boundary. The trail will, on occasion, wander beyond these cairns, but in every case it soon curves back in bounds.

At about 1 mile from the bridge (not counting the Jail spur), the track crosses a wash just before it approaches a gravel pit. This wide, sandy wasteland is left over from one of the many times the Verde has wiggled in its course. Contrast with nearby Pecks Lake, another remnant of a course change. Some game trails proceed across the sand, but don't be fooled. Keep to the left (west) side of the bank, following a side wash around a wooded shelf until the trail becomes obvious once more.

Up the bank from the wash runs a dirt road designated Tuzigoot Vista. It will dead-end in private driveways, so stay in the wash.

Soon after, the trail comes to the steep banks of the Verde River itself, 50 yards wide at this point. The trail follows the high bank for another 0.33 mile before coming across an irrigation-diversion trench extending from a pipeline crossing the river.

Here ends the hike. Return the way you came.

Nearby Attractions

The touted historical part of downtown Cottonwood stretches along a section of Main Street that cuts north from the Lion's Park and Blowout Creek to just past the curve heading west toward Clarkdale. In this section you'll find a number of cafés, wine bars, book and antiques shops, bars and grills, and the eclectically shabby Sun Dial Motel ([928] 634-8031). For lunch, the Old Town Cafe ([928] 634-5980; **oldtownroaster.com/cafe**) serves coffee and sandwiches, and the Old Town Red Rooster Café ([928] 649-8100; **oldtownredroostercafe.com**) offers more-traditional restaurant fare. Both places run $8–$15 a plate. All are within 0.25 mile of the Jail Visitor Center.

Directions

In Cottonwood, follow AZ 260 west until it becomes Main Street, past the intersection with AZ 89A. Main Street proceeds north but then curves west again in about 1 mile. Shortly after this curve, turn right (north) on 10th Street and continue a block until Riverfront Drive. Turn right (east) on Riverfront, which will dead-end at the park of the same name.

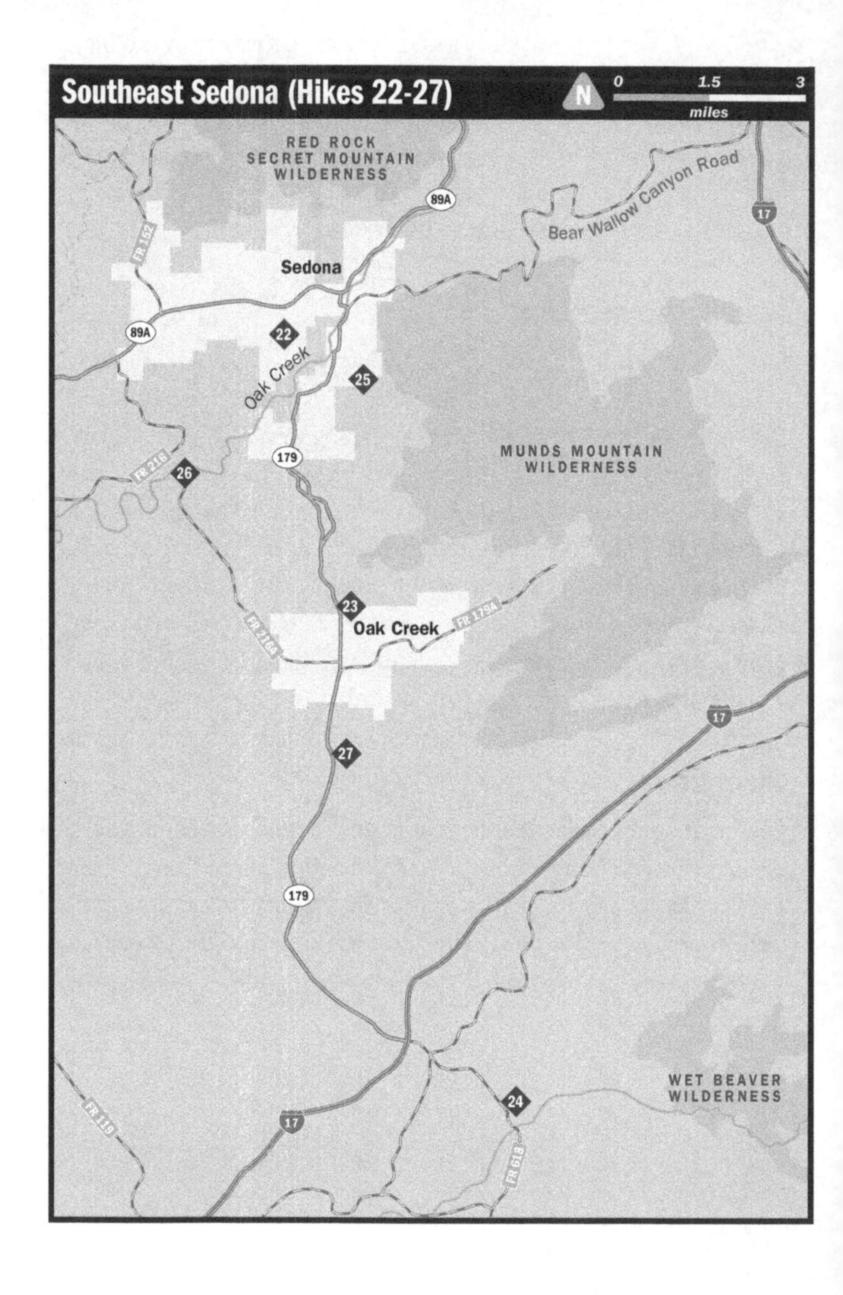
Southeast Sedona (Hikes 22-27)
N
0
1.5
3
miles
RED ROCK
SECRET MOUNTAIN
WILDERNESS
89A
Bear Wallow Canyon Road
17
FR 152
Sedona
89A
22
Oak Creek
25
179
MUNDS MOUNTAIN
WILDERNESS
FR 216
26
23
Oak Creek
FR 179A
FR 216A
17
27
179
WET BEAVER
WILDERNESS
24
FR 119
17
FR 618

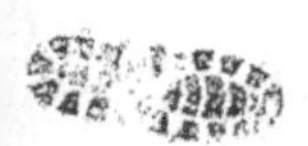

Southeast Sedona

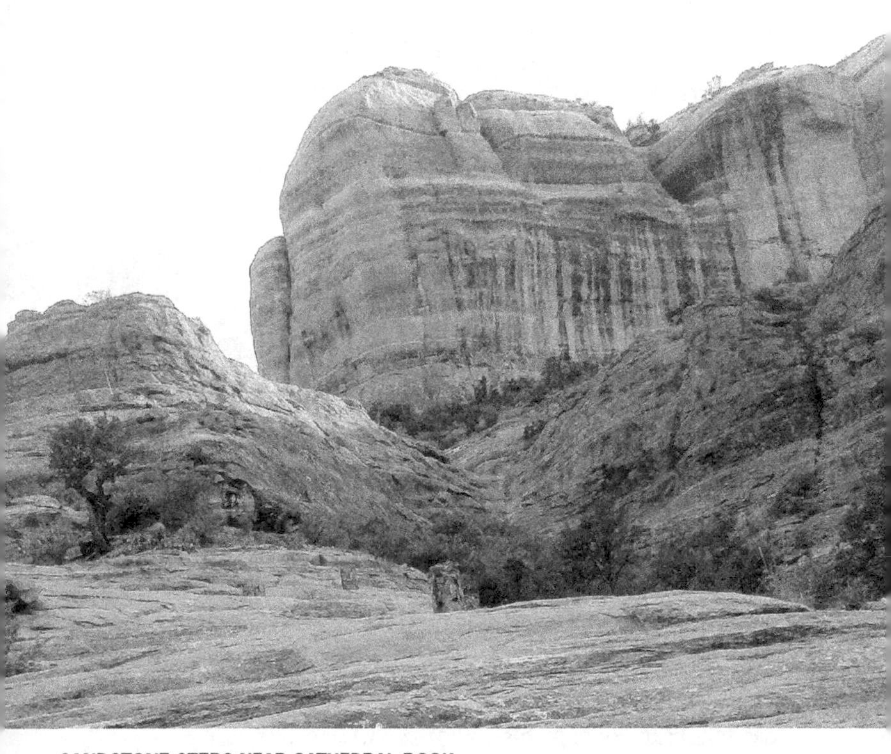

SANDSTONE STEPS NEAR CATHEDRAL ROCK

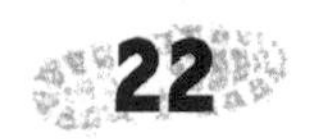

22 Airport Mesa

SCENERY: ★★★★
TRAIL CONDITION: ★★★★★
CHILDREN: ★★★★
DIFFICULTY: ★★
SOLITUDE: ★★

CAIRN ART ON AIRPORT MESA

GPS TRAILHEAD COORDINATES: N34° 51.344' W111° 46.803'

DISTANCE & CONFIGURATION: 3.5-mile loop

HIKING TIME: 2 hours

HIGHLIGHTS: Scenic vistas all the way around Sedona and vortex site

ELEVATION: 4,567 feet at trailhead to 4,722 feet at the top of the mesa

ACCESS: Requires a Red Rock Pass

MAPS: USGS Sedona

FACILITIES: None

WHEELCHAIR ACCESS: None

COMMENTS: Optional spur across Table Top Trail adds 1 mile and 30 minutes. Very little shade.

CONTACTS: Coconino National Forest, Red Rock Ranger District, P.O. Box 20429, Sedona, AZ 86341; (928) 282-4119; **www.fs.fed.us/r3/coconino/recreation/red_rock/airport-loop-tabletop-tr.shtml**

Overview

This hike circumnavigates what is properly known as Table Top Mesa, though because of its current use, everyone calls it Airport Mesa. The loop starts and ends at a vortex site but along the way provides sightseers and photographers with broad vistas of Sedona's famous rock formations.

Route Details

From the parking area, all trails head up the little rise. To your immediate east (left) is the rocky prominence around which a vortex can be felt. This is why the trailhead is so crowded. The vortex isn't centered on any particular part of the outcrop, but it does seem stronger on the south side.

Three other trails spring from this trailhead: Yavapai Loop, Overlook Point, and Brewer Loop. These are all short little tramps. Ignore them and continue up to the top of the saddle, the Courthouse Butte Overlook, which provides a spectacular angle on its titular formation across the valley.

Airport Mesa Loop Trail 211 takes off to the right (southwest) of this, following a ledge of the red-rock mesa through stunted piñon pines and twisted juniper trees. The slopes are further adorned with scrub oaks and prickly pear cacti, as well as a scattering of cairns, not all of which will be helpful. The trail, though, will be starkly obvious throughout the hike.

As you cross the various sandstone terraces, you can see the valley spreading to the east. Visible are both Oak Creek and AZ 179 cutting their various paths through the valley, one bringing life and the other bringing money.

At 0.8 mile, the sandstone terraces yield to stark red cliffs. The junipers tend to grow bigger through here, and occasionally yuccas or ocotillos will poke through the large groves of prickly pear cacti.

At 1.2 miles, the trail bends a little to the south and climbs. From here you may start hearing the noise from the airport traffic. The climb

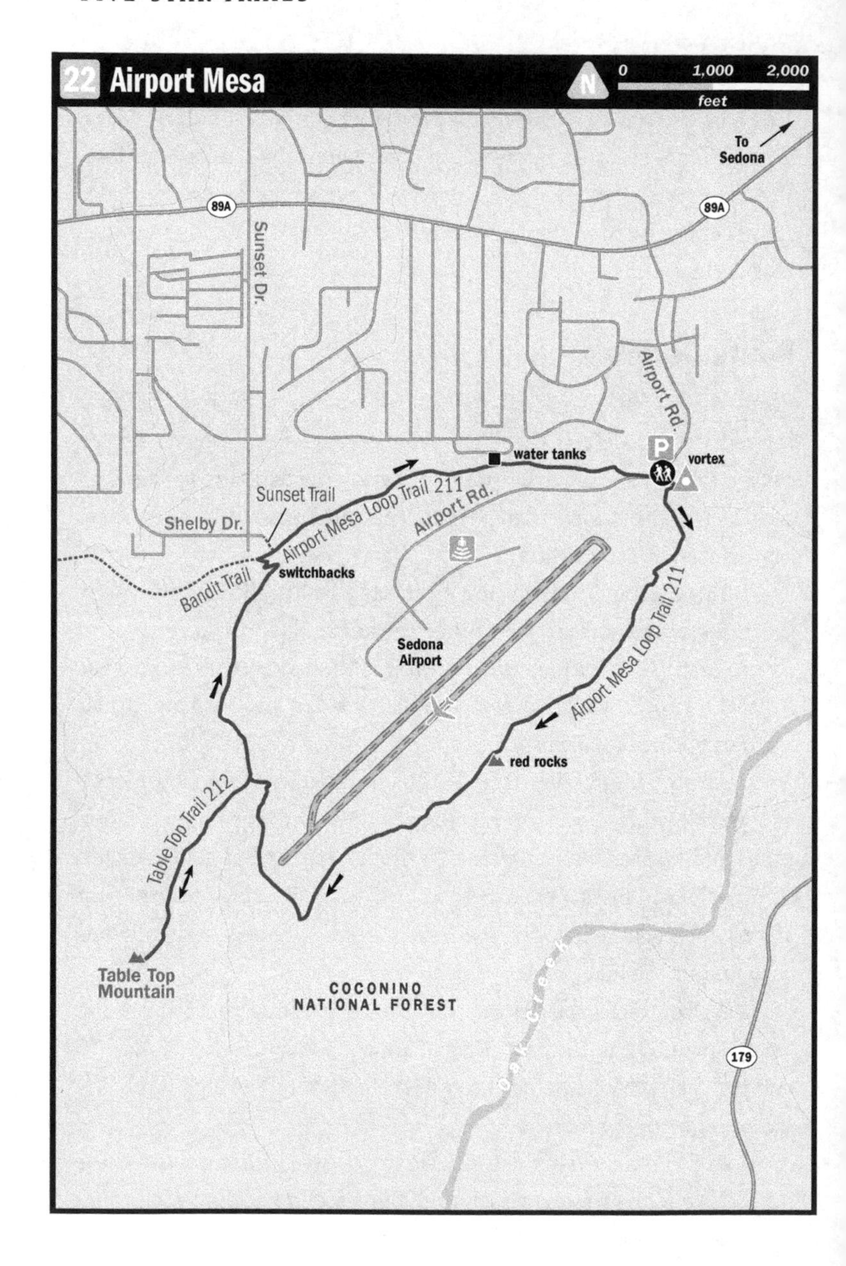
22 Airport Mesa
N
0 1,000 2,000
feet
To Sedona
89A
89A
Sunset Dr.
Airport Rd.
P
vortex
water tanks
Airport Mesa Loop Trail 211
Airport Rd.
Sunset Trail
Shelby Dr.
switchbacks
Bandit Trail
Sedona Airport
Airport Mesa Loop Trail 211
red rocks
Table Top Trail 212
Table Top Mountain
COCONINO NATIONAL FOREST
Oak Creek
179

continues for 0.25 mile until the top of the butte, at 4,722 feet, where the trail makes a U-turn through the stand of junipers. The trail surface has transitioned now from sidewalk-consistency red rock to asphalt-consistency black dirt.

The U-turn bends the trail roughly northwest, where it soon follows along the airport fence. The new chain-link hurricane fence follows the barbed-wire fence that marked the boundary in earlier decades. Signs caution you to watch for low-flying aircraft, but they won't really buzz that close; you'll still get a good look at their undersides from time to time. Also watch for hawks circling about.

Soon you come to a T-intersection with Table Top Trail 212, which winds through the agaves, following the finger ridge southwest out to its end. This sidetrack adds just under a mile to the hike out-and-back. A trace trail continues down the ridge toward Carroll Canyon, but that's not part of this hike.

Returning to Airport Mesa Loop 211 and continuing north, you can see Scheurman Mountain towering over the high school, the broad prairie stretching beyond AZ 89A, and, as you move farther north, Bear Mountain and the rest of the Secret Mountain Wilderness behind it.

Right at the corner of the airfield, the route hits a wash filled with boulders. These rocks were deposited by Oak Creek, or rather its ancient predecessor, before the modern creek cut its way down a fault to the east.

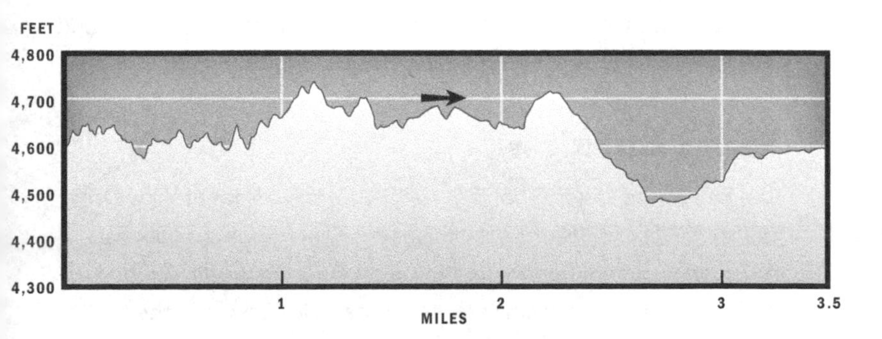

Just beyond the ancient creek bed, you begin a small climb. While crossing the top, look for the artistic cairn someone built. Its delicately balanced stones defy gravity. Sedona has cairn artists in the way New York City has graffiti artists—except that cairns are generally legal. Don't be the hiker who knocks the cairn over.

Past this, the main view of Sedona becomes more and more dominant. You can see the roads and churches and playgrounds and strip malls and housing developments that make up the small city, and beyond that the numerous rock formations that make up its reputation for beauty.

From roughly west to east you can spot Chimney Rock, Capital Butte, Coffee Pot Rock, Brins Mesa, the more distant Wilson Mountain, and, finally, Steamboat Rock.

As the trail continues northeast around the butte, it descends via some brief switchbacks. At the bottom you come to junctions with Bandit Trail and, shortly thereafter, Sunset Trail, both of which feed into the Carroll Canyon trail network.

From here the trail dips toward town (or the town creeps up the mesa, depending on your perspective). Every so often you'll see a spur trail heading downslope, probably heading for a cul-de-sac. These spurs may or may not cross private property (but they probably do) and should not be used as secret access points. By the time you pass the big green water tanks, you are heading roughly east. Within 0.25 mile of this landmark, the path climbs briefly to emerge behind the traffic barricade across the street from the trailhead.

Nearby Attractions

The Red Planet Diner (1655 W. AZ 89A, on the corner of View Drive; [928] 282-6070) features good burgers, outstanding breakfasts, a full-service bar, and decor that is cheesy on a cosmic level. The laid-back vibe sometimes translates to slow service, so while the food is generally worth the wait, don't come here if you're watching your watch. Expect to pay $8–$15 a plate.

Directions

From the Y in Sedona, take AZ 89A south less than a mile before turning left (roughly south) onto Airport Drive. The trailhead is halfway up the mesa. It has space for about eight cars, but frequently a dozen or more will cram in. Parking at the airport overlook, about 0.5 mile farther up the butte, is plentiful and free, but there is no designated pedestrian path to the trail. You take your chances on a narrow, winding road full of tourists. Parking at this trailhead requires a Red Rock Pass; a solar-powered vending machine on-site dispenses the passes for cash or credit.

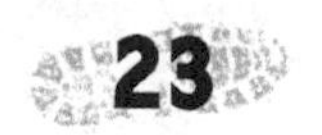

23 Bell Rock

SCENERY: ★★★★
TRAIL CONDITION: ★★★★
CHILDREN: ★★★★
DIFFICULTY: ★★
SOLITUDE: ★

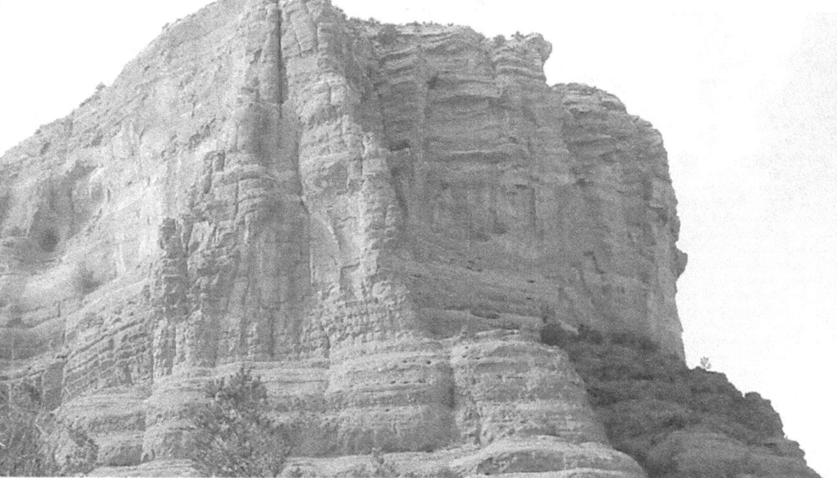

BELL ROCK FROM THE SOUTH SIDE

GPS TRAILHEAD COORDINATES: N34° 47.487' W111° 45.692'

DISTANCE & CONFIGURATION: 4.6-mile loop; adventure option (see page 166) is a 10-mile car shuttle

HIKING TIME: 2–3 hours; 5–6 hours with adventure option

HIGHLIGHTS: Views, geology, and vortex site

ELEVATION: 4,180 feet at trailhead to approximately 4,545 feet or higher on Bell Rock

ACCESS: Requires a Red Rock Pass

MAPS: USGS Sedona and Munds Mountain

FACILITIES: Trash cans

WHEELCHAIR ACCESS: None

COMMENTS: On weekends with good weather, Bell Rock may have amusement park–type crowding. No water available. Very little shade; this is a hot hike in the summer months. See note following "Route Details" on combining this hike with Broken Arrow Trail (see page 174) as a car shuttle.

CONTACTS: Red Rock Ranger District, P.O. Box 20429, Sedona, AZ 86341; (928) 282-4119; **www.fs.fed.us/r3/coconino/recreation/red_rock/bell-rock-pathway.shtml**

Overview

This hike circumnavigates two of the most famous rock formations around Sedona. Going counterclockwise, it uses Courthouse Butte Loop Trail to circumnavigate that rock formation, passing in and out of the Munds Mountain Wilderness in the process. A series of short trail connections leads to Bell Rock, one of the signature rock formations of Sedona. The wide, easy Bell Rock Pathway leads back to the trailhead.

Route Details

Start out from the trailhead toward Bell Rock Pathway—the way everyone else will be going. Take the first trail going right (east): the southern leg of Big Park Loop. Within sight of this junction, take the spur trail heading left (north). This doesn't have a name, but it connects the north and south legs of Big Park Loop. When you reach that north leg in 0.5 mile, turn right (east) again.

These trails wander through classic transition scrubland dominated by three different kinds of junipers. In and around the junipers, you'll find prickly pear cacti, scrub oaks, manzanitas, and occasional yuccas. This is all lovely, but the attraction is the rocks.

The smaller tower of red rock to the west is Bell Rock. From most angles you can see its namesake shape. To the east, the larger formation is Courthouse Butte. Stay straight (east) on Big Park, following the base of the butte, past a second connector spur going right (south) until, at 1.2 miles, it crosses a sizable wash. Across the wash is a caged cairn with a wooden sign. Here you turn left (north) onto Courthouse Butte Loop Trail following the wash. Big Park Loop continues its journey south across the desert.

Caged cairns mark Courthouse Butte Loop Trail as it makes its way around the east side of its namesake. At 1.5 miles, you pass the wilderness boundary, marked by a metal post warning mountain bikers of fines. Soon after, the route crosses a wash lined with sandstone. Stay left (west) to find the next cairn.

While the butte dominates the west, the tall cliffs to the east

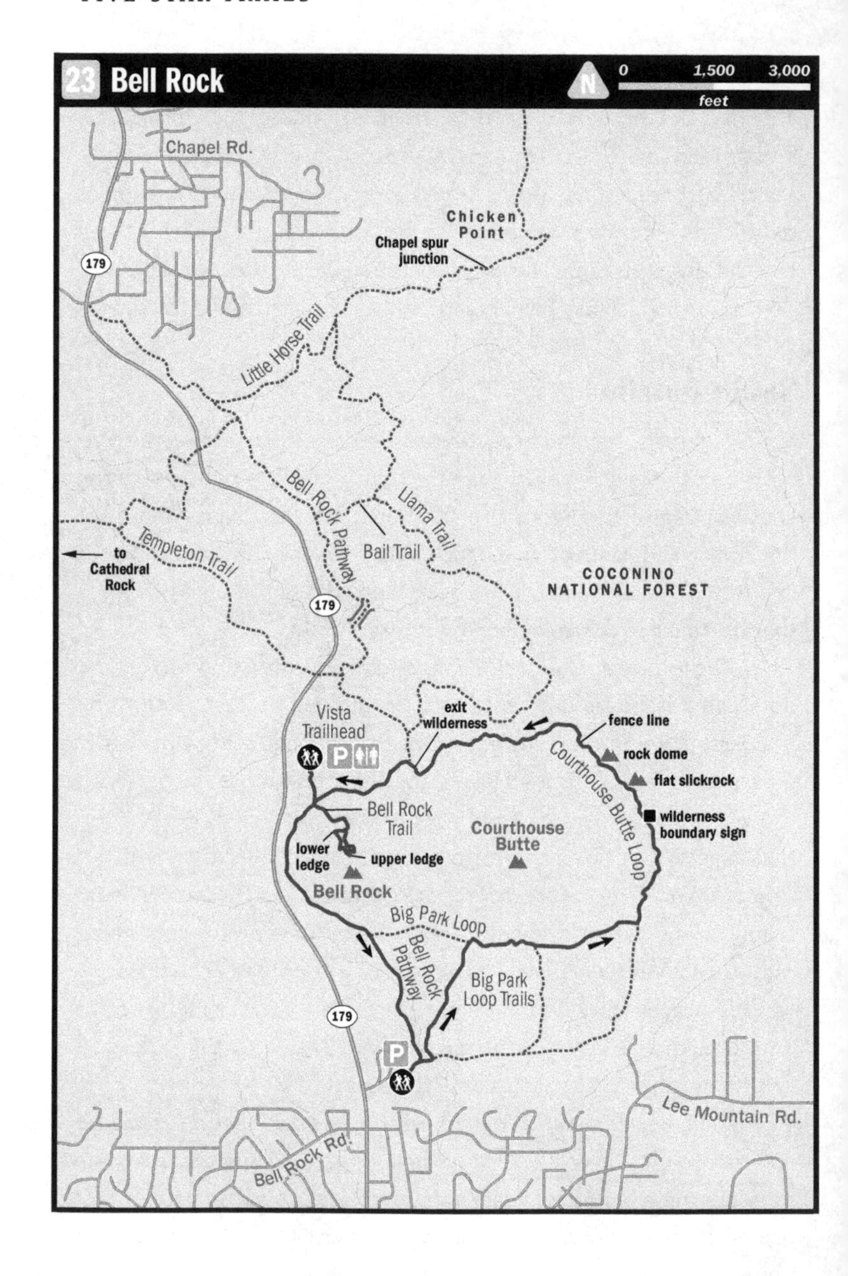
23 Bell Rock
0
1,500
3,000
feet
Chapel Rd.
179
Chicken Point
Chapel spur junction
Little Horse Trail
Bell Rock Pathway
Llama Trail
Bail Trail
Templeton Trail
to Cathedral Rock
COCONINO NATIONAL FOREST
179
exit wilderness
Vista Trailhead
fence line
rock dome
flat slickrock
wilderness boundary sign
Courthouse Butte Loop
Bell Rock Trail
Courthouse Butte
lower ledge
upper ledge
Bell Rock
Big Park Loop
Bell Rock Pathway
Big Park Loop Trails
179
Lee Mountain Rd.
Bell Rock Rd.

are part of Lee Mountain, a southern finger of the Mogollon Rim.

The next curiosity is a house-sized rock dome. The trail passes this at 1.75 miles. Then, beyond a fence line, the trail starts bending west, continuing around the butte. It will continue this way until, at 2.5 miles, the path exits the wilderness and almost immediately comes to the junction with the Llama Trail. While the Llama heads right (north), stay straight and you soon come to a second intersection, this time with Bell Rock Pathway. By now, as you continue left (east) toward Bell Rock, you will have company.

The Bell Rock formation is 500 feet of bright-orange sandstone formed from the sand of a windswept, tide-slapped beach some 280 million years ago, when Sedona looked a lot like modern-day Namibia. The top of the formation is crowned with 10 feet of limestone and dolomite, the Fort Apache Member, formed when the sea advanced to place Sedona under water. These same formations run through Courthouse Butte, though they're not as striking.

Bell Rock is also considered a major vortex: a spiral of spiritual force centered on the rock formation itself. And you can climb it.

The signs on the Pathway indicate a Big Bell Rock Trail and a Little Bell Rock Trail, but both lead to essentially the same slickrock ledge about a third of the way up the formation. Once you make your way up, you have a good view of Twin Buttes and other points north. The cairned route goes only a few hundred feet up the terraces, but

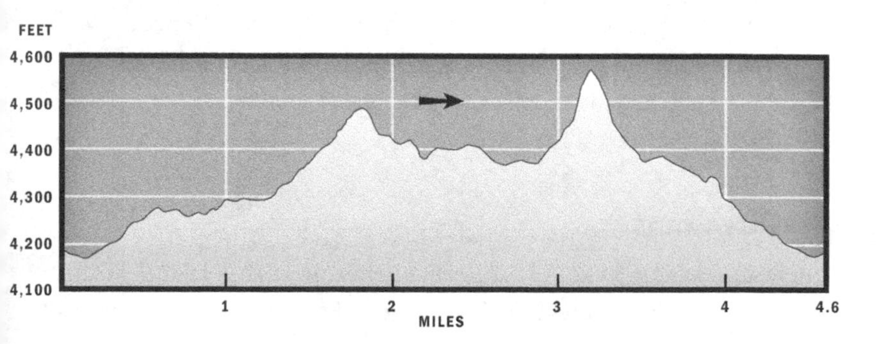

you can continue to climb as far as your skill and nerves will allow.

When you come down, Bell Rock Pathway will continue winding west, then south, around the rock, so go left. You will pass a signed junction with Big Park Loop, but keep straight. The Pathway will lead directly back to the trailhead.

Adventure option: You can combine this with the Broken Arrow Trail (see page 174) to create a memorable car-shuttle hike. The route as far as Chicken Point is shown on the map for this hike.

Once you climb down from Bell Rock, go right (north) on Bell Rock Pathway. Continue north past a spur to the Llama Trail, a spur to Bell Rock Vista Trailhead (where there are restrooms), and the junction with the Templeton Trail, which heads west across the desert, eventually reaching Cathedral Rock. At about 4.5 miles, the Pathway crosses a bridge. At 0.25 mile later, you'll see a spur trail heading right (east). Take it.

The Bail Trail, as it's called, will T with the Llama Trail within 0.5 mile. Go left (north) on the Llama until it in turn comes to a T with the Little Horse Trail 61 at around 6 miles. Turn right (northeast) on Little Horse as it angles toward Twin Buttes. You will pass a junction with the Chapel Trail, which follows the base of the buttes for 0.7 mile to the famous Chapel of the Holy Cross, but stay straight on Little Horse.

At about 7 miles, you come to Chicken Point, a series of smooth ledges lining the wash. On top of these ledges is the junction with both Broken Arrow Trail 125 and Broken Arrow Road. Either will lead you to the Broken Arrow Trailhead in about 3 miles (see page 178 for information past this point).

Directions

From Sedona, take AZ 179 south about 3 miles (past Bell Rock). The highway will divide and then rejoin. Look for the turnoff to the trailhead just past where the highway rejoins. If you reach the Village of Oak Creek, you've gone too far. There is ample parking.

24 Bell Trail

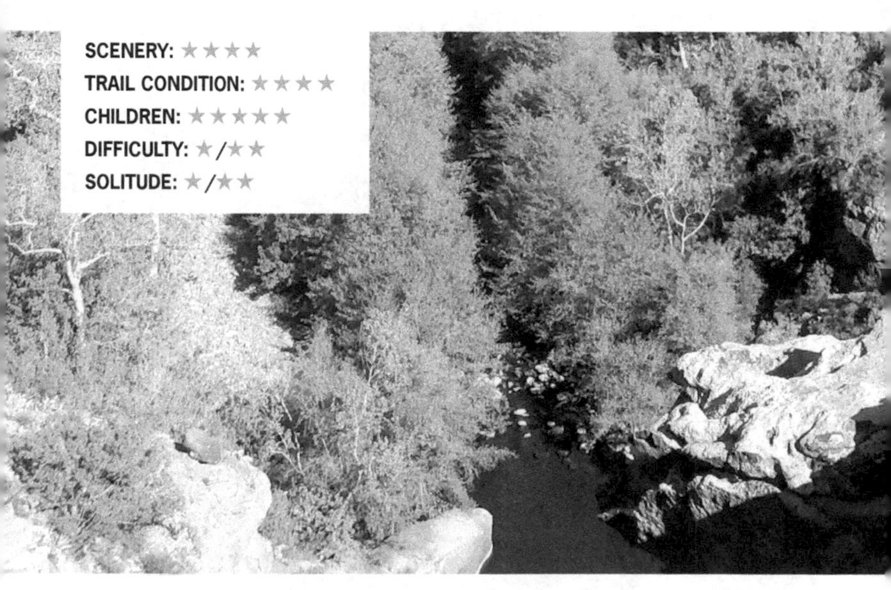

SCENERY: ★★★★
TRAIL CONDITION: ★★★★
CHILDREN: ★★★★★
DIFFICULTY: ★/★★
SOLITUDE: ★/★★

WET BEAVER CREEK FROM HIGH ON THE CANYON WALL

GPS TRAILHEAD COORDINATES: *Bell Trailhead:* N34° 40.466' W111° 42.798'

Brockett Trailhead: N34° 40.746' W111° 43.047'

DISTANCE & CONFIGURATION: 8 miles out-and-back; 5 miles out-and-back for easy version

HIKING TIME: 4 hours plus splash time for the full hike; 2.5 hours plus splash time for the easy hike

HIGHLIGHTS: Riparian glades, rock formations, swimming, and wading

ELEVATION: 3,876 feet at trailhead to 4,242 at the red cliffs to 4,125 feet at Bell Crossing

ACCESS: Requires a Red Rock Pass

MAPS: USGS Walker Mountain

FACILITIES: Restroom at trailhead

WHEELCHAIR ACCESS: None

COMMENTS: The easy version of this hike takes the Wier Trail to the swimming hole by the gauging station. The regular version goes farther into the canyon, to where the trail crosses the creek. Popular swimming hole, crowded during warm weather. Water in the creek is unsafe to drink. Poison ivy can grow close to the creek. Portions of the trail pass

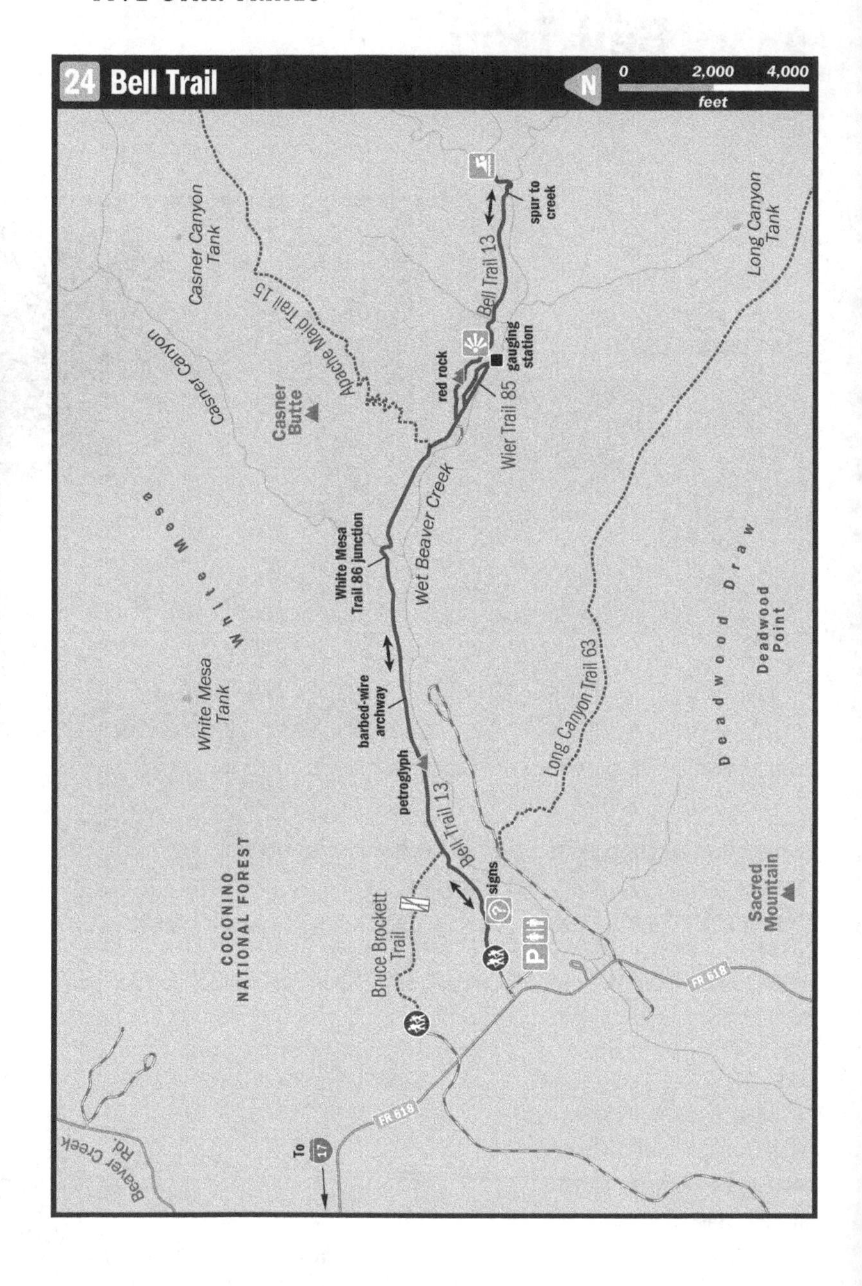
24 Bell Trail
N
0
2,000
4,000
feet
Casner Canyon Tank
Apache Maid Trail 15
Casner Canyon
Casner Butte
White Mesa
White Mesa Tank
COCONINO NATIONAL FOREST
spur to creek
Bell Trail 13
gauging station
red rock
Wier Trail 85
Wet Beaver Creek
White Mesa Trail 86 junction
barbed-wire archway
petroglyph
signs
Bruce Brockett Trail
Long Canyon Trail 63
Long Canyon Tank
Deadwood Draw
Deadwood Point
Sacred Mountain
FR 618
To 17
Beaver Creek Rd.

through private property (see "Route Details"). Do not confuse this with Bell Rock Trail (see page 162).

CONTACTS: Red Rock Ranger District, P.O. Box 20429, Sedona, AZ 86341; (928) 282-4119; **www.fs.fed.us/r3/coconino/recreation/red_rock/bell-tr.shtml**

Overview

The canyon ecosystem goes from high chaparral on the slopes to deep riparian glades along the creek. The farther you go, the fewer the people and the better the scenery. The easy hike takes Bell Trail 13 to Wier Trail 85, leading to the gauging station, swimming holes, and springs. The long hike takes Bell Trail 13 all the way up to Bell Crossing, where it finally crosses Wet Beaver Creek 4 miles up the canyon.

Route Details

Bell Trail 13 begins as a wide dirt road (indeed, it still sees some traffic from service vehicles) heading east from the trailhead into the high chaparral. Healthy stands of prickly pear cacti and a scattering of stumpy mesquite trees line the red-dirt track.

Unless it is snowing, you will have company on this road: hikers of all ages, mountain bikers, and dogs. The crowds will thin out as you walk, but it might be wise to use the restroom at the trailhead. You'll never have suitable privacy on the trail.

Shortly, the road passes through a fence line, where signs

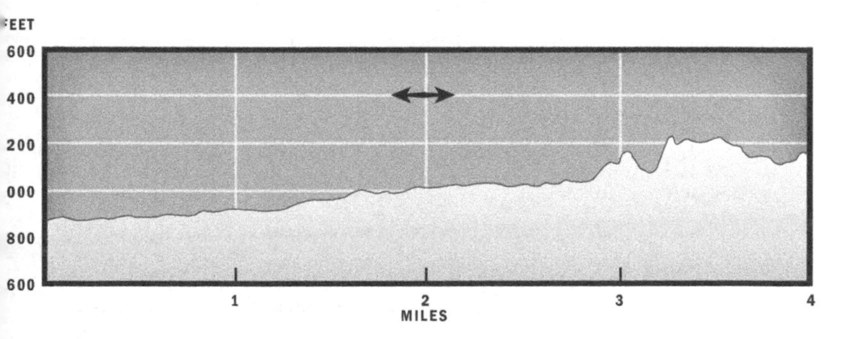

1) declare the land beyond to be private property; 2) describe the history of the Bell Trail; and 3) give distances to the junction with Apache Maid Trail 15 (2 miles) and to Bell Crossing (4 miles).

The old ranch property is now owned by Southwestern Academy, a private college-preparatory boarding school. Hikers on the Bell Trail 13 have the academy's permission to pass through—on the trail, that is. Beyond the trail, the land toward the creek (thus south) is still private property, even though this restriction, judging from the number of spur trails going to the creek, is clearly and widely ignored.

About 0.5 mile later, a pile of huge logs marks an intersection of sorts. To the right (east), a heavily used spur trail leads to the river, despite signs warning about private property. You'd be on your own with that. To your left (west), the spur trail to the Bruce Brockett Trailhead joins the Bell; it's an alternate trailhead for equestrians (see page 173).

At 0.8 mile you pass a wilderness-area boundary sign and another indicating no camping or campfires.

At 100 feet farther, look for the basalt boulder with petroglyphs. This is the work of the southern Sinaguan tribe circa 600–800 years ago, when they left such markings all over the valley they once inhabited (see "Nearby Attractions").

As you go on, a wide pasture opens between the trail and the river, crossed with inviting spur trails. These are all nicer than the trail you're on, but legally on private property. The main trail is the only legal corridor. Beyond the pasture, the tall, pointed junipers mark the location of the school campus. As you walk past it, you'll pass under a barbed-wire archway.

The climb becomes a little more noticeable as you pass several pools below the trail. Red-rock ledges line the pools on the near side, and a thicket of cottonwoods and Arizona sycamores crowds the far bank.

Soon you come to the well-marked junction with White Mesa Trail 86, which does indeed go up and over the mesa upon whose eastern flanks you have been hiking for some time. Soon after that, you come to a similarly marked junction with Apache Maid Trail 15. It goes over Casner Butte, the one on the right-hand slope to your north. Both of these trails are hard scrambles uphill to reach isolated cattle tanks, and of little interest to recreational hikers. In both cases, the sign-in stations are for those using these trails. The sign-in for the Bell Trail 13 is yet to come.

Less than 0.25 mile past that junction, you come to the Y-junction where Wier Trail 85 splits off to the south of the Bell Trail 13. This, too, is marked with numerous signs and another sign-in log for those continuing on the Bell Trail 13. This is also a more accurate marking of the wilderness boundary, and the turnaround point for any mountain bikes.

The Wier Trail 85 continues a short distance farther to a gauging station, which monitors the river's flow between a deep swimming hole downstream and a spring-fed wading pool upstream. Here, all manner of trees—ash, cottonwoods, sycamores, willows, and Arizona walnuts—line the banks of Wet Beaver Creek. Wild grape chokes the spring on the far side. Look out also for poison ivy, which you may see along the banks. Nothing prevents you from playing around on the gauging-station platform except good manners and common sense. This is the turnaround for the easy hike.

If you're going onward, sign the logbook and begin the climb—a real climb now—farther up the Bell Trail 13. This ascent, steep but short, takes you to the base of the towering red-rock formation you've been staring at for the past 2 miles, and you spend another 0.25 mile walking around its edge. This is an exposed section of Supai sandstone, the remnant of an ancient seabed deposited more than 250 million years ago. About 200 feet below, you'll see the gauging station. About 200 feet above, you see the top of Casner Butte. Beyond for several miles you see the rest of the canyon, where Wet Beaver Creek flows through a wall of broad-leafed trees.

Past the red rocks, the trail flattens out a bit, content to let the river rise up to it as it follows the edge of the butte through stunted junipers and expansive prickly pear cacti. At just over 3.5 miles, the trail turns to switchback down a hundred feet or so to the creek. Wet Beaver Creek still drains through cattle country, so don't drink the water. And again, watch out for poison ivy.

Bell Trail 13 crosses the creek about a hundred feet downstream, to continue steeply up the mesa. You would be on your own with that.

Go back up the switchback and follow the (unofficial) trail farther up the canyon (roughly north). Within 0.1 mile you will come to a larger swimming hole lined with huge red-rock formations. The local kids like to dive off these rocks, even though the depth below the opaque green water varies from as little as 5 to as much as 20 feet. You're better off finding your way down to the gravelly bank just downstream and slipping quietly in.

When you have satisfied your curiosity and sufficiently lowered your body temperature, return the way you came.

Nearby Attractions

The V-V Ranch heritage site, just down the forest road from the Bell Trailhead, showcases the remains of the original Bruce Brockett homestead. More important, it is the location of a cliff face where the Sinaguan people carved an intricate series of petroglyphs over and around those left by earlier peoples. The towering chimney is all that stands from the old Brockett place, but by following the easy (wheelchair grade) 1.5-mile trail, you reach the petroglyph site. It is astonishingly well preserved, largely because Brockett did not approve of vandals. A ranger will interpret the symbols for you according to the most recent theories regarding their meaning. Access to the site requires a Red Rock Pass, and the visitor center sells all sorts of things, including bottled water and a ranch guidebook.

Directions

The Bell Trail 13 can be found about 2 miles east of I-17 on FR 618. Take I-17 to its junction with AZ 179, Exit 298. At that junction, turn right (west) onto the dirt road instead of east onto the state highway.

Head east; then, on FR 618, you'll cross a bridge, then come to a four-way stop before you pass the turnoff for the Brockett Trailhead (see below) just before reaching the Bell Trailhead, the right turn next to the U.S. Forest Service work center. If you reach Wet Beaver Creek Campground, you've gone too far.

Alternate access, Bruce Brockett Trailhead: The turnoff for this trailhead comes 0.25 mile before the Bell Trailhead. Besides an expansive parking lot (suitable for maneuvering horse trailers), a corral, and a vault toilet, you'll also find a sign extolling Mr. Brockett, the longtime rancher for whom the trailhead is named. Brockett Trail starts at the eastern edge of the trailhead, next to the chain-link gate guarding the water-reclamation tank, and continues up the hill, through a gate at the top of the saddle, and down again to join the Bell Trail 13 less than a mile from the main trailhead, making it a slightly shorter and far less crowded alternative.

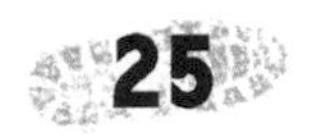

25 Broken Arrow

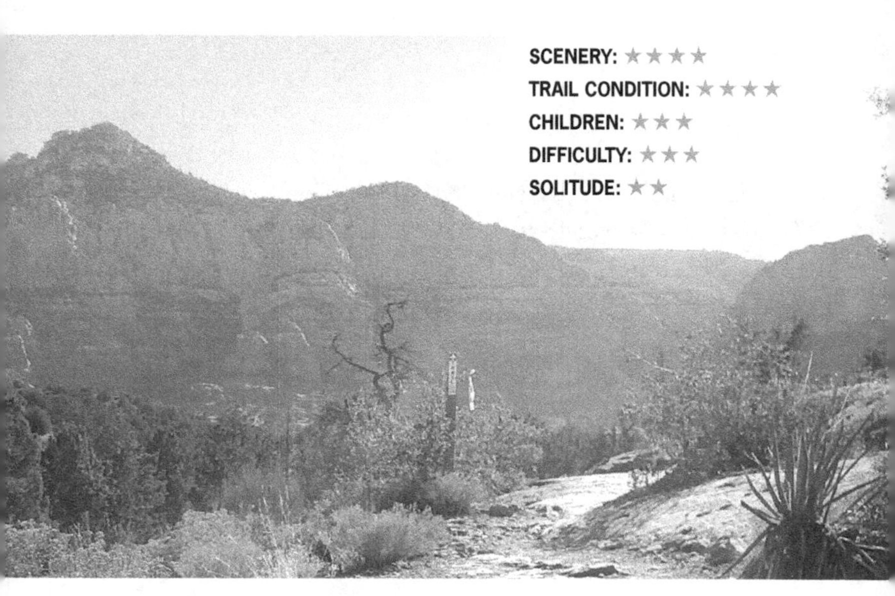

SCENERY: ★★★★
TRAIL CONDITION: ★★★★
CHILDREN: ★★★
DIFFICULTY: ★★★
SOLITUDE: ★★

TRAIL MARKER FOR BROKEN ARROW

GPS TRAILHEAD COORDINATES: N34° 50.727' W111° 45.409'

DISTANCE & CONFIGURATION: 4 miles for basic hike; 6 miles with spur to Submarine Rock; adventure option (see page 178) is 10-mile car shuttle

HIKING TIME: 2–3 hours; 5–6 hours for adventure option

HIGHLIGHTS: Scenic views, sinkhole, and rock formations

ELEVATION: 4,278 feet at trailhead to 4,674 feet about 0.5 mile north of Chicken Point

ACCESS: Requires a Red Rock Pass

MAPS: USGS Sedona

FACILITIES: None

WHEELCHAIR ACCESS: None

COMMENTS: Parts of the trail, popular with mountain bikers, intersect with a jeep road. Almost no shade; this will be a hot hike during the summer. No water available. Can be combined with Bell Rock as a car shuttle; see notes following "Route Details."

CONTACTS: Red Rock Ranger District, P.O. Box 20429, Sedona, AZ 86341; (928) 282-4119; **www.fs.fed.us/r3/coconino/recreation/red_rock/broken-arrow-tr.shtml**

Overview

This short, easy hike follows the east base of the Twin Buttes formation, wandering through the low junipers to pass several well-known geologic oddities, including a sinkhole, the distinctive Submarine Rock, and the scenic vistas from Chicken Point.

Route Details

From the trailhead, cross the road near the big sign, following Broken Arrow Trail 125 west. A sign-in log is within sight of the road. Soon after, the rocky path turns south.

The trail meanders across the orange rocks and around the low junipers, following cairns and fiberglass signs. It is most evident, however, from bicycle tracks, as this path is heavily used by mountain bikers. On a weekend with good weather, you've already encountered a few by this point.

A low slickrock hill rises to the west, while across the canyon to the east, Munds Mountain, a southern finger of the Mogollon Rim, towers more impressively. Ahead, the trail goes toward the Twin Buttes, two neighboring structures that seem to mirror each other from certain angles. Before you get there, though, at 0.5 mile, the trail turns abruptly east. Look for the cairn across the sandstone wash (complete with pools if there's been any rain). Do not be fooled by the bike tracks continuing south.

The turn starts a short, sharp descent down to Devil's Dining Room, a 30-foot-wide sinkhole going down 60–90 feet. It's hard to see the bottom because of the fence surrounding it, but you can hear your voice echo on the sheer stone walls. The sinkhole is also adjacent to the jeep trail, and there is a pullout for jeeps to park. You can expect company here. As a sign explains, the sinkhole is a collapsed cavern formed when water hollowed out the red-wall limestone beneath the ground here. It is also a bat habitat.

The trail continues south from the sinkhole, wandering over ridges toward the Twin Buttes. Just shy of 1 mile, the trail splits in

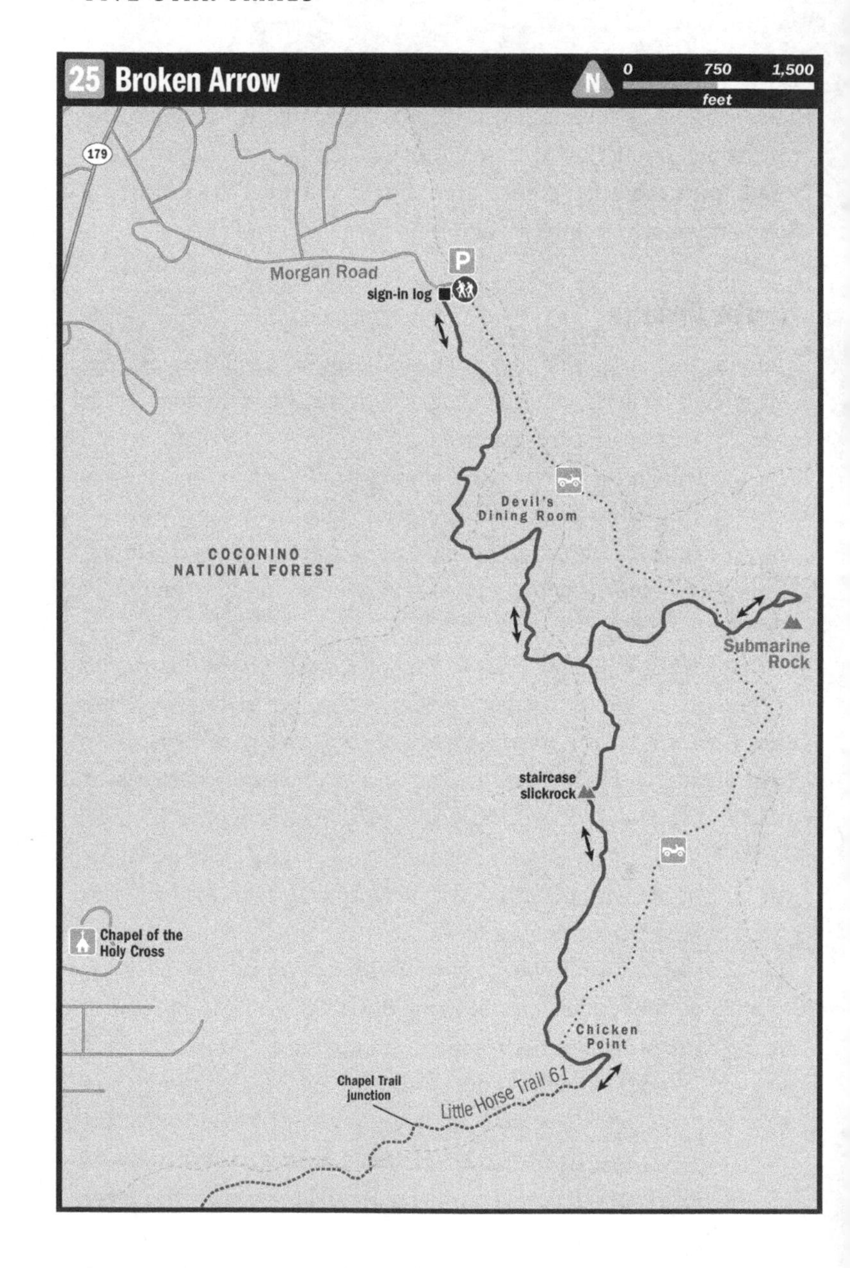
25 Broken Arrow
N
0
750
1,500
feet
179
Morgan Road
sign-in log
Devil's
Dining Room
COCONINO
NATIONAL FOREST
Submarine
Rock
staircase
slickrock
Chapel of the
Holy Cross
Chicken
Point
Chapel Trail
junction
Little Horse Trail 61

a Y. To the left (east), a spur goes to Submarine Rock, while straight and right (south), Broken Arrow continues on.

The spur to Submarine Rock is optional but worth it, either on the way in or on the way back. The spur to the formation, about 1 mile round-trip, will take 30 minutes or so to complete, depending on how long you dawdle on the rock.

SUBMARINE ROCK: Go left (east) at the Y. The trail proceeds down the ridge, across a wash lined with slickrock, and then up and around a hill to the road. This jeep road is also called Broken Arrow. It is strictly a four-wheel-drive route, with most of its traffic coming from commercial jeep tours. The trail continues directly across the road, where it drops into a deep wash. On the far side of the wash, you wind through a hundred feet of junipers before coming to the northern tip of Submarine Rock.

Submarine Rock is a long pile of terraced, orange sandstone that from a distance indeed looks more like a submarine than, say, a cow pie. You can climb it, of course. There is no particular route up, but the climb is not particularly challenging from most angles. A thin trail circumnavigates the formation as well. The junipers on the far side may be the only reliable shade on the entire hike.

On the south side is a pullout for jeep parking, so jeep tourists climb about like ants on a hill. When you have satisfied your curiosity, return to Broken Arrow Trail 125.

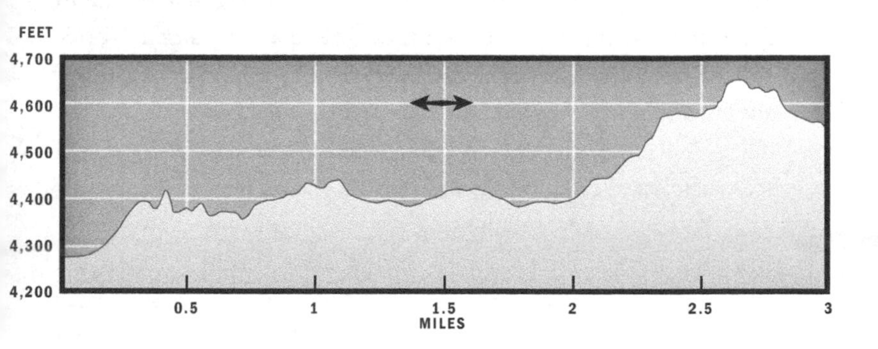

SOUTH TO CHICKEN POINT: From the Submarine Rock Y, continue south on Broken Arrow Trail 125. In about 0.25 mile, the trail emerges from the chaparral to cross a slickrock shelf the size of a soccer field. Two spurs from the jeep trail lead here, the easy one coming up the hill and the technical one going down called the "staircase." As a result, the rock is scarred with tire marks. Look for the caged cairn on the upslope corner of the formation on the other side.

Beyond the staircase slickrock, Broken Arrow cuts an easy, if rocky, path along the base of the buttes, gently climbing as it does so. After just over 0.5 mile from the staircase rock, or just under 2 miles from the trailhead (not including the Submarine Rock spur), you come to a slickrock shelf at the southeast corner of the butte: Chicken Point. From here you can see two sandstone pillars to the immediate west, called the Sisters or the Nuns. Looking farther out, you can view Bell Rock and Courthouse Butte prominently in the distance, the Seven Sisters formation across the highway to the west, and beyond, the Village of Oak Creek.

The Broken Arrow jeep trail also terminates on this rock shelf. Nearby, following the caged cairns across the wash, you find the trail continues as Little Horse Trail 61. This is the turnaround, though, for this hike. Return the way you came.

Adventure options: On the east side of the wash at Chicken Point, an informal cairned path called the Jim Bryant Trail continues east into the Munds Mountain Wilderness Area. This is not a maintained U.S. Forest Service trail, so while it can be easily followed by keeping an eye out for cairns, it can be a rough route, going steeply up and down the ridges. It continues for at least 0.5 mile to the boundary and then 0.5 mile past that, though it becomes thinner and rougher as it goes.

You can also extend this hike as a car shuttle down to Bell Rock. That full route covers 10 miles (including the entirety of Broken Arrow) and would take 5–6 hours.

Continue south on Little Horse Trail 61, past the stone pillars called the Nuns, and past the junction with the Chapel Trail, which leads to the Chapel of the Holy Cross. Turn left (south) at the junction with the Llama Trail, and then turn right (west) at its junction with the Bail Trail. The Bail Trail soon comes to a T with Bell Rock Pathway, where you want to continue left (south) toward Bell Rock.

The entry on Bell Rock (see page 162) has more details and a map of this connecting hike, so refer to that hike profile to continue.

Directions

From the Y in Sedona, go south on AZ 179 for 1.4 miles to the roundabout with Morgan Road. Take Morgan Road east for 0.5 mile, where the pavement ends. Continue on the beginning of the rough jeep road (a passenger car can get through it with care) about a hundred yards to the trailhead on the left side. The driveway into the trailhead is about a hundred feet and strictly one lane. Be certain that it is empty before turning, or there will be drama. No services. Parking here requires a Red Rock Pass.

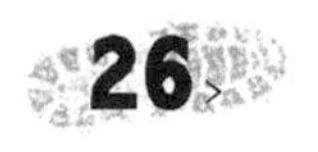

Cathedral Rock

SCENERY: ★★★★★
TRAIL CONDITION: ★★★★
CHILDREN: ★★★
DIFFICULTY: ★/★★★ *(Baldwin and Templeton/Cathedral Rock)*
SOLITUDE: ★

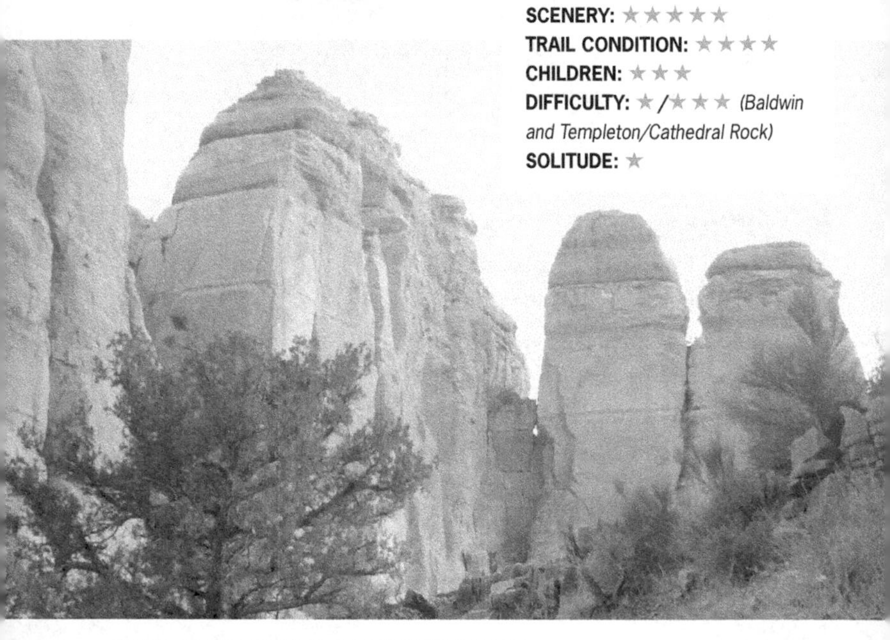

TOWERS NEAR THE TOP OF CATHEDRAL ROCK

GPS TRAILHEAD COORDINATES: *Baldwin Trailhead:* N34° 49.322' W111° 48.436'
Cathedral Rock Trailhead: N34° 49.508' W111° 47.309'

DISTANCE & CONFIGURATION: 3.6 miles out-and-back

HIKING TIME: 3 hours

HIGHLIGHTS: Scenic views, rock formations, riparian groves, seasonal swimming holes, and vortex site

ELEVATION: 3,992 feet at creek access to 4,660 feet at the saddle

ACCESS: Red Rock Pass required for either trailhead

MAPS: USGS Sedona

FACILITIES: None

WHEELCHAIR ACCESS: None

COMMENTS: Bring your own drinking water.

CONTACTS: Red Rock Ranger District, P.O. Box 20429, Sedona, AZ 86341; (928) 282-4119; **www.fs.fed.us/r3/coconino/recreation/red_rock/templeton-baldwin-trs.shtml**

Overview

This route is wildly popular because it combines the best of Sedona in a compact, accessible package. The hike drops to the banks of Oak Creek before climbing through classic red-rock desert to wind up Cathedral Rock, one of the signature rock formations of Sedona. Near a vortex site, it is one of the most visited and photographed locations in Sedona.

Route Details

From the Baldwin Trailhead go left (roughly northeast), following the wider dirt path. The path to the right (south) is the other side of the Baldwin Loop, and not part of this hike. The trail crosses a wash before descending into the main drainage of Oak Creek, where the creek bends westward south of Sedona.

Once down on the bank, you soon come to a T-intersection in a wide, grassy clearing. To your right (east), Baldwin continues toward Cathedral Rock. To the left (west), a social trail follows the north side of the shallow canyon to join Oak Creek at Baldwin Crossing. This popular swimming hole and access site is across the creek from the Crescent Moon Recreation Area. Go right (east). As you cross the canyon, a number of spur trails go north through the grass to the creek.

As the walls of the canyon push in, you come to a second T. To the right (south), Baldwin Loop climbs a ravine to circle the rock formations back to the trailhead. Straight ahead, Templeton Trail continues east toward Cathedral Rock. Continue east on Templeton.

The trail goes up and down the rocky slope, winding through boulders and trees (mostly junipers and Arizona walnuts) before descending to Oak Creek. You arrive at the first of two good swimming holes separated by a small rapid.

Sources conflict, or are simply unclear, regarding whether the vortex is centered on the rock formation or on this bend in the creek. Most agree, however, that the energies are strong enough to feel

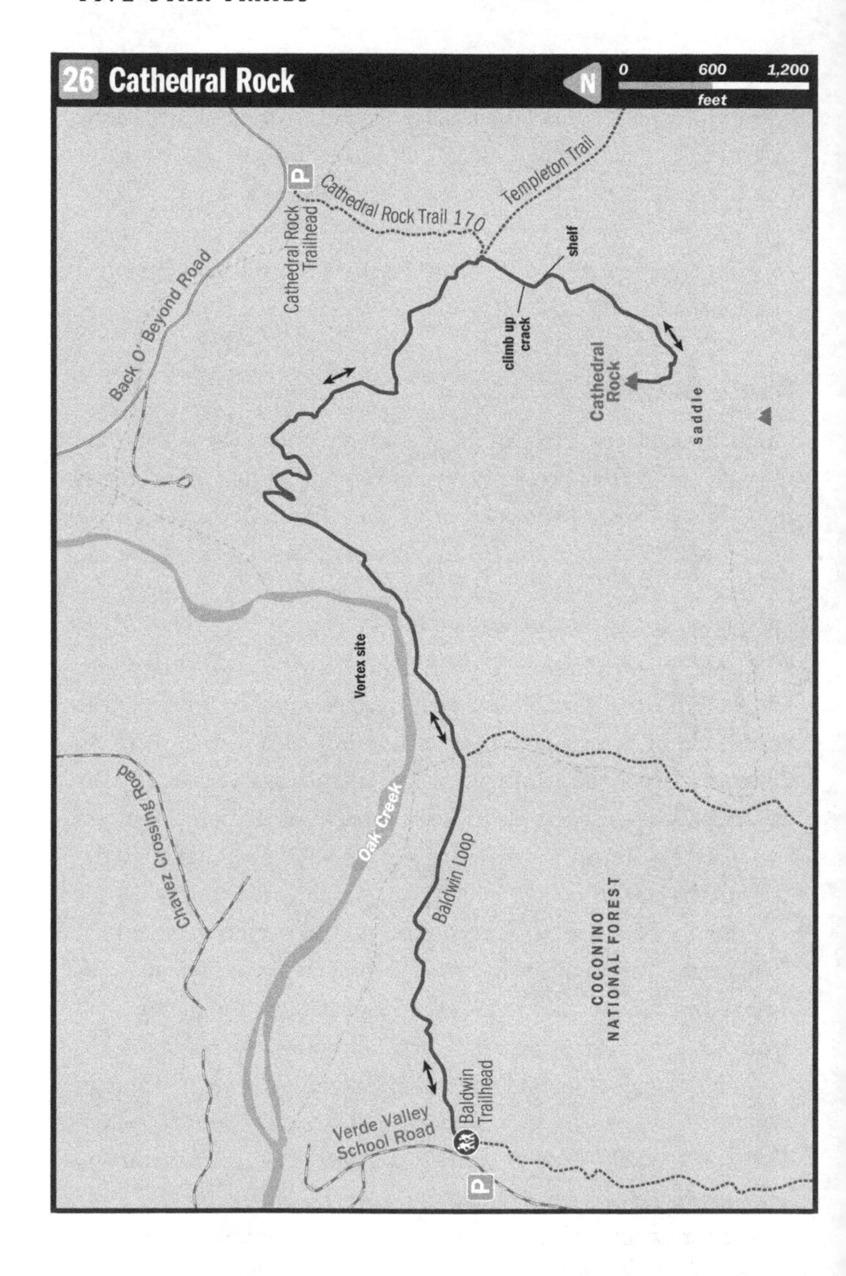
26 Cathedral Rock
N
0 600 1,200
feet
Templeton Trail
Cathedral Rock Trail 170
Cathedral Rock Trailhead
Back O' Beyond Road
shelf
climb up crack
Cathedral Rock
saddle
Vortex site
Chavez Crossing Road
Oak Creek
Baldwin Loop
COCONINO NATIONAL FOREST
Verde Valley School Road
Baldwin Trailhead
P

from Crescent Moon, so you would presumably be in the midst of the vortex from here on out.

Past the second swimming hole, the trail enters a deep and varied riparian forest. Wild grapes grow around towering cottonwoods and sycamores. The sandy track continues through the deep shade until the 0.8-mile mark.

Switchbacks begin leading you up and out of the canyon. Within 0.25 mile, you will find yourself standing in the transition desert, staring down at the trees you were recently staring up at. A private-property fence marks the end of the switchbacks. Now Templeton Trail winds southeast, around the base of Cathedral Rock. Keep an eye out for prickly pear cacti, century plant agaves, and ocotillos, as fine specimens grow along these slopes. This is what Sedona is supposed to look like.

The trail winds loosely southwest around the slopes of Cathedral Rock for 0.4 mile until it intersects with the Cathedral Rock Trail 170, marked by a sign and large, caged cairns. To the right (south), the path goes up into the rock formation. To the left (north) is an 0.5-mile spur to the Cathedral Rock Trailhead. Go right up the steep stairs of sandstone.

Note: If all you want to do is climb the rock formation, you could make a much shorter hike (about 2.5 miles round-trip) by starting at the Cathedral Rock Trailhead, about 0.33 mile north from this junction.

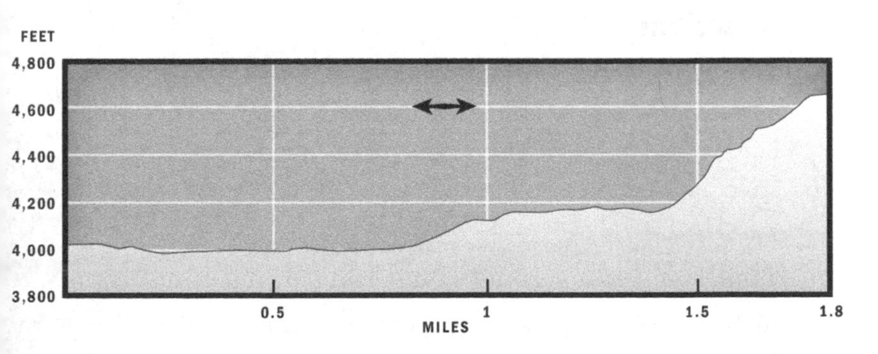

The U.S. Forest Service is trying to revegetate this area, so it is important to stay on the trail, even if it's just a series of cairns leading up the slickrock. A lattice of microorganisms holds this desert soil together, and it does not respond well to boot prints.

In about 500 feet, you come to the crack, the longer of only two rock scrambles on this hike. Someone has chiseled some footholds, which are convenient for going up and vital when coming down. At the top of this, you will reach a shelf with postcard-quality views of the rock formations southeast of Sedona. Seriously, every gift shop in Sedona has a postcard with a photo taken from, at, or near this shelf.

Another short but steep scramble up slickrock follows. Then the trail cuts left, following the ridge to next little climb. While the remaining rock scrambles are easier after this, the pattern will repeat several times until the final climb to the saddle.

At 4,660 feet, the saddle is the end of the hike. This bridge of sandstone separates canyons to the north and south and two towering stone prominences to the east and west. Social trails go off to either side for further exploration. To the west, if you squeeze through the prickly pears, you can pick your way to a ledge affording vistas to the south. Following the trail east, you can explore the spaces between the stone spires. When you have satisfied your curiosity, return the way you came.

Directions

To Baldwin Trailhead: From Sedona, go south on AZ 179 about 6 miles to the Village of Oak Creek. Turn west on Verde Valley School Road (one of the roundabouts) and continue another 4 miles to the trailhead. The road will become graded dirt for the last mile. Some older U.S. Forest Service publications warn of no parking, but there is now a bare-dirt parking lot across the road from the trailhead.

To Cathedral Rock Trailhead: In Sedona, take AZ 179 south to Back O' Beyond Road. Go west from the roundabout for about 2 miles. The trailhead is a small parking area on the left.

27 Woods Canyon Trail

SCENERY: ★★★★ (★★★ *if dry*)
TRAIL CONDITION: ★★★★
CHILDREN: ★★★★/★★★
DIFFICULTY: ★★/★★★
SOLITUDE: ★★★/★★★★

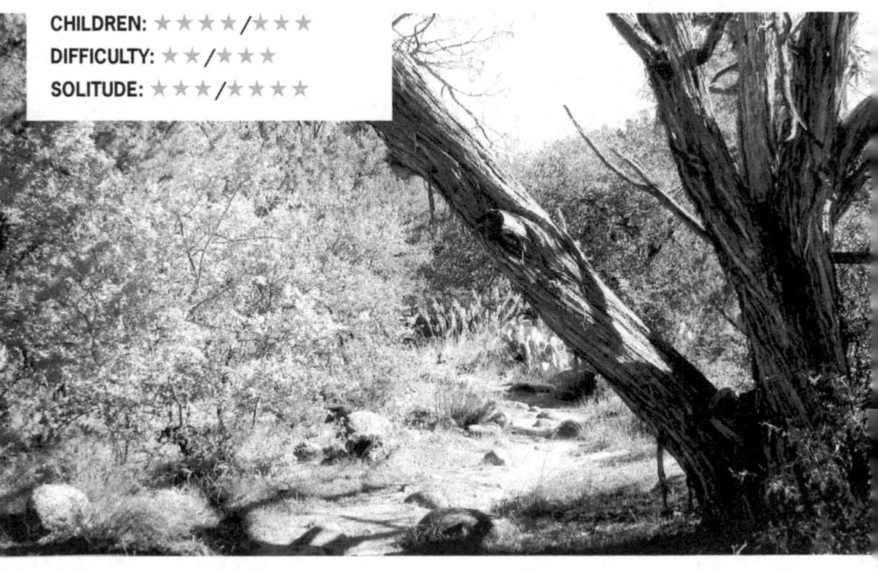

BRUSH CLOSING IN ON THE TRAIL

GPS TRAILHEAD COORDINATES: N34° 45.368' W111° 45.801'

DISTANCE & CONFIGURATION: 10.8 miles out-and-back; easy option is 5.6 miles out-and-back; medium option is 7.5 miles out-and-back

HIKING TIME: 5.5 hours for the full hike; 3 hours for the easy hike; 4 hours for the medium hike

HIGHLIGHTS: Riparian habitat, birds, geology, and seasonal swimming holes

ELEVATION: 3,937 feet at trailhead to 4,307 feet at trail's end

ACCESS: No fees or restrictions

MAPS: USGS Munds Mountain and Sedona

FACILITIES: No official services here, but the visitor center has restrooms, water, trash cans, and vending machines.

WHEELCHAIR ACCESS: None

COMMENTS: This hike has easy and medium-length alternatives. Best in spring or after recent rains, when Dry Beaver Creek is actually running.

CONTACTS: Red Rock Ranger District, P.O. Box 20249, Sedona, AZ 86341; (928) 282-4119; **www.fs.fed.us/r3/coconino/recreation/red_rock/woods-canyn-tr.shtml**

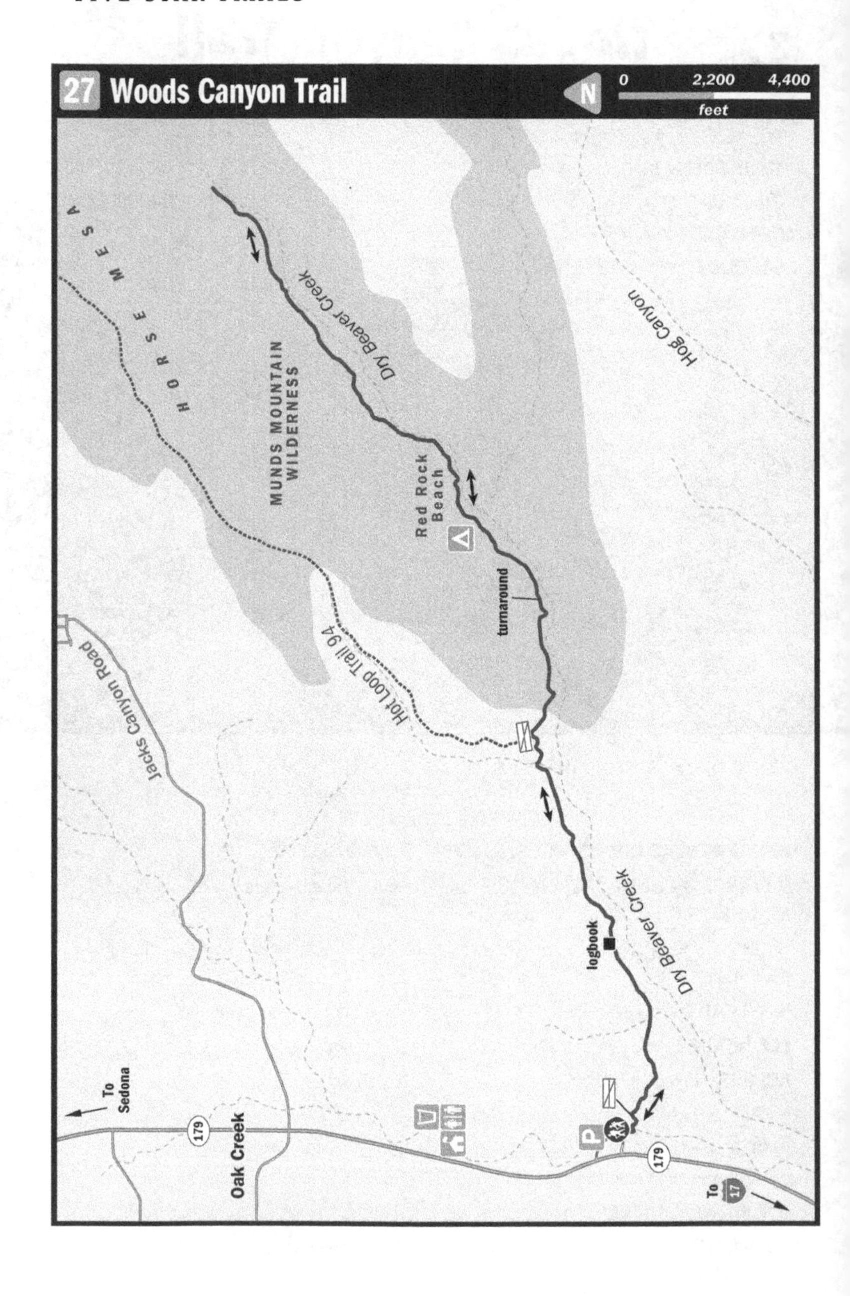
27 Woods Canyon Trail
N
0
2,200
4,400
feet
HORSE MESA
MUNDS MOUNTAIN WILDERNESS
Dry Beaver Creek
Hog Canyon
Red Rock Beach
turnaround
Hot Loop Trail 94
Jacks Canyon Road
logbook
Dry Beaver Creek
To Sedona
179
Oak Creek
179
To 17

Overview

This is a relatively easy hike into a pretty but often overlooked canyon. In early spring or after recent rains (but not during the rain due to flash-flood dangers), you can find substantial swimming holes. In midsummer, this route is too dry and hot to be considered a five-star experience.

Route Details

Woods Canyon Trail 93 begins in the corner of the parking lot, where the sidewalk ends. Take the dirt path downhill into the grass, not uphill (to the storage lot). Some cut-metal signs will guide you.

The trail winds into and through the Jacks Canyon Exclosure Area. Yes, ***exclosure*** is a real word, and it means, in this context, no vehicles allowed. The area includes the riparian strip the trail passes through immediately beyond the parking lot. Little trails riddle the exclosure, so look for the official route bending to the south before crossing the normally dry creek bed.

Past the exclosure, the trail climbs the sandy hills and continues through a gate that you must open and close. A sign warns that the Jacks Canyon and Hot Loop trails are not casual day hikes. Don't worry about that; this hike is far easier. Past the gate you quickly cross a wash, and then follow the remnant jeep trail up

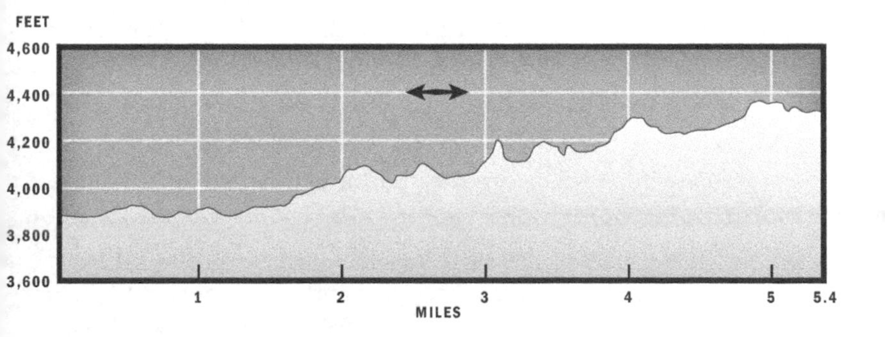

toward the mouth of the canyon. Junipers, acacias, and pines poke through the red dirt until grass replaces it as you enter the wide mouth of the canyon proper.

At just past 1 mile in, you come to the logbook, which you should sign. Past this, the trail crosses Dry Beaver Creek several times, winding beneath the birds pursuing their busy agendas among the juniper branches. Most of the year, this creek lives up to its name, and even in wetter times it may still be dry this far down the hill. As the trail winds through the wash, alternating between singletrack and boulder-strewn drainage, bigger trees, mostly cottonwoods, provide more substantial shade.

The trail starts climbing the bluff to the north at 1.8 miles, following the red canyon walls. Hummingbirds might be dashing around the agave cacti and smokethorn paloverde trees on top of the rim. At 2.2 miles, a gate marks the official wilderness boundary. Soon thereafter you come to the junction with Hot Loop Trail 94, which heads off on a long journey up Horse Mesa to the north. Stay right (east). The trail descends from the bluff to follow a broad shelf lined with paintbrush bushes, manzanitas, and prickly pear cacti. After 0.5 mile of this, the trail climbs another bluff and then crosses another shelf. This pattern will repeat for most of the hike.

Before it climbs, though, the route curves into a drainage lined with red sandstone and decorated with agaves. This is as pretty a spot as you're going to find in the lower canyon; it's the halfway marker for the full hike and the turnaround for the easy hike. The remaining hike, though, is not much more difficult.

On the second bluff, you'll pass a campsite at 3.25 miles. The climb up the next bluff is thin, rough, and often clogged with boulders. The red cliffs begin to close in as you pass the confluence with Rattlesnake Canyon.

Just past that confluence, you'll find a broad shelf of ochre rock lining a wide swimming hole (if water is present at all). This is Red Rock Beach, and the turnaround for the medium hike. A tumble of boulders blocks the east end of this shelf; you will have to climb over or around these rocks before reaching the skinny goat trail that continues up the canyon.

Take note that the trail will remain on the north wall of Woods Canyon for the remainder of the hike.

Large basalt boulders, some the size of cars, decorate the shelf past Red Rock Beach. Beyond this shelf the trail climbs again, nearly to the top of the canyon, leveling out along the Supai sandstone–basalt cap boundary before dropping down into a shelf blanketed with prickly cat's-claw. From this shelf, you drop down into a glade filled with grass, pine trees, and several dozen deer trails. Stay to your left (the north side of the wash) and look for cairns.

Past the glade you begin a long climb, plowing through a dense thicket composed of every single type of plant you have seen so far on the journey. (The trail itself is actually pretty clear.) Past this thicket, the trail drops down toward Dry Beaver Creek once more. If any water has run, you may pass a series of wide swimming holes, or perhaps just depressions filled with gravel. Past these, at 5.4 miles, the trail empties into the boulder highway of Dry Beaver Creek. A single large red boulder the size of a garden shed stands in the middle of the wash, signaling that this is the end of the trail. Return the way you came.

Directions

The Red Rock Ranger District Visitor Center is on AZ 179 about 9 miles south of Sedona. The trailhead is at the southwest corner of the administrative parking lot—the building and lot south of the visitor center.

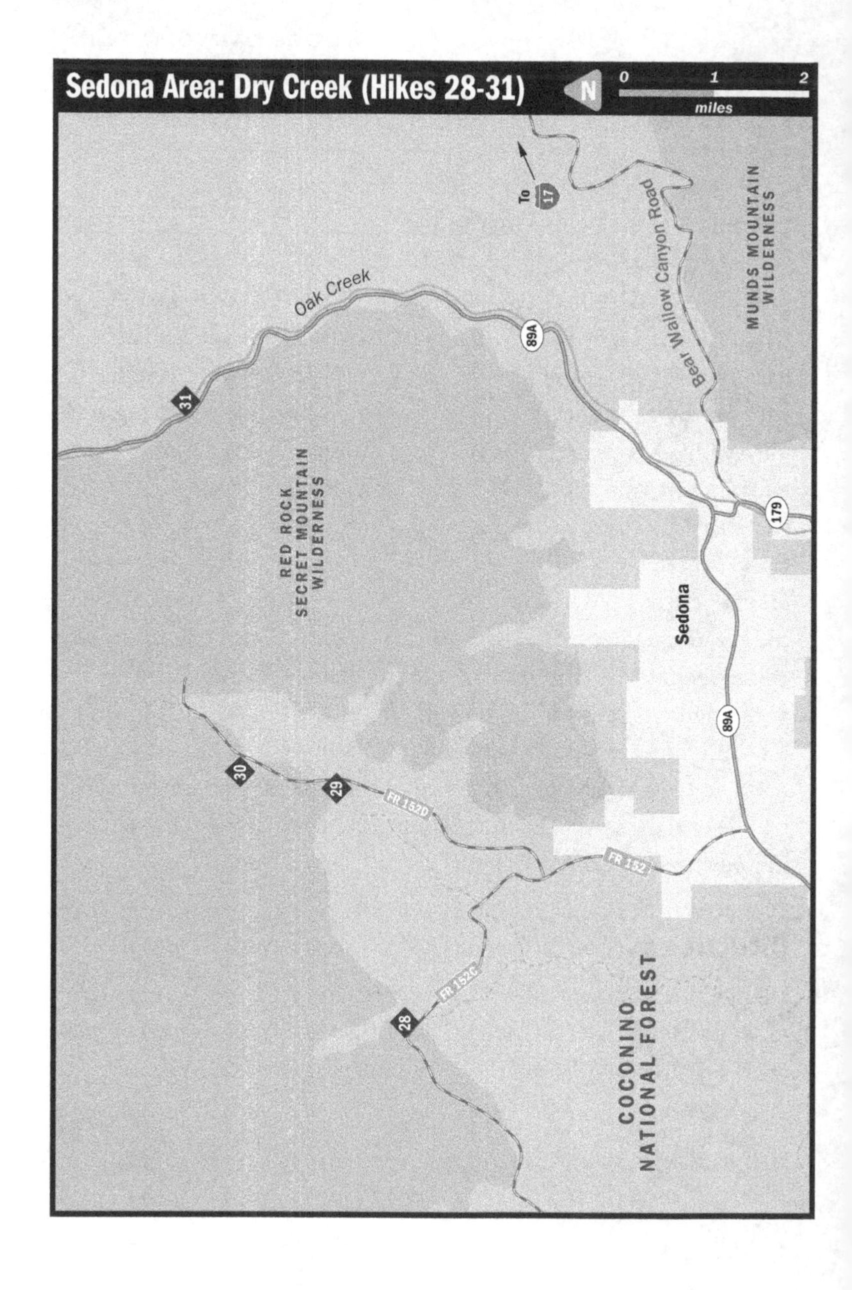

Sedona Area: Dry Creek (Hikes 28-31)
N
0
1
2
miles
To
17
Oak Creek
89A
Bear Wallow Canyon Road
MUNDS MOUNTAIN
WILDERNESS
31
RED ROCK
SECRET MOUNTAIN
WILDERNESS
179
Sedona
89A
30
29
FR 152D
FR 152
FR 152C
28
COCONINO
NATIONAL FOREST

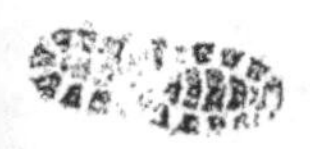

Sedona Area: Dry Creek

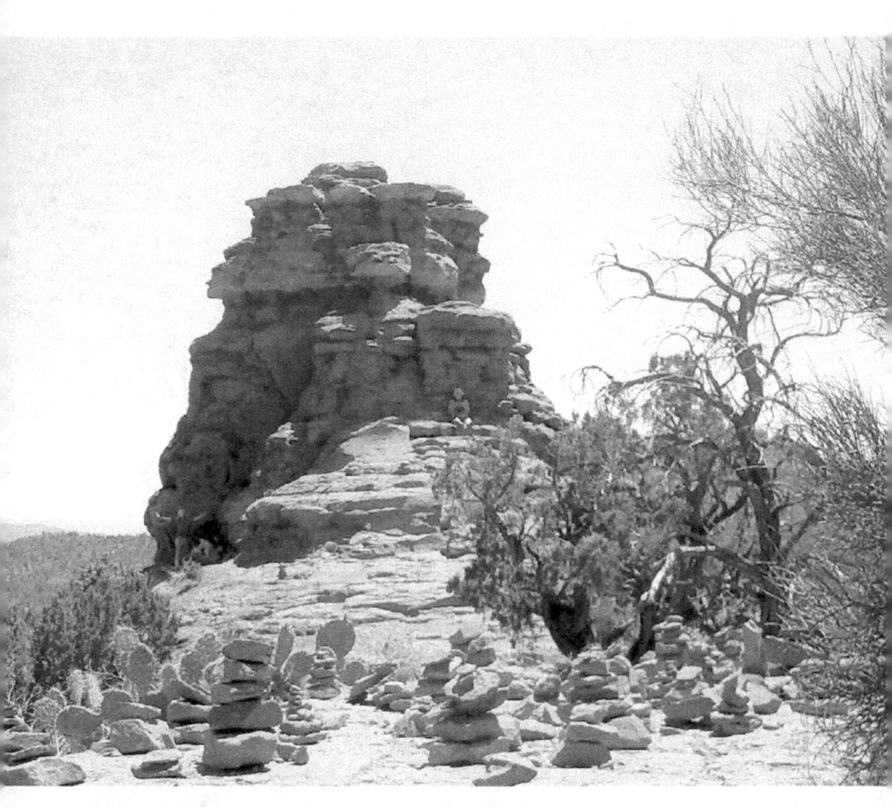

KACHINA WOMAN AND CAIRNS NEAR BOYNTON CANYON

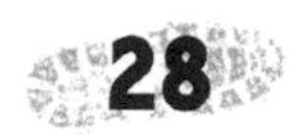

28 Boynton Canyon Trail

SCENERY: ★★★★
TRAIL CONDITION: ★★★★
CHILDREN: ★★★★★/★★★
DIFFICULTY: ★/★★★
SOLITUDE: ★

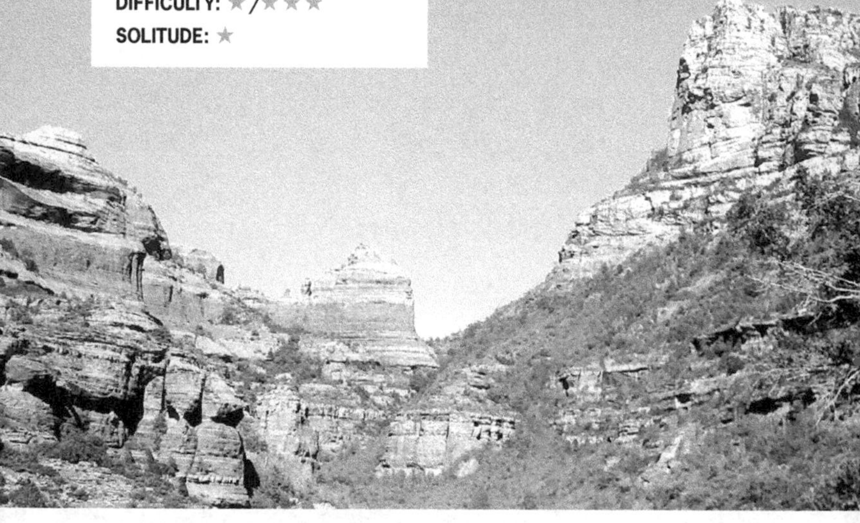

CLIFFS CLOSING IN ON UPPER BOYNTON CANYON

GPS TRAILHEAD COORDINATES: N34° 32.667' W111° 30.551'

DISTANCE & CONFIGURATION: 7 miles out-and-back; easy hike is 5.7 miles out-and-back

HIKING TIME: 3 hours for full hike; 2 hours for easy hike

HIGHLIGHTS: Vortex site, red-rock geology, scenic vistas, stand of ponderosa pines, Sinaguan ruins off-trail, and waterfall in season

ELEVATION: 4,525 feet at trailhead to 4,800 feet at the easy terminus or 5,200 feet at the top of the canyon

ACCESS: Requires a Red Rock Pass

MAPS: USGS Wilson Mountain and Loy Butte

FACILITIES: Vault toilets

WHEELCHAIR ACCESS: None

COMMENTS: You will pass, but do not try to park at or enter, the private Enchantment Resort. No water is available on this trail.

CONTACTS: Red Rock Ranger District, P.O. Box 20429, Sedona, AZ 86341; (928) 282-4119; **www.fs.fed.us/r3/coconino/recreation/red_rock/boynton-tr.shtml**

Overview

Boynton Canyon Trail 47 combines every virtue of hiking in Sedona into a single trail. The well-defined trail winds up through manzanita scrub and then shady pines, all surrounded by stunning rock formations dotted with Native American ruins and a vortex. You'll also find all the usual complaints: crowds and development right up to the edge of the wilderness. The easy hike turns around before the stiff climb to the end of the trail.

Route Details

Take the only trail from the trailhead, across from the vault toilets at the entrance to the trailhead. The red-gravel path descends into and out of a wash lined with piñon pines. Just past the wash, a signed junction indicates where Deadmans Pass Trail splits to the right (east) from the Boynton Canyon Trail 47 going roughly north, into the canyon. Stay straight on Boynton Canyon Trail 47.

In less than 0.5 mile up the trail, you'll pass the wilderness-boundary sign and shortly thereafter encounter the junction with Vista Trail, a 0.7-mile hike up the rock dome to your east. This trail is steep but well constructed. As you reach the slabs of slickrock near the top, look for footpaths to your right (or just march up the rocks if you're confident in your soles). Kachina Woman, a tall smokestack of a rock tower, rises to your north, while a shorter knob juts up to the south. In the rocky saddle between them, a sign announces the end of the trail, though many trace trails continue around Kachina Woman.

Besides the Sedona-wide views that give the Vista Trail its name, the path is also the home of a vortex, a supposed swirl of geomagnetic energy. Many locals and some visitors consider these sites sacred, and it is poor form to be loud and unruly in such places. Treat the area as if you were in a church because that's how many of your fellow hikers feel about it.

There are varied reports of the effects of being in a vortex, but

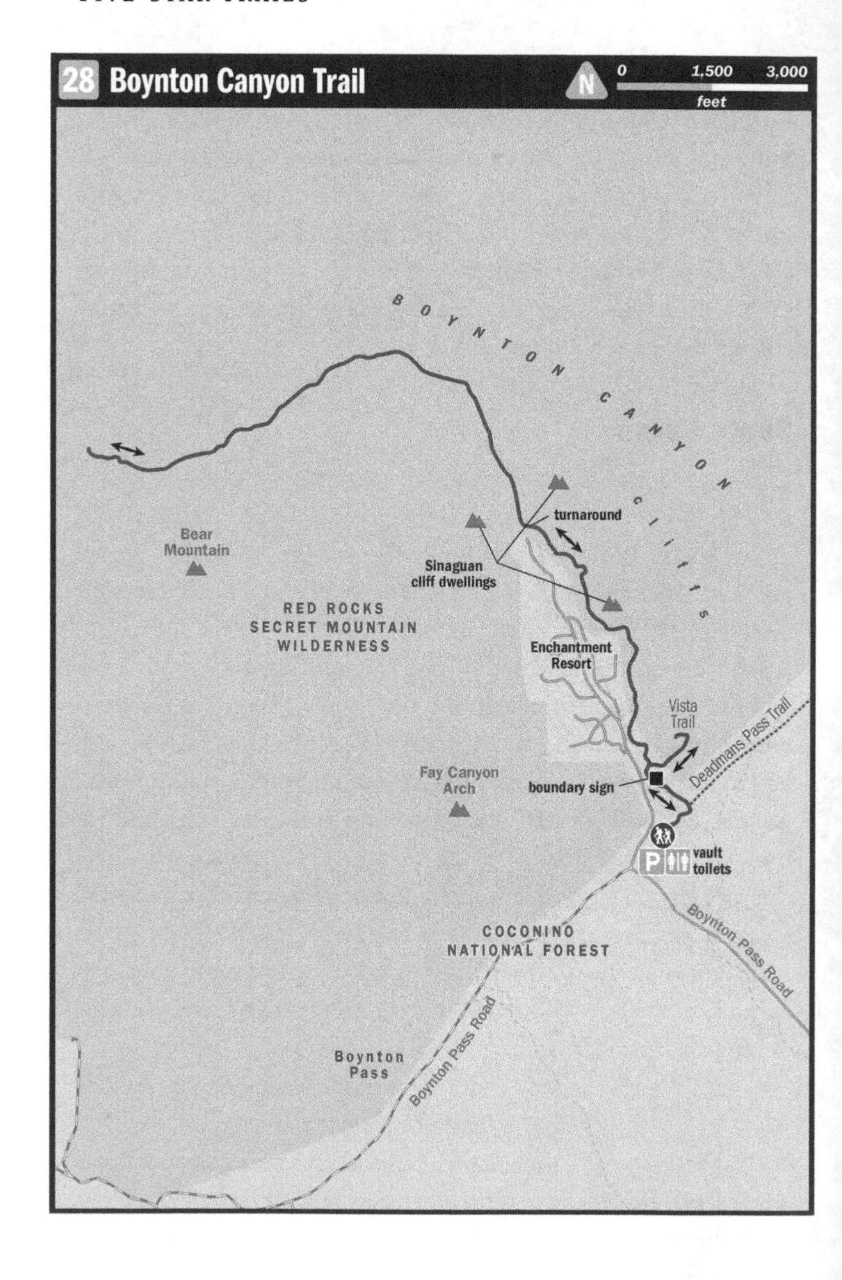

28 Boynton Canyon Trail
N
0
1,500
3,000
feet
BOYNTON CANYON cliffs
turnaround
Bear Mountain
Sinaguan cliff dwellings
RED ROCKS SECRET MOUNTAIN WILDERNESS
Enchantment Resort
Vista Trail
Deadmans Pass Trail
Fay Canyon Arch
boundary sign
P
vault toilets
COCONINO NATIONAL FOREST
Boynton Pass Road
Boynton Pass
Boynton Pass Road

one of them, among some visitors, clearly, is an uncontrollable urge to build rock cairns, as more than a dozen are clustered in the center of the saddle. When you've had your fill of peace, head back down to the Boynton and keep going right (north).

The trail climbs the east side of the canyon, to shoot the narrow gap between the red-walled cliffs and the private Enchantment Resort. Consequently, you'll have fine views of the resort and a couple of mansions built on the far side of the canyon. To your left, some spur trails lead to the resort. Don't take them; the resort does not care for visitors not registered as guests.

To your right, a few, thinner trails cut through the manzanitas toward Sinaguan cliff dwellings. The U.S. Forest Service does not advertise these dwellings, but they are well known locally and indicated on USGS topographic maps. If you find them, look but don't touch. Climbing around in the ruins degrades them for future visitors and is against federal law to boot. Hike these trails with care.

After 1.5 miles, the trail bends past the northeast corner of the resort. Near the wrought-iron fence, you'll see several brightly colored wooden crosses. These are used for a Yavapai-Apache ceremony that the resort sponsors annually in late February. Look the other direction (north) to find the sign delineating Boynton Canyon Trail 47 from the numerous spur trails that wander from the northern end of the resort.

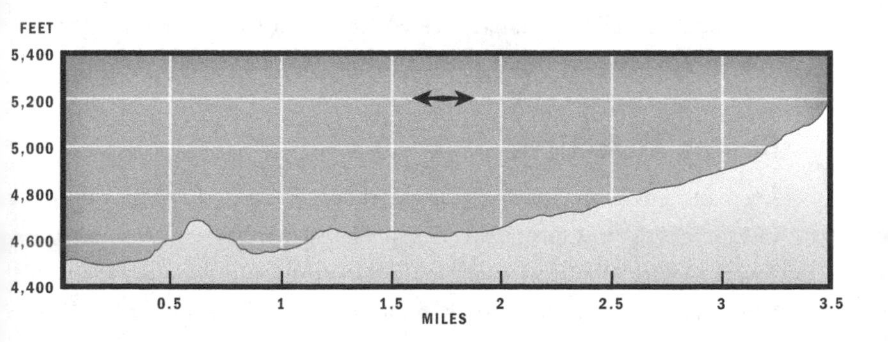

Past this point, the trail changes in character from a hard and rocky path up and down the side of the canyon to a sandy trench burrowing through the manzanitas that fill the middle of the canyon. Soon you start following the creek, as pines, junipers, and oaks provide scattered bits of shade.

If the creek has water, you can expect the waterfalls later on, but it and the falls above are typically dry.

At about 2.5 miles, the trail closes in on the western cliffs, and then starts climbing as both the trail and the canyon bend to the west. As you climb, you'll find yourself in a stand of Gambel oaks and a scattering of Texas mulberry trees. The trail continues to climb, and the oaks yield to pines, both piñon and the occasional ponderosa. By now you've curved around so that you are heading southwest, and have climbed about 400 feet from the trailhead.

Many species of birds chirp and carry on throughout these trees. You may spot white-tailed deer on rare occasions in the upper canyon, while jackrabbits are commonly seen throughout.

The wash crossing at about 3 miles marks the turnaround for the easy hike. If the water is falling, it does so through here.

After this the climb becomes much steeper and rockier (as in climb-over-boulders rockier). The last 0.5 mile gains almost as much elevation (500 feet) as the rest of the previous hike combined.

At the top of the scramble, a sign announces the end of the trail, next to a slab of orange rock where you can sit and admire the canyon you just came through. Return the way you came.

Nearby Attractions

Enchantment Resort (**enchantmentresort.com**) hosts two well-regarded restaurants open to the public. One is the AAA Four Diamond–rated Yavapai, which offers fine dining for breakfast and dinner (reservations and business-casual attire required for the latter). Expect to pay $24–$42 per person (exclusive of alcohol). Less formal, and less expensive, is the Enchantment's Tii Gavo bar and grill, open 2:30–10:30 p.m.

For a more structured encounter with Sinaguan ruins, visit the Palatki Heritage Site in Coconino National Forest. Reservations are recommended for seeing the multistoried cliff dwellings and a wall of petroglyphs. No pets are allowed, and a Red Rock Pass is required. From the Boynton Canyon Trailhead, continue west for 3 miles on Boynton Pass Road (FR 152C), which will become graded dirt. Turn right (north) on FR 795 and continue another 2 miles to the site. Call (928) 282-3854 between 9:30 a.m. and 3 p.m., or visit **www.fs.fed.us/r3/coconino/recreation/red_rock/palatki-ruins.shtml.**

Directions

From the Y in Sedona, go west on AZ 89A, turning right on Dry Creek Road (the intersection has a traffic signal). Follow this paved road—which becomes Boynton Pass Road after Dry Creek Road splits off to become a dirt track—to the T-intersection. Go left (roughly west) and follow the signs to the trailhead. There is parking for a dozen cars, but frequently twice that number squeeze in.

29 Brins Mesa–Soldier Pass Loop

SCENERY: ★★★★
TRAIL CONDITION: ★★★★
CHILDREN: ★★
DIFFICULTY: ★★★
SOLITUDE: ★★

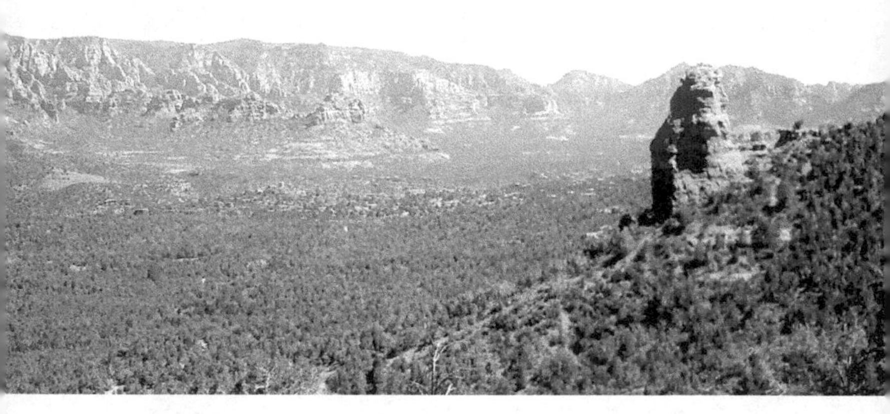

UPTOWN SEDONA FROM BRINS MESA

GPS TRAILHEAD COORDINATES: *Brins Mesa Trailhead:* N34° 55.010' W111° 48.512'

DISTANCE & CONFIGURATION: 9.5-mile lasso loop; easy hike is 4.2 miles

HIKING TIME: Full hike is 5 hours; easy hike is 2 hours

HIGHLIGHTS: Brins Mesa, scenic vistas, Devil's Kitchen sinkhole, Seven Sacred Pools, and huge arches

ELEVATION: 4,600 feet at trailhead to 5,100 feet at top of mesa

ACCESS: Requires a Red Rock Pass

MAPS: USGS Wilson Mountain

FACILITIES: Restrooms and trash cans at Jim Thompson Trailhead

WHEELCHAIR ACCESS: None

COMMENTS: No water available anywhere on the hike, and this route can be quite hot.

CONTACTS: Red Rock Ranger District, P.O. Box 20429, Sedona, AZ 86341; (928) 282-4119; **www.fs.fed.us/r3/coconino/recreation/red_rock/brins-mesa-tr.shtml; www.fs.fed.us/r3/coconino/recreation/red_rock/soldier-pass-tr.shtml**

Overview

This lasso loop combines several different trails: Brins Mesa Trail 119 east to the Jim Thompson Trailhead, where you take two Sedona North Urban trails—Cibola Pass and the Jordan Trail—to reach Soldier Pass Trail 66. You pass a sinkhole, pools, and a spur to three arches before crossing the pass and rejoining Brins Mesa Trail 119.

Route Details

Brins Mesa Trail 119 starts eastward toward its namesake as a wide, red-dirt track lined with scrub oaks, manzanitas, and prickly pear cacti. Climb a little bump of a hill, cross the wash, and then cross the first wilderness boundary. Junipers and piñon pines provide some scattered shade.

The abandoned jeep route follows the drainage, crossing a couple of times for about 0.5 mile, finally pulling away through the spruce–oak forest until you come to the second wilderness-boundary sign. Shortly after this sign, the remnant road, now filled with stumble-rocks, starts a moderate but noticeable climb up the mesa.

On top of Brins Mesa, the forest spreads out a bit, as the pines and junipers are shorter and farther apart, still separated by manzanitas and scrub oaks. To your left (north) tower the white rock slopes of Wilson Mountain. To your right Sedona sprawls below the mesa.

At 1.4 miles, you will come to the junction with Soldier Pass Trail 66. You'll revisit this by the end of the hike, but for now keep going straight (roughly southeast) on Brins Mesa. As you go, you can catch glimpses on your right of many of Sedona's famous rock formations: Coffee Pot Rock, the Sphinx, and the knob on Brins Mesa itself, dead ahead.

As you approach this rise, you pass through a burn area, the scar from the 2006 Brins Fire. The naked corpses of the junipers, sad as they are, do deliver a small upside: The views of the surrounding rock formations open up considerably. If that is insufficient, several

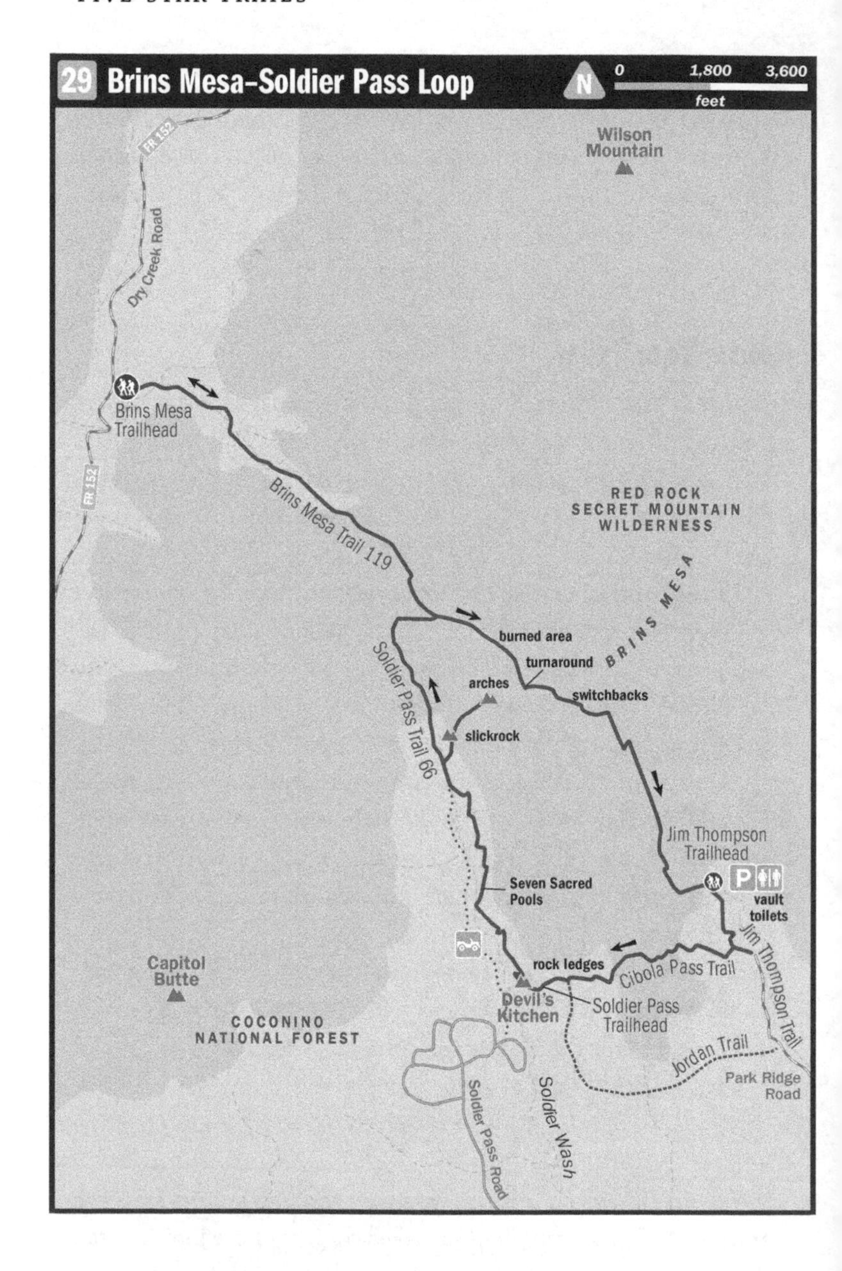

29 Brins Mesa–Soldier Pass Loop
N
0
1,800
3,600
feet
Wilson Mountain
FR 152
Dry Creek Road
Brins Mesa Trailhead
FR 152
Brins Mesa Trail 119
RED ROCK
SECRET MOUNTAIN
WILDERNESS
BRINS MESA
burned area
turnaround
switchbacks
arches
slickrock
Soldier Pass Trail 66
Jim Thompson Trailhead
P
vault toilets
Seven Sacred Pools
Jim Thompson Trail
rock ledges
Cibola Pass Trail
Capitol Butte
Devil's Kitchen
Soldier Pass Trailhead
COCONINO
NATIONAL FOREST
Jordan Trail
Park Ridge Road
Soldier Pass Road
Soldier Wash

shutterbug spurs wind off to your right to better views at the southern edge of the mesa.

Just past the knob, the mesa ends abruptly, though the trail goes on in a series of switchbacks. You are 2.1 miles in at this point and at the height of your journey, namely 5,100 feet. This is the turnaround for the easy hike.

A well-defined spur trail heads north from this point, providing views of upper Mormon Canyon. The main hike, however, goes down from here, and down steeply.

The trail switchbacks down the slope, goes over and around a couple of ridges, and finally descends into pine-filled Mormon Canyon, where the now-remnant road receives regular shade.

About 1.5 miles past the start of the switchbacks (3.5 miles total), you will reach the bright-gray gravel parking lot of the Jim Thompson Trailhead. The vault toilet here may be a welcome convenience (but there is no water). Several trails depart from here; the junction with the one you want, Cibola Pass, is back to the west. You would have passed it before entering the parking area.

Take the right turn onto Cibola Pass Trail, which bends immediately back toward the northwest. This scenic connector trail climbs steeply but shortly up and across Cibola Pass (the top of which is indicated by a fence).

On the far side of the butte, Cibola Pass Trail winds down to

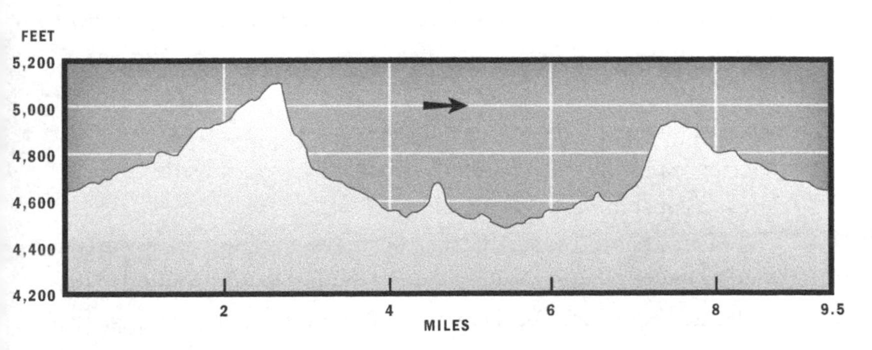

join the Jordan Trail. You have traveled about 0.7 mile from the Jim Thompson Trailhead, and just over 4 miles total at this point. Soon after, the trail follows a ledge of red slickrock. No discernible path crosses the rocks, but a series of caged-rock cairns will guide you easily enough.

These soon lead you to the intersection of Jordan and Soldier Pass trails, which you will take north, through Soldier Pass, back to the Brins Mesa Trail 119. First, though, immediately past the junction, look for a giant sinkhole named the Devil's Kitchen.

The U.S. Forest Service, showing remarkable restraint, has not built any useful barricade around the 50-foot-deep sinkhole, formed as water wore away the underlying limestone. You can see where rocks the size of houses simply sheared themselves off the cliff face to tumble into the hole. Obviously, there's nothing safe about climbing around in there. Don't be the hiker who prompts the U.S. Forest Service to build a railing after all.

Soldier Pass gives its name to both a foot trail and a jeep trail—a muddy-blue road running in parallel with the trail up the canyon—and they share some real estate near the sinkhole. If you follow the edge of the sinkhole to your left (west), though, you will easily find the singletrack footpath.

Soldier Pass Trail 66 marches (get it?) up another 0.7 mile through the pine forest deeper into the canyon, toward a famous attraction called the Seven Sacred Pools. At one time, these pools were a primary water source for the natives who lived here. Nowadays, with a lower water table, they are less impressive, being primarily a series of pits in the slickrock filled with stagnant water. Nonetheless, the jeep trail, which arrives on the opposite (west) side of the wash, brings a constant flow of visitors.

Less than 0.25 mile farther up the trail, you make your last encounter with the jeep trail, where the road must turn around at the wilderness boundary. Past here, the trail winds peacefully through the tall pines, but keep an eye out for a spur trail on your right (east).

This spur takes you toward those huge arches and caves that you have glimpsed occasionally through the trees. The 0.5-mile journey is steep and poorly defined in places. When you cross the large slickrock, follow the seam across the rock and then look for the trail on the left. This advice works for both directions. Closer to the arches, the trail starts to braid according to different hikers' opinions on how best to make the final climb. The shallow caves are also huge arches, 70–100 feet tall. The goat trail continuing around the cliff face is pretty sketchy; your safest bet is to return to Soldier Pass Trail 66 the way you came.

Once you are back on Soldier Pass, you will soon start a steep climb out of the canyon. This is the only really challenging climb of the hike as you trudge up and then around a butte. When you pause for breath during this climb, turn around. To your left you can see the arches, then the Sphinx, then downtown Sedona, then Coffee Pot Rock, and then the butte you're climbing. Over the butte, you level out in a thicket of manzanitas and live oaks. The trail wanders through this for about 0.1 mile before its junction with Brins Mesa Trail 119. A left (west) turn here takes you back the way you came.

Alternate access: This loop could also be done from the Jim Thompson Trailhead or the Soldier Pass Trailhead, about 0.25 mile south from the junction of Soldier Pass and the Jordan Trail. Such loops, omitting the western half of the Brins Mesa Trail 119, would encompass about 7.5 miles. In either case, travel clockwise to avoid going up the switchbacks in Mormon Canyon. Soldier Pass on its own is also an easy and popular little hike.

Directions

From the Y in Sedona, go west on AZ 89A past downtown Sedona to turn right (north) at the intersection with Dry Creek Road (there is a traffic signal). After about 1 mile, turn off on the dirt road, Vultee Arch Road (FR 152). This very bumpy dirt road can be traversed in a passenger car with patience, diligence, and a bit of nerve. You travel about 1.5 chattering miles before you reach the Brins Mesa Trailhead.

30 Secret Canyon–Bear Sign Canyon Loop

SCENERY: ★★★★
TRAIL CONDITION: ★★★★
CHILDREN: ★★
DIFFICULTY: ★★★
SOLITUDE: ★★★

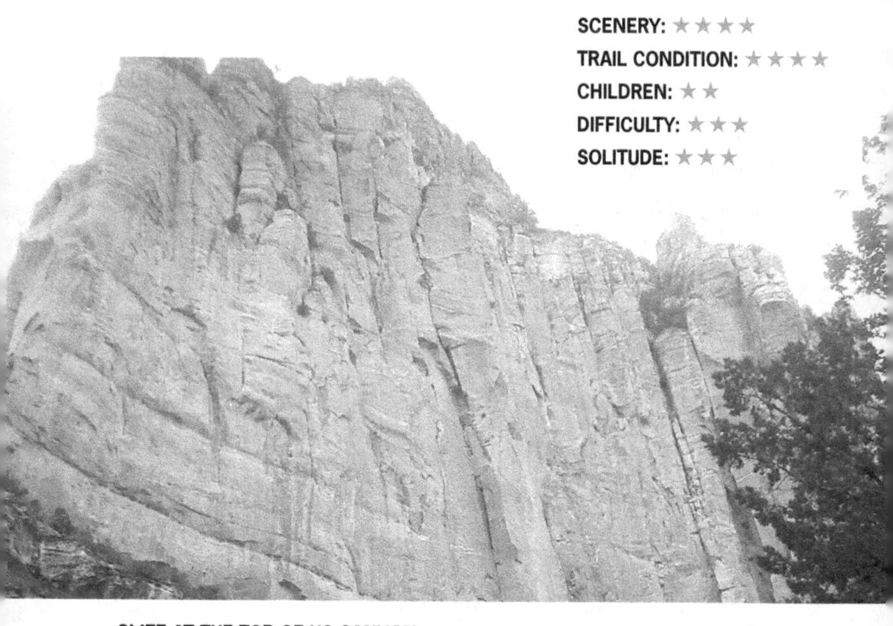

CLIFF AT THE TOP OF HS CANYON

GPS TRAILHEAD COORDINATES: *Secret Canyon Trailhead:* N34° 55.806' W111° 48.405' *Dry Creek Trailhead:* N34° 56.235' W111° 47.660'

DISTANCE & CONFIGURATION: 7-mile loop; 10.2 miles with HS Canyon spur

HIKING TIME: 4–6 hours

HIGHLIGHTS: Scenic views, rock formations, wildlife, and foliage

ELEVATION: 4,676 feet at trailhead to 5,467 feet at Miller Saddle

ACCESS: High-clearance vehicle recommended; requires Red Rock Pass

MAPS: USGS Wilson Mountain

FACILITIES: None

WHEELCHAIR ACCESS: None

COMMENTS: No water available on the hike. Portions of the Secret Canyon leg have little shade and can be hot during the summer.

CONTACTS: Red Rock Ranger District, P.O. Box 20429, Sedona, AZ 86341; (928) 282-4119; **www.fs.fed.us/r3/coconino/recreation/red_rock/secret-cyn-dry-creek-loop.shtml**

Overview

This loop hike uses four different trails and a forest road to explore the Secret Mountain Wilderness. Starting northwest up Secret Canyon Trail 121, past the optional spur into HS Canyon, the route breaks north to cross a saddle on the David Miller Trail. On the other side, it goes down Bear Sign Canyon to Dry Creek Trail. That in turn leads to Dry Creek Road, and then back to the trailhead.

Route Details

There's no secret, of course; it's right there on the map. Yet this route remains one of the less frequently traveled trails in the Sedona area. That doesn't mean you won't have company, but you are unlikely to face crowds.

Cross the boulder field of Dry Creek Wash (which normally reflects its name). A sign-in log at the wilderness boundary waits on the far side. You may have to veer a bit to the right to find it.

Secret Canyon Trail 121 follows an old roadbed across the chaparral toward the canyon. Junipers grow from the sandy soil, while sandstone cliffs rise up to either side. The sand on the trail holds footprints: mostly of your fellow hikers (and their dogs) but sometimes of other critters as well. The canyon is a known habitat for deer and javelina (also known as peccary).

At 0.5 mile in, you cross a large wash, the drainage from Secret Canyon. At 0.25 mile beyond, a spur going up HS Canyon goes off to the left (west). This spur adds 3 miles and just over an hour to the journey.

HS CANYON: HS Canyon Trail 50 starts climbing along the slickrock-lined wash. It then climbs up to a shelf, where vistas of the mountains, particularly Wilson Mountain to the south, open up. Thereafter, it drops back down to the wash. Oaks and manzanitas line its slopes. In some spots, the manzanitas grow taller than the oaks.

At 0.5 mile past the junction, the climb starts getting steeper

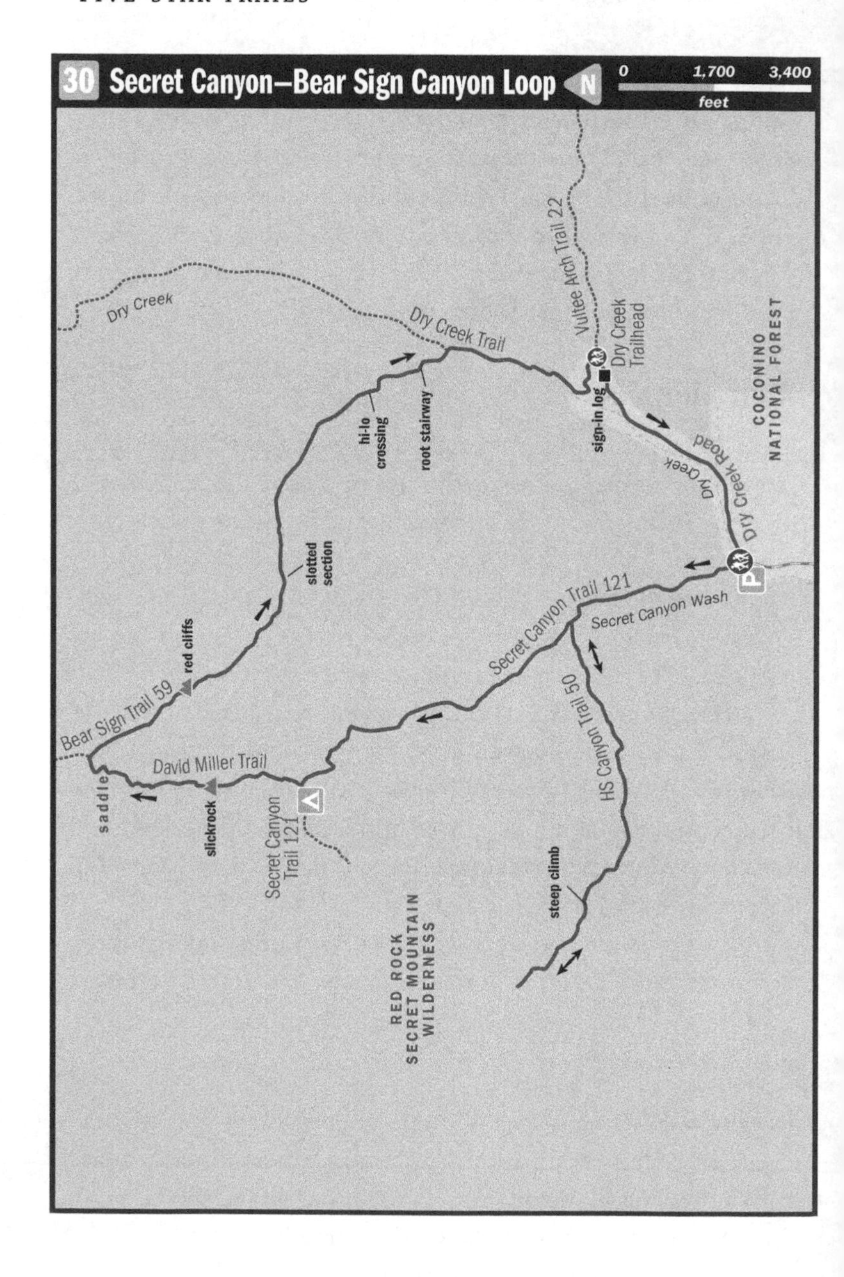
30 Secret Canyon–Bear Sign Canyon Loop
N
0
1,700
3,400
feet
Vultee Arch Trail 22
Dry Creek
Dry Creek Trail
Dry Creek Trailhead
sign-in log
COCONINO NATIONAL FOREST
Dry Creek
Dry Creek Road
hi-lo crossing
root stairway
slotted section
red cliffs
Bear Sign Trail 59
Secret Canyon Trail 121
Secret Canyon Wash
HS Canyon Trail 50
David Miller Trail
saddle
slickrock
Secret Canyon Trail 121
steep climb
RED ROCK SECRET MOUNTAIN WILDERNESS
P

along with the canyon. Near the 1-mile mark, the trail might seem to dead-end in the middle of the wash, but push through the Gambel oak saplings a bit, and small cairns will lead you onward. HS Canyon digs into Maroon Mountain, and the towers and cliffs of this sandstone edifice rise on either side by now.

As you climb, alligator junipers replace the manzanitas. At about 1.6 miles from the junction, and 5,300 feet, the path ends in a tiny clearing. It is, of course, possible to keep climbing up into the canyon, but you're on your own with that. When you're satisfied, return to Secret Canyon Trail 121.

THE REST OF SECRET CANYON TRAIL: Secret Canyon Trail 121 continues across the relatively flat chaparral into the mouth of the canyon. The old road thins to a dirt singletrack. Oaks displace some of the junipers. Every time you turn a corner, you'll see a different pile of hoodoos, or eroded rock.

You cross the wash again at 1.5 miles (not counting the HS Canyon spur). On the far side, the trail becomes rockier, and the fossilized sand castles of Secret and Maroon mountains rise higher before you. Manzanitas take over for the oaks, providing some color but not much shade.

The trail crosses the wash a third time at 2.16 miles; look for the cairn across the slickrock. There, rocky steps lead steeply up the

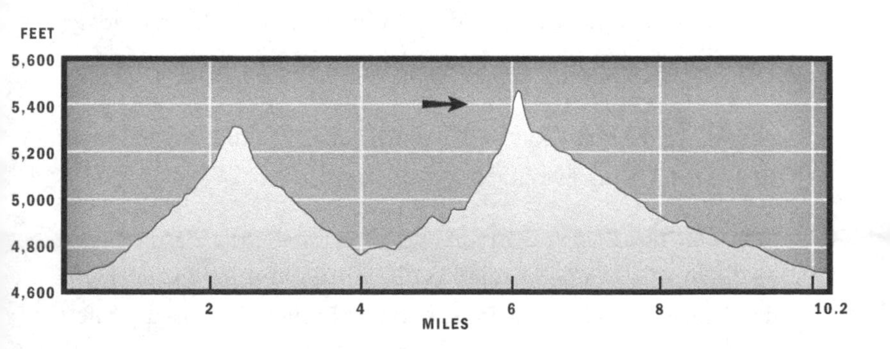

hill, leveling out at a tiny clearing with a tiny campsite. The trail keeps going through the grass and yuccas about halfway down the hill to Y at the junction with the David Miller Trail.

To the west (left), Secret Canyon Trail 121 drops the rest of the way to the wash, and then continues into the canyon another 2.5 miles or so. To the right (east), David Miller Trail climbs up a ridge of Little Round Mountain. A small stand of oaks surrounding a campsite near the junction provides a fine resting spot. Take the right, up the David Miller Trail.

DAVID MILLER TRAIL: Named for a longtime forest ranger, the David Miller Trail climbs from the junction through the junipers, following a small canyon. About 0.3 mile up, the trail crosses a slab of slickrock that lines that drainage. Head upstream 50 feet toward the alligator junipers to find the track. Past this crossing you start climbing steeply through tree-sized manzanitas.

The climb becomes switchbacks, often stair steps of pavestone-quality sandstone. From the junction, you will have climbed 900 feet in about 0.75 mile, so at the saddle you stand at 5,467 feet and about 3 miles in.

On the far side of the saddle, the landscape turns instantly from manzanita scrub to tall pines and spruces. The trail itself transforms to soft dirt and pine needles, winding steeply around orange boulders down the north slope of the ridge. Within 0.25 mile, the trail crosses a wash to T-bone with the Bear Sign Trail 59, within the canyon of the same name. To the left, loosely north, the trail continues up the canyon. To the right (south), the trail heads down the canyon toward Dry Creek. Go right (south) down the trail.

BEAR SIGN TRAIL: Don't worry about the name—there hasn't been a bear sighted in the Sedona area for more than 50 years. You might see deer, however. This easygoing dirt track through the mixed conifers heads down the canyon. Sandstone pillars line the walls to the left, while sandstone terraces make the wall to the right. All along the trail, the twisted oaks and alligator junipers compete for sunlight with the spear-straight piñons and ponderosas. Closer to the drainage, which you will cross several times, Arizona sycamores and some wild grape also join the fight.

About 0.5 mile past the junction, the trail crosses the wash, and then follows a base of red-rock cliff for about 20 feet before becoming a dirt track once more. Soon after, you pass by a stone pillar standing by itself near the bottom of the drainage.

At 1 mile past the junction, about 4 miles total, you pass a slotted portion of the wash, which will have falls and pools if the water is running. By this time, tall gray junipers will have supplanted the pines. At 1.8 miles past the junction, you must take the low road. The old route climbed a bluff here, but it is now blocked with logs, prompting you to take the trail through the wash. You have to duck under some deadfall and step around the boulders. At 0.25 mile later, a root stairway leads you down to the confluence of Bear Sign and Dry Creek trails, and to the signed junction with Dry Creek Trail.

DRY CREEK TRAIL & DRY CREEK ROAD: Dry Creek Trail runs north–south along its namesake. Head right (south). You'll have to pick your way across the blue boulders in the wash for the first few hundred yards, but then it climbs out onto dirt. It continues as a bright-orange path through the transition scrub. That dirt might hold tracks of rabbits, raccoons, and javelina.

At 0.5 mile past the confluence of boulders, you cross the wash once more. Soon after, within 0.25 mile, you pass the wilderness boundary, nearly within sight of the Dry Creek Trailhead (also called the Vultee Arch Trailhead; see page 211). It is a rough dirt cul-de-sac similar to the one from which you started.

This is actually the north terminus of Dry Creek Road (FR 152), so go south down the road, which isn't a five-star experience (but easy enough) and leads back to your car.

Directions

To Secret Canyon Trailhead: Take AZ 89A south through Sedona to Dry Creek Road on the west edge of town. Turn right (north) and continue 2 miles until you reach FR 152 (still called Dry Creek Road here). Continue north on FR 152 about 3.3 miles to the trailhead, where a rough, narrow driveway leads to a small dirt lot on the left (west) side.

To Dry Creek Trailhead: Continue about 1 mile farther up Dry Creek Road to reach this alternate trailhead.

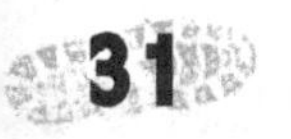

31 Vultee Arch & Sterling Pass

SCENERY: ★★★★
TRAIL CONDITION: ★★★★
CHILDREN: ★★★/★
(Vultee Arch/Sterling Pass)
DIFFICULTY: ★★/★★★
SOLITUDE: ★★★

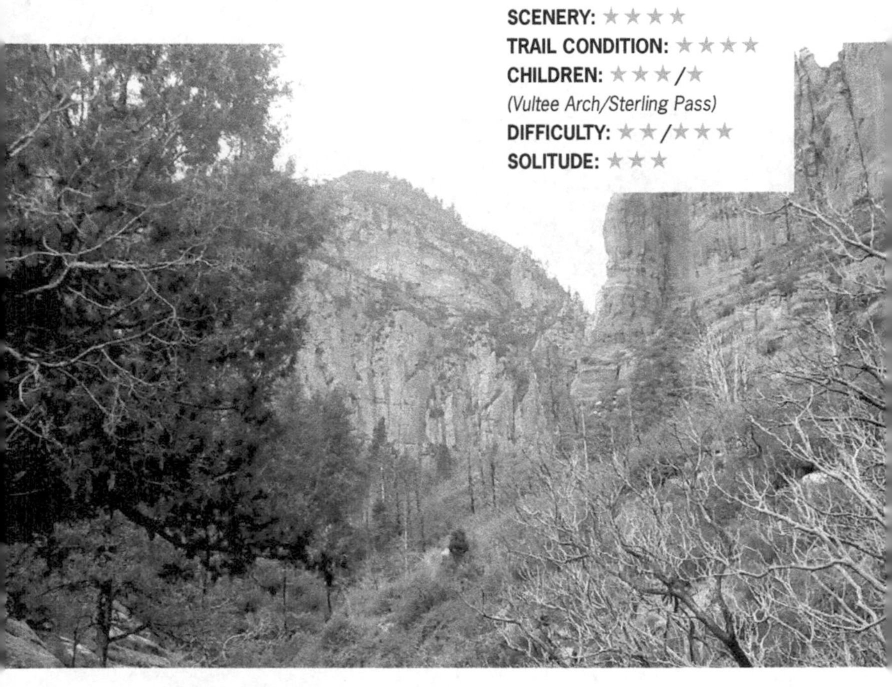

DEEPER INTO STERLING CANYON ON THE VULTEE ARCH TRAIL

GPS TRAILHEAD COORDINATES: *Sterling Pass Trailhead:* N34° 56.196' W111° 44.826'
Vultee Arch Trailhead: N34° 56.235' W111° 47.660'

DISTANCE & CONFIGURATION: 10.5 miles out-and-back; two easier options, taking just one trail or the other, would be 4 or 5 miles.

HIKING TIME: 5 hours; 2–3 hours for the easier options

HIGHLIGHTS: Geology, foliage, Vultee Arch, and wildlife

ELEVATION: 4,830 feet at Vultee Arch Trailhead, 5,325 feet near the arch, and 5,948 feet at the top of Sterling Pass

ACCESS: High-clearance vehicle recommended for Vultee Arch Trailhead. Requires Red Rock Pass for parking at both trailheads and for anywhere on FR 152.

MAPS: USGS Wilson Mountain and Munds Park

FACILITIES: None

WHEELCHAIR ACCESS: None

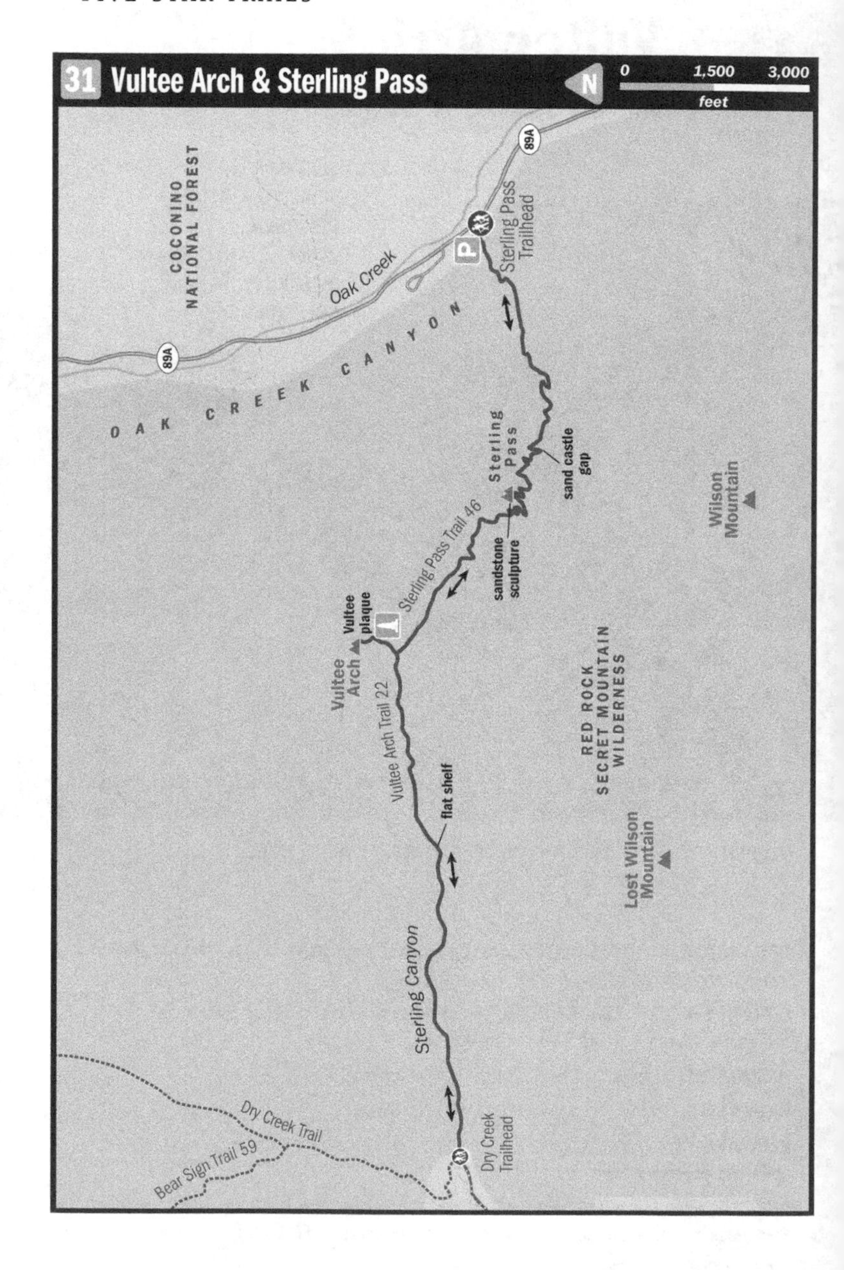

31 Vultee Arch & Sterling Pass
N
0
1,500
3,000
feet
COCONINO NATIONAL FOREST
89A
Sterling Pass Trailhead
P
Oak Creek
OAK CREEK CANYON
Sterling Pass
sand castle gap
Wilson Mountain
Sterling Pass Trail 46
sandstone sculpture
Vultee plaque
Vultee Arch
Vultee Arch Trail 22
RED ROCK SECRET MOUNTAIN WILDERNESS
flat shelf
Lost Wilson Mountain
Sterling Canyon
Dry Creek Trail
Bear Sign Trail 59
Dry Creek Trailhead

COMMENTS: No water available. Poison ivy and poison oak grow in the area.

CONTACTS: Red Rock Ranger District, P.O. Box 20429, Sedona, AZ 86341; (928) 282-4119; **www.fs.fed.us/r3/coconino/recreation/red_rock/sterling-pass-tr.shtml; www.fs.fed.us/r3/coconino/recreation/red_rock/vultee-arch-tr.shtml**

Overview

This hike consists of two trails that go to the same destination from different directions. Sterling Pass Trail 46 goes west from AZ 89A, climbing up and over its namesake to drop into the canyon and winding down to Vultee Arch. Vultee Arch Trail 22 goes east from Dry Creek, following the drainage up the canyon to reach its namesake, one of the largest arches in the area.

Route Details

There is no question that Vultee Arch Trail 22 is easier than Sterling Pass, but there's also no question that the Sterling Pass Trailhead is far easier to reach. You could set up a super-easy car shuttle, but you would spend more time driving up and down Dry Creek Road than you would hiking on the trail.

STERLING PASS TRAIL: Sterling Pass Trail 46 wastes no time. It climbs steeply up the hill away from a deep gully and the highway. You soon cross a red-rock-lined wash, and the climb levels out slightly after that.

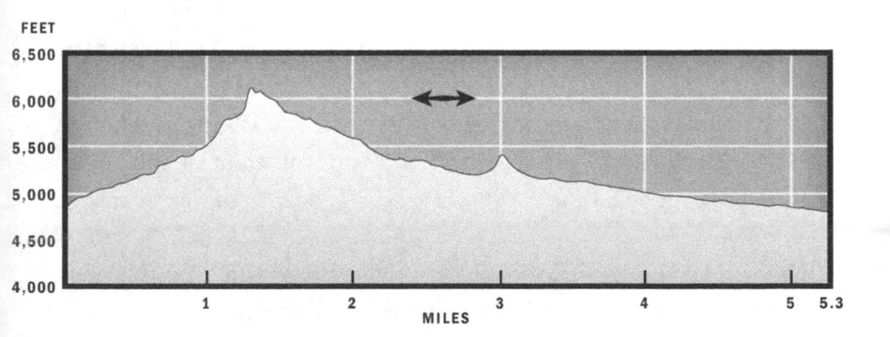

The climb follows the ravine up toward the towering cliffs of Wilson Mountain and similar formations to its north. You soon approach the edges of the 2006 Brins Fire. The underbrush has grown back prolifically around the vertical corpses of trees. Here and there, though, a stand of ponderosas still grows rust and green. Dominant canyon walls composed of various layers of Paleozoic seabed are exposed for your viewing pleasure.

The switchbacks, and there are many of them, start at 0.9 mile. Toward the top they become staircase-steep. In fact, many passages are rocks piled on top of each other as stairs.

As you climb, it is worth sticking your head through the gap between two pillars of sandstone to gaze upon the sheer drop into the canyon beyond. This is one of several points where this trail brings you into touch with the geology. All of this sandstone was laid down in the Paleozoic era, the age before the dinosaurs, as essentially fossilized sand dunes. The area that would someday become Sedona was, 250–280 million years ago, a coastal desert much like modern-day Namibia or Yemen. Erosion has carved these rocks into monstrous sand castles.

At 1.5 miles, and 5,340 feet, you reach Sterling Pass, a narrow gap between two towering Paleozoic structures filled in with Gambel oaks, dwarf maples, and other brush. Many locals who do this hike just for the exercise turn around at this point.

To reach Vultee Arch, a full mile of switchbacks waits on the other side of the pass. Here and there, Gambel oaks bend across the trail. Keep an eye out for a sandstone sculpture on your right about 0.33 mile down from the pass. Every switchback brings a different view of Sterling Canyon as it stretches out in front of you. These slopes light up during wildflower season and when the leaves change colors in the fall.

By the 2.5-mile mark, the switchbacks end. The trail now follows the drainage closely, crossing several times. Around you, particularly to the south, are remains of the 1996 Arch Fire. Within 0.5 mile, you come to a metal sign marking the junction with the

Vultee Arch Trail 22 (which continues west). Take the short spur that heads north, toward the arch.

VULTEE ARCH TRAIL: A short, blocked-off jeep trail connects the trailhead with the wilderness boundary. Past this sign and sign-in log, a footpath continues west, following the drainage through the juniper and piñon-pine scrub forest. Live oaks, manzanitas, and prickly pear cacti also line the trail.

The trail soon closes in on the wash and will stay close to it throughout, crossing the normally dry drainage many times. This is deer country, and on rarer occasions javelina have been sighted here as well. Ravens and hawks frequently patrol overhead.

At the 1-mile mark, the dusty track crosses a flat shelf. Pines start replacing junipers, and the red-rock walls start closing in on the trail. Wild grape lines the wash.

As the canyons narrow, you enter the remnants of the Arch Fire, with the skeletons of trees poking from the thick brush that crowds the trail. That thin track goes up and down but mostly up, following the wash toward the junction.

At the signed junction, at 1.7 miles, the trail continues eastward as Sterling Pass Trail 46, while a spur trail breaks left (north) to head for the arch. Take the left, of course.

VULTEE ARCH: That short spur winds north from the junction through the oaks. Within a hundred yards, cairns lead you up wide shelves of orange slickrock to a plaque commemorating aviation icon Gerard "Jerry" Vultee and his wife, Sylvia Parker, who died in a 1938 plane crash. Vultee Arch is visible on the north slope beyond. This is the best view of that sandstone arch available without fighting your way up the canyon walls. Cairns continue north, though, if you're up for that.

At the bottom of the ravine, cairns lead you across to a trail that seems to go straight up the hill. You may hesitate, though, because the footpath bends westward to continue following the ravine. You might think the path bends around the ravine somewhere, providing an easier route to the arch, or that it perhaps goes to the site of the plane crash—and you would be wrong on both counts. In about 0.2 mile, that footpath will disintegrate, becoming so washed-out and overgrown that you might as well be bushwhacking. It is, however, a lovely stroll through the woods while it lasts.

To reach the arch, take the goat trail up the slope. Cairns lead you most of the way. You will have to scramble up rocks, push through thickets of live oaks and manzanitas, and dodge some inconvenient prickly pears. Success brings you to the arch in a hard 0.5 mile. (Or you could save yourself the scratches and take pictures from the plaque.) When you have satisfied your curiosity, return the way you came.

Nearby Attractions

Less than 1 mile up the road is Slide Rock State Park, a water-recreation site where you can wade in the swimming holes or slide down the water across the chunk of slickrock for which it was named. The entrance fee is $20 per vehicle in summer (Memorial Day–Labor Day) and $10 per vehicle the rest of the year, and still the parking lot fills quickly on weekends with warm weather. Call (928) 282-3034 or visit **azstateparks.com/Parks/SLRO.**

A little farther up the road, at 9351 N. AZ 89A, between Slide Rock and Call of the Canyon Day Use Area, you can enjoy lunch or dinner at the Junipine Cafe. Expect to pay $10–$20 a person for burgers, seafood, and other casual fare, not counting drinks from the full-service bar. Call (928) 282-7406 or visit **junipine.com.**

Directions

To Sterling Pass Trailhead: Take AZ 89A north from Sedona about 5.5 miles. Just past mile marker 380, there will be a small, unmarked pullout on the left (west) side. It's about 100 yards north of the Manzanita Campground (on the east side), though you cannot park there unless you pay for a campsite. If you reach Slide Rock State Park, you've gone too far. Be wary on summer weekends, as the pullout is often used as unofficial overflow parking for the state park.

To Vultee Arch (also called Dry Creek) Trailhead: Take AZ 89A south through Sedona to Dry Creek Road on the west edge of town. Turn right (north) and continue 2 miles until you reach FR 152 (still called Dry Creek Road here). Continue north on FR 152 about 4.3 miles to its termination at the trailhead. FR 152 is a rough dirt road but is passable in passenger vehicles if you take your time. A high-clearance vehicle, though, will go easier on the nerves.

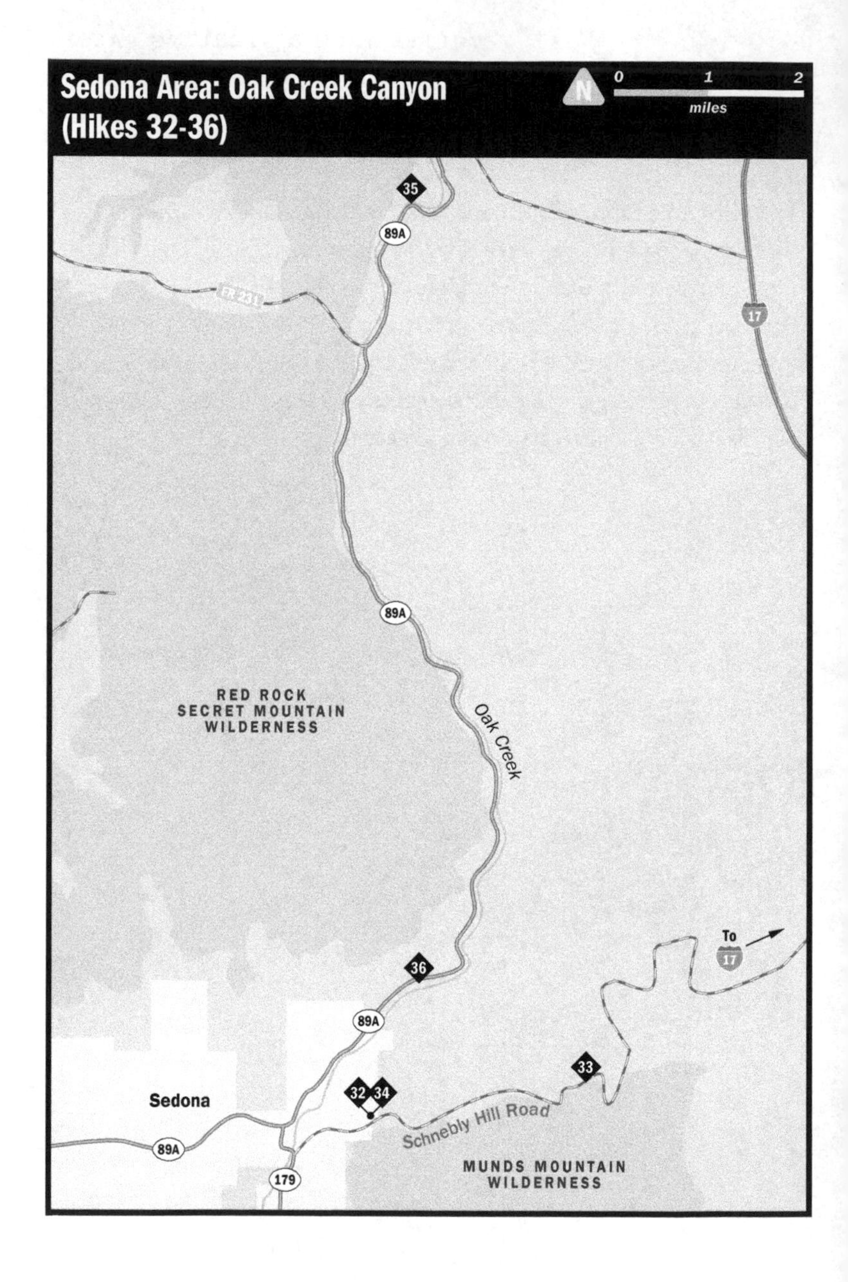

Sedona Area: Oak Creek Canyon
(Hikes 32-36)
N
0
1
2
miles
35
89A
FR 231
17
89A
RED ROCK
SECRET MOUNTAIN
WILDERNESS
Oak Creek
To
17
36
89A
33
32
34
Sedona
Schnebly Hill Road
89A
179
MUNDS MOUNTAIN
WILDERNESS

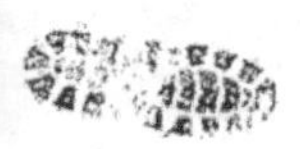

Sedona Area: Oak Creek Canyon

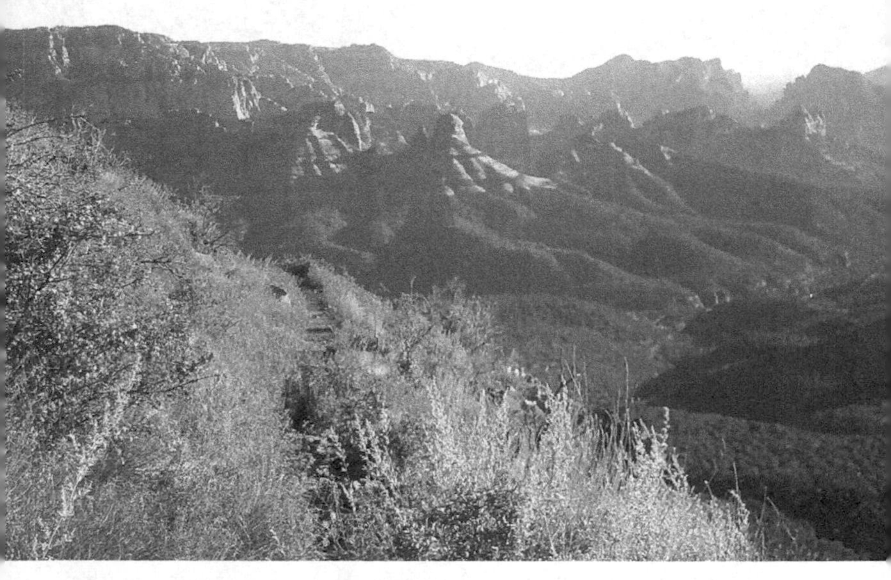

SOUTH ALONG THE SLOPE OF WILSON MOUNTAIN

32 Huckaby Trail

SCENERY: ★★★★
TRAIL CONDITION: ★★★★
CHILDREN: ★★★
DIFFICULTY: ★★★
SOLITUDE: ★★

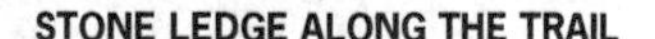

STONE LEDGE ALONG THE TRAIL

GPS TRAILHEAD COORDINATES: *Schnebly Hill Trailhead:* N34° 52.004' W111° 44.940'
Midgely Bridge Trailhead: N34° 53.133' W111° 44.494'

DISTANCE & CONFIGURATION: 6.4 miles out-and-back; 5.2 miles out-and-back to just Oak Creek; adventure option (see page 224) is an 11-mile loop

HIKING TIME: 3 hours; 6–7 hours for adventure option

HIGHLIGHTS: Scenic views, geology, old homestead, and creek access

ELEVATION: 4,463 feet at trailhead to 4,290 feet at Bear Wallow Creek to 4,514 feet at Midgely Bridge

ACCESS: Requires a Red Rock Pass for both trailheads

MAPS: USGS Munds Park, Munds Mountain, and Sedona

FACILITIES: Restrooms at Schnebly Hill Trailhead; picnic tables at both trailheads

WHEELCHAIR ACCESS: None

COMMENTS: No drinkable water on the trail. Southern portion offers very little shade and can be very hot in summer. Do not attempt to cross Oak Creek at high water levels. Can be combined with other trails to form an 11-mile loop; see adventure option following "Route Details."

CONTACTS: Red Rock Ranger District, P.O. Box 20249, Sedona, AZ 86341; (928) 282-4119; **www.fs.fed.us/r3/coconino/recreation/red_rock/huckaby-tr.shtml**

Overview

This recently constructed trail crosses in and out of Bear Wallow Canyon and then follows the south rim of Oak Creek Canyon, affording views of the canyon from uptown Sedona to the bend past Indian Gardens. The trail then drops down to pass through the old Huckaby homestead before reaching Oak Creek. If you desire to cross the creek, the trail continues up the opposite wall to Midgely Bridge.

Route Details

Huckaby Trail 161 starts from the northwest end of the Schnebly Hill parking area. Follow the caged cairns and wooden signs on the wide path through transition juniper country. You soon pass the junction with Marg's Draw. Keep straight. The wooden signs and cairns disappear as the trail winds down into Bear Wallow Canyon. You cross the creek in a wide slickrock channel, and then start steeply up. And up. The trail keeps climbing, winding up the ridge, sometimes quite steeply.

A bench marks the halfway point of this 0.5-mile climb. Take a moment to notice the different kinds of junipers; the bright-green, long-needled prickly pear cacti; the profusion of manzanitas; and the scrub oaks and sumacs.

Then keep climbing as views of uptown Sedona and the buttes behind it open behind you. Near the top of the climb, also near the 1-mile mark, the trail bends as it circumnavigates the edge of Mitten Ridge. As you head north you will see Wilson Mountain, and then, completing your way around to the northeast, Oak Creek Canyon stretching up ahead. The latter vista includes the Midgely Bridge, the terminus for this trail.

The trail follows the ridgeline for 0.3 mile before switchbacks make their way down to Oak Creek. At their end, you walk between a pair of enormous junipers to emerge close to Oak Creek. The trail now

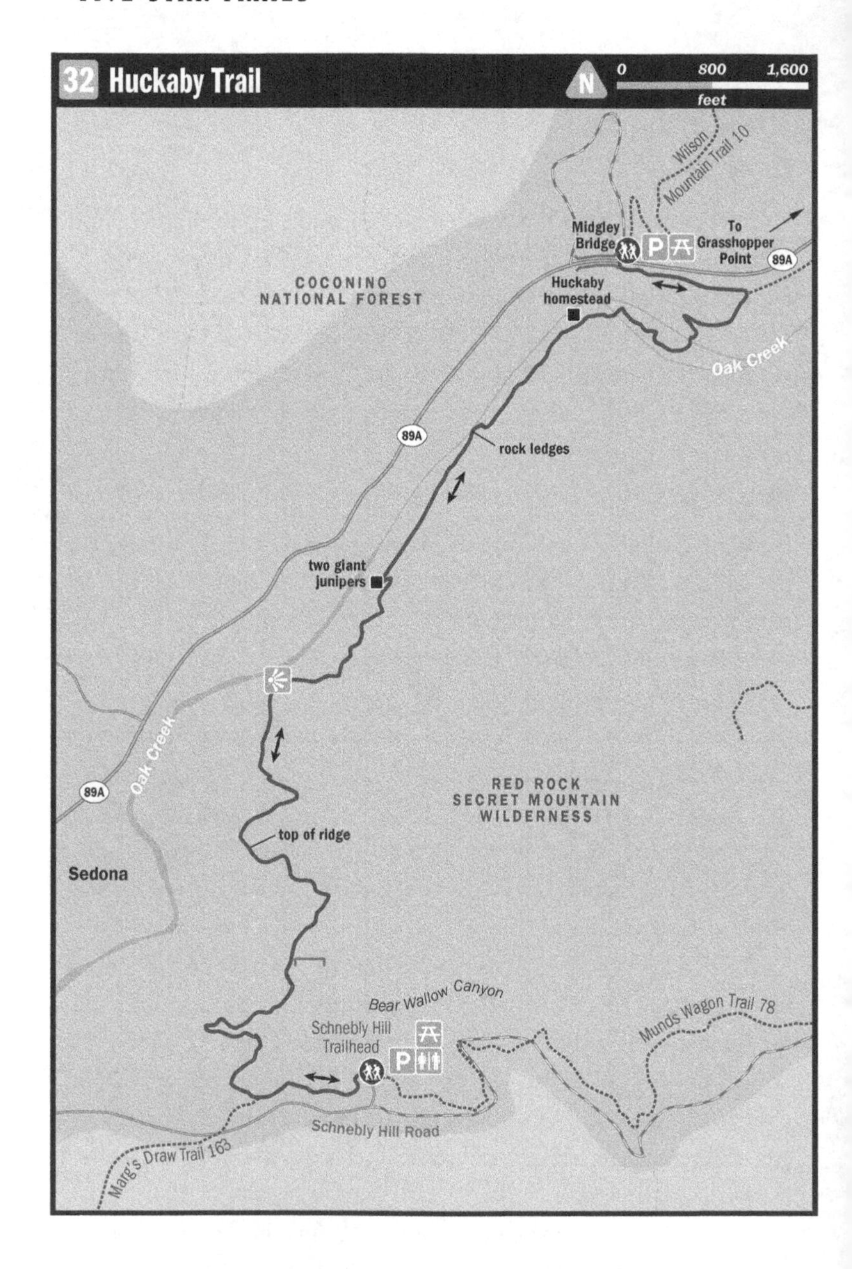

32 Huckaby Trail
N
0
800
1,600
feet
Wilson Mountain Trail 10
Midgley Bridge
To Grasshopper Point
89A
COCONINO NATIONAL FOREST
Huckaby homestead
Oak Creek
89A
rock ledges
two giant junipers
Oak Creek
89A
RED ROCK SECRET MOUNTAIN WILDERNESS
top of ridge
Sedona
Bear Wallow Canyon
Munds Wagon Trail 78
Schnebly Hill Trailhead
Schnebly Hill Road
Marg's Draw Trail 163

follows that creek upstream. A wide, rocky shelf separates you from the water as the trail hugs the base of the limestone cliffs lining the canyon wall. In two distinct stretches, the trail is a wide stone ledge jutting out from those cliffs. Wader trails lead from the main trail through the junipers, maples, and sycamores to the banks of the creek.

After 0.5 mile, the trail drifts away from the cliff to cross an open, sandy shelf. This was the residence of Bill Huckaby, the trail's namesake and a state highway worker who lived here with his family in the late 1930s. What little trail remains is buried beneath the Indian paintbrush, creosote, and wild grapes that grow rampant across the shelf. Toward the north end, an old well is the most visible remnant.

Just past the well, the trail returns to the cliffside and follows that closely to the boulder-strewn banks of Oak Creek, at 2.4 miles. This is a fine turnaround point. It's only another 0.5 mile to Midgely Bridge, but most of that is switchbacks up the gravelly canyon wall.

If you wish to continue, two crossings are involved: The first and widest is here and goes to the southern tip of an island in the creek. Then you follow the cairns and well-trodden footpath northward to a second, smaller crossing. Your spot is marked most reliably by a 1-inch-thick wire rope left over from engineerings past. Many times locals will have slapped together makeshift bridges, but these typically wash downstream every spring.

Across the creek, Huckaby is again an abandoned road, this

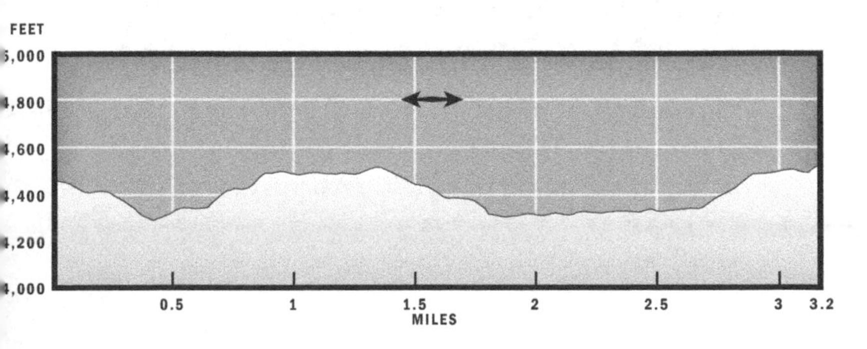

time a series of steep, wide, gravelly switchbacks plowing up the side of the canyon. You pass a spur going to the Grasshopper Point Day Use Area, after which the climb lessens. Soon you find yourself walking through a chute of barbed-wire fence containing both sides of the trail. You will have company by now: Tourists crowd Midgely Bridge at about any hour during daylight.

This long tourist chute climbs to a railing-line overlook, and then turns to pass beneath the steel bridge, finally climbing a series of stone steps to the trailhead.

Adventure option: To form a loop, you may combine the Huckaby Trail 161 with Munds Wagon Trail 78 and the Mitten Ridge Trail (see page 231 and opposite page). Such a loop would be best done counterclockwise, which would mean taking Huckaby in the opposite direction than described here. Plan on hiking 11 miles over 6–7 hours for the entire loop. A more detailed account of this route can be found following the Munds Wagon Trail description (see page 235).

Directions

To Schnebly Hill Trailhead: In Sedona, Schnebly Hill Road is on AZ 179 on the roundabout just south of the creek crossing, or 0.3 mile south of the Y intersection of AZ 179 and AZ 89A. Turn left onto Schnebly Hill Road and go 0.8 mile to the trailhead on the left side. The pavement ends just past the trailhead, so if your tires hit dirt, you've just missed it. There is room for a couple dozen vehicles.

To Midgely Bridge Trailhead: Take AZ 89A north from Sedona for 1.9 miles until you cross Midgely Bridge, the first bridge you come to. The trailhead is on the left side immediately north of the bridge. There are parking spaces for about eight vehicles, but people routinely and creatively cram many more vehicles into this turnout.

33 Mitten Ridge Trail

SCENERY: ★★★★
TRAIL CONDITION: ★★★
CHILDREN: ★★★
DIFFICULTY: ★★★
SOLITUDE: ★★★

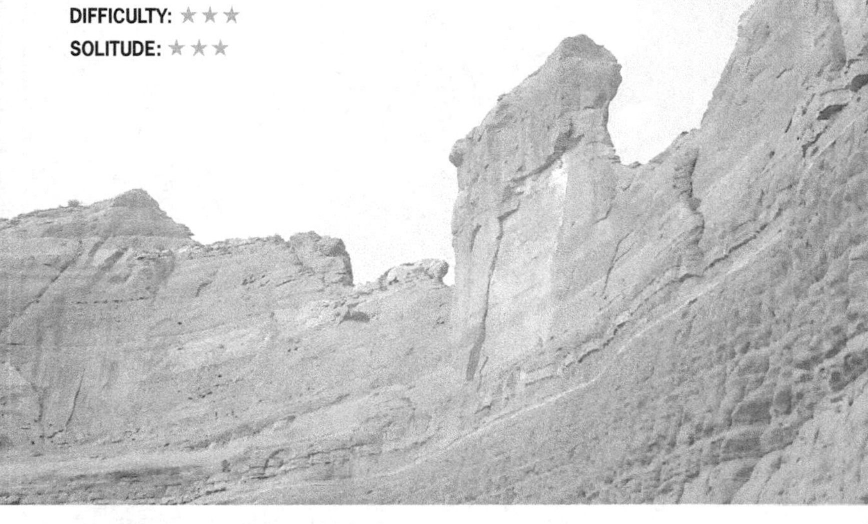

ROCK FORMATIONS CROWN MITTEN RIDGE.

GPS TRAILHEAD COORDINATES: *Three Mile Trailhead:* N34° 52.329' W111° 42.783'

DISTANCE & CONFIGURATION: 10.4 miles out-and-back; easy version (just the west fork) is 5.2 miles out-and-back; adventure option (see page 230) is 11-mile loop; 5.2 miles as a car shuttle

HIKING TIME: 6 hours for main hike; 2.5 hours for easy hike or car shuttle; 6–7 hours for adventure loop

HIGHLIGHTS: Scenic vistas, rock formations, creek access, and vortex site

ELEVATION: 5,047 feet at Three Mile Trailhead to 4,443 feet at Grasshopper Point and 5,243 feet at Mitten Saddle

ACCESS: Three Mile Trailhead requires a high-clearance vehicle and a Red Rock Pass. Grasshopper Point Day Use Area charges $8 a vehicle. There are some discounts available for various pass holders, but these rules are changing, so just bring $8. Grasshopper Point also charges $2 for pedestrian access.

MAPS: USGS Munds Park, Munds Mountain, and Sedona

FACILITIES: Grasshopper Point has toilets, trash cans, and picnic tables; none at Three Mile

WHEELCHAIR ACCESS: Accessible toilets and picnic tables at Grasshopper Point. Nothing is accessible at Three Mile Trailhead.

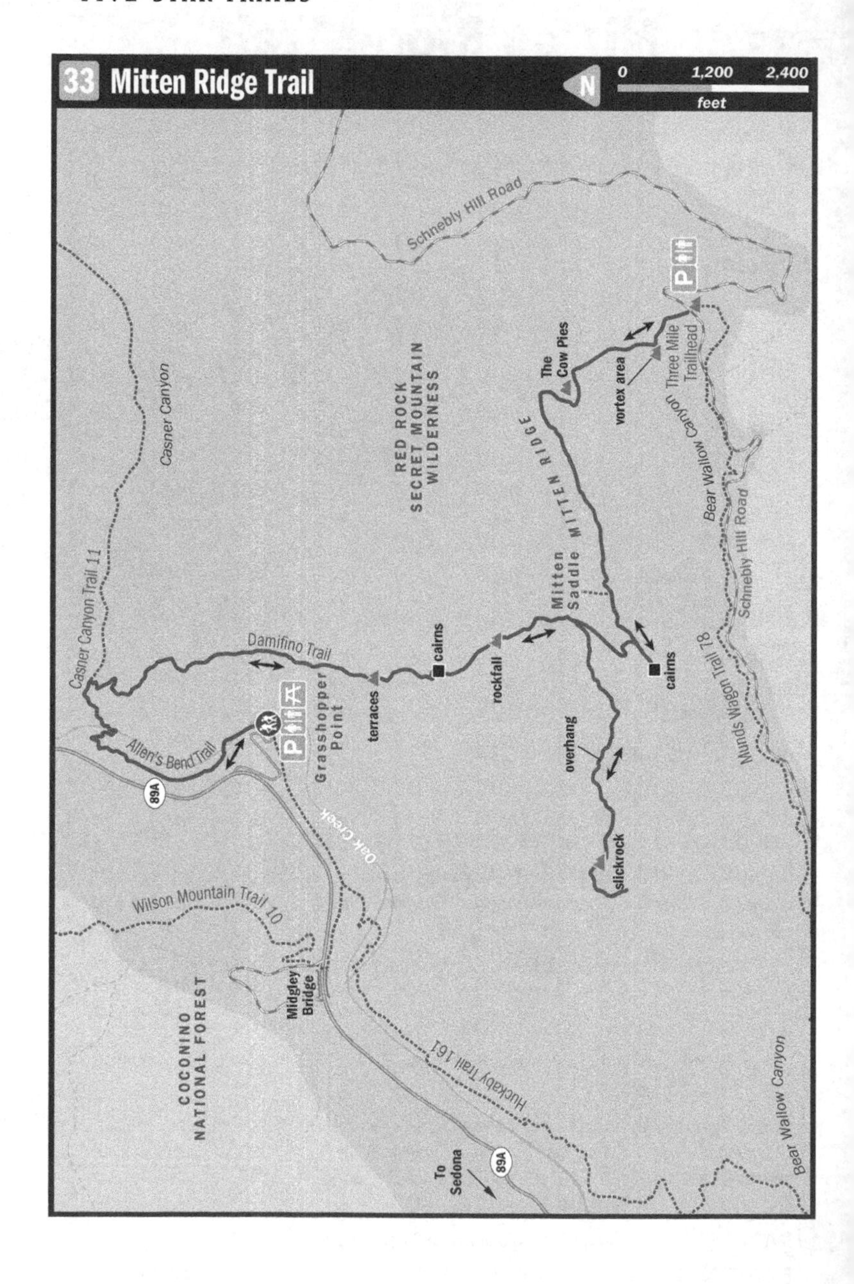
33 Mitten Ridge Trail
N
0
1,200
2,400
feet
Schnebly Hill Road
Casner Canyon
Casner Canyon Trail 11
RED ROCK
SECRET MOUNTAIN
WILDERNESS
The
Cow Pies
vortex area
Three Mile
Trailhead
Bear Wallow Canyon
MITTEN RIDGE
Mitten
Saddle
Schnebly Hill Road
Munds Wagon Trail 78
Damifino Trail
cairns
rockfall
cairns
terraces
Grasshopper
Point
Allen's Bend Trail
89A
overhang
slickrock
Oak Creek
Wilson Mountain Trail 10
Midgley
Bridge
COCONINO
NATIONAL FOREST
Huckaby Trail 161
To
Sedona
89A
Bear Wallow Canyon

COMMENTS: Not a designated U.S. Forest Service trail. Very little shade; hiking can become quite hot in the summer. Do not attempt to cross Oak Creek at high water levels. The North segment is sometimes known as the Damifino "damn if I know" Trail. Several possible routing options—see notes following "Route Details." Can be combined with other trails to form an 11-mile loop.

CONTACTS: Red Rock Ranger District, P.O. Box 20249, Sedona, AZ 86341; (928) 282-4119; **www.fs.fed.us/r3/coconino/recreation/red_rock/grasshopper-pic.shtml**

Overview

Unofficial and largely unmarked, this hike is a combination of routes that run along or across Mitten Ridge and all the way down to Oak Creek if you desire. The hike crosses a vortex site and the Cow Pie rock formations before reaching the ridge and crossing a saddle between two cliffs. One route then runs west along the rest of the ridge, while another descends to the creek. See notes following the hike description about route options.

Route Details

THE COW PIES & THE SADDLE: The wooden sign across the road from the trailhead simply says COW PIES next to an arrow. This is the only place the trail is marked. Cross the road, following the dirt path through the junipers and across the wash to the first large slickrock formation, less than 0.25 mile away. This is considered a vortex site,

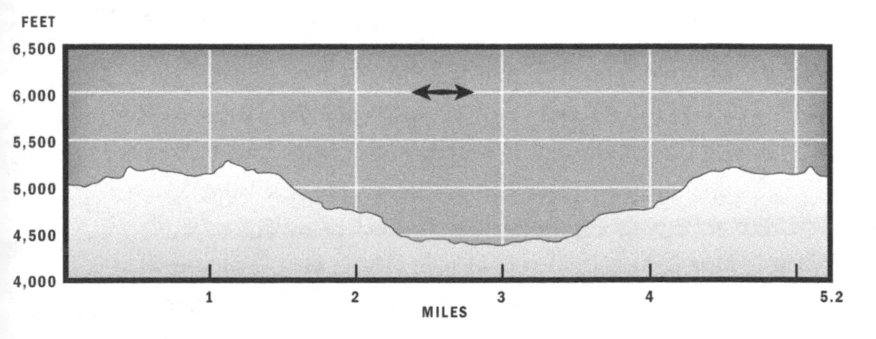

and locals have used the lava rocks scattered across its surface to form cairns and medicine wheels.

The actual Cow Pie formation is the expanse of terraced sandstone the size of a baseball diamond another 0.25 mile north up the trail. Its similarity to its namesake is more obvious from a distance. You might have noticed it from the road.

On the north side, the trail continues up onto Mitten Ridge, turning westward in the process. From either the Pies or the ridge, you have outstanding vistas of Bear Wallow Canyon and uptown Sedona beyond. More impressive are the sheer sandstone walls that tower above you. Follow the cairns along the base of these walls. There may be multiple paths. Do your feet a favor and take the higher path, which is usually the most level.

It is possible to follow cairns along the ledges for the better part of a mile, but within 0.5 mile you pass beneath a low spot in the cliffs: the saddle of Mitten Ridge. Spur trails to the east or west side climb to the top of this saddle (the one to the west is shown on the map). This wide sandstone shelf separates two of the giant rock formations that crown the ridge and provides a spectacular vantage point for the views on either side.

At the northeast corner, a thin dirt trail leads down via a couple of short, steep switchbacks. Within a few hundred feet it splits: One track goes north while the other goes west. Both trails were created by and for local mountain bikers, but they are great for hikers as well.

THE WESTERN LEG: Cross the ledge beneath the saddle to find the dirt track beyond. This track will follow the base of the cliffs for the duration. Junipers and pines grow out of the downslope side, and occasional rock overhangs crowd the upslope side. When space clears, Casner Canyon and Schnebly Hill stretch below and beyond.

At 0.5 mile past the saddle, you'll pass beneath an overhang that clearly doubles as a waterfall when it rains. In another 0.25 mile, the trail hits a wide ledge of slickrock. Keep going—there is dirt track again about 100 feet farther. Soon after, the track starts hooking south around the towering rock formation at the end of the ridge. It will wind around nearly 180 degrees, until you are actually facing southeast, before it evaporates into a series of cairns across the rocks, cutting sharply back west, down and across the slickrock. Mountain bikers have marked the route below with cairns and white paint, but it's not as much fun on foot. This is the turnaround for the easy hike, or the point for returning to the split if you wish to do the other half.

THE NORTH LEG (ALSO KNOWN AS THE DAMIFINO TRAIL): From the split, take the dirt track north through the live oaks and the prickly pears. In about 0.2 mile, the track is wiped out by a rockfall, but the slab left behind can still be crossed with a bit of caution. At about 0.4 mile from the split, the dirt evaporates into slickrock, and you must follow the cairns around the ridge on top of the sandstone ledge.

As the cairns lead you down the rock formation, you will be able to see the parking area for Grasshopper Point in the distance. If you angle your approach toward the right edge of the parking area, the cairns, which generally identify the path of least peril, will be easier to locate. If you do not see them or they conflict, head down whichever way seems safest. Take your time and think your steps through, because while this isn't mountaineering, the rocks are as slick as their reputation suggests.

It's only about 500 feet vertically or horizontally between the end of the ledge above and the beginning of the dirt track below. That track darts across another couple sections of slickrock before becoming a red-gravel path heading northwest through the juniper scrub. The formations of Mitten Ridge form a geologic skyline to the south, while Oak Creek Canyon stretches out ahead and to the north.

At 1.7 miles past the saddle, you reach the edge of the finger ridge and the trail bends sharply north. This is your turnaround unless you want to reach Oak Creek or have a car waiting at Grasshopper Point.

CASNER CANYON TO GRASSHOPPER POINT: The trail winds around to switchback down the north side of this ridge and then meet Casner

Canyon Trail 11, 0.5 mile into the canyon of the same name. Continuing left (northwest) along that trail, you reach Oak Creek. Should you cross Oak Creek, you come to Allen's Bend Trail, heading south for 0.5 mile to Grasshopper Point. Much of Allen's Bend is actually a stone walkway shaded by both limestone cliffs and riparian trees. Return the way you came unless you left a car here.

Going north to south: If you start at Grasshopper Point, here are a few things to help you out: Look for the Damifino Trail to cut off from the Casner Canyon Trail 11 just past the power lines. As you climb the ridge, some of the terraces give the illusion of a Y in the trail. There is no Y—stay to the right (west) in every case.

As you climb the slickrock, pull out your GPS, look for the ledge at 5,110 feet, and follow it south around the ridge. This will lead you around to the trail.

Adventure option: The Mitten Ridge Trail can be combined with the Huckaby Trail 161 and the Munds Wagon Trail 78 (see page 220 and opposite page) to form a loop. Such a loop would be best done counterclockwise. Plan on hiking 11 miles over 6–7 hours for the entire loop, excluding the west segment of the Mitten Ridge Trail. A more detailed account of this route can be found on page 235.

Directions

To Three Mile Trailhead: Schnebly Hill Road is within Sedona on AZ 179 on the roundabout just south of the creek crossing, or 0.3 mile south of the Y—the intersection of AZ 179 and AZ89A. Three Mile Trailhead is, in fact, nearly 3 miles east up this road, which becomes a very rough dirt road after 0.8 mile. The parking area is a wide rock shelf on the left side.

To Grasshopper Point: From Sedona, take AZ 89A north for about 2 miles, about 1 mile past the Midgely Bridge, to the signed turnoff for Grasshopper Point Day Use Area on the right.

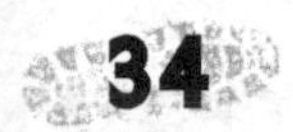

34 Munds Wagon Trail

SCENERY: ★★★★
TRAIL CONDITION: ★★★★
CHILDREN: ★★★
DIFFICULTY: ★★★
SOLITUDE: ★★

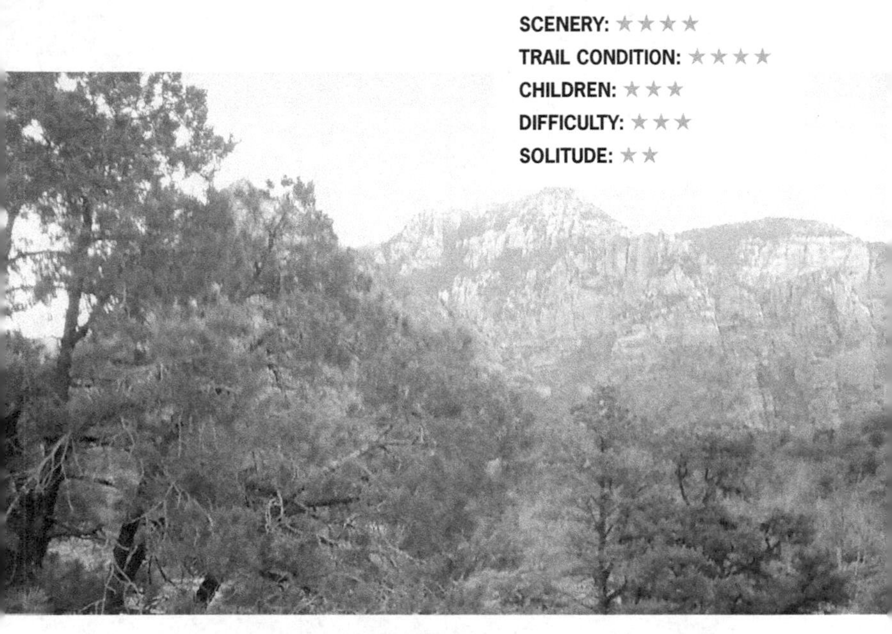

MUNDS MOUNTAIN FROM THE SOUTH TERMINUS OF MUNDS WAGON TRAIL

GPS TRAILHEAD COORDINATES: *Schnebly Hill Trailhead:* N34° 52.004' W111° 44.940'
Three Mile Trailhead: N34° 52.329' W111° 42.783'

DISTANCE & CONFIGURATION: 6 miles out-and-back; adventure option (see page 235) is an 11-mile loop

HIKING TIME: 3 hours; 6–7 hours for adventure option

HIGHLIGHTS: Scenic views, little falls and rapids if Bear Wallow Creek is flowing, and historical route

ELEVATION: 4,459 feet at Schnebly Hill Trailhead to 5,090 feet near Three Mile Trailhead

ACCESS: Three Mile Trailhead requires a high-clearance vehicle, and both trailheads require a Red Rock Pass for parking.

MAPS: USGS Munds Park, Munds Mountain, and Sedona

FACILITIES: Restrooms and picnic tables at Schnebly Hill Trailhead; no services at Three Mile Trailhead

WHEELCHAIR ACCESS: None

COMMENTS: Water in Bear Wallow Creek must be treated before drinking. Also known as Old Munds Trail. Munds Wagon Trail is a different trail from Munds Mountain Trail. Can

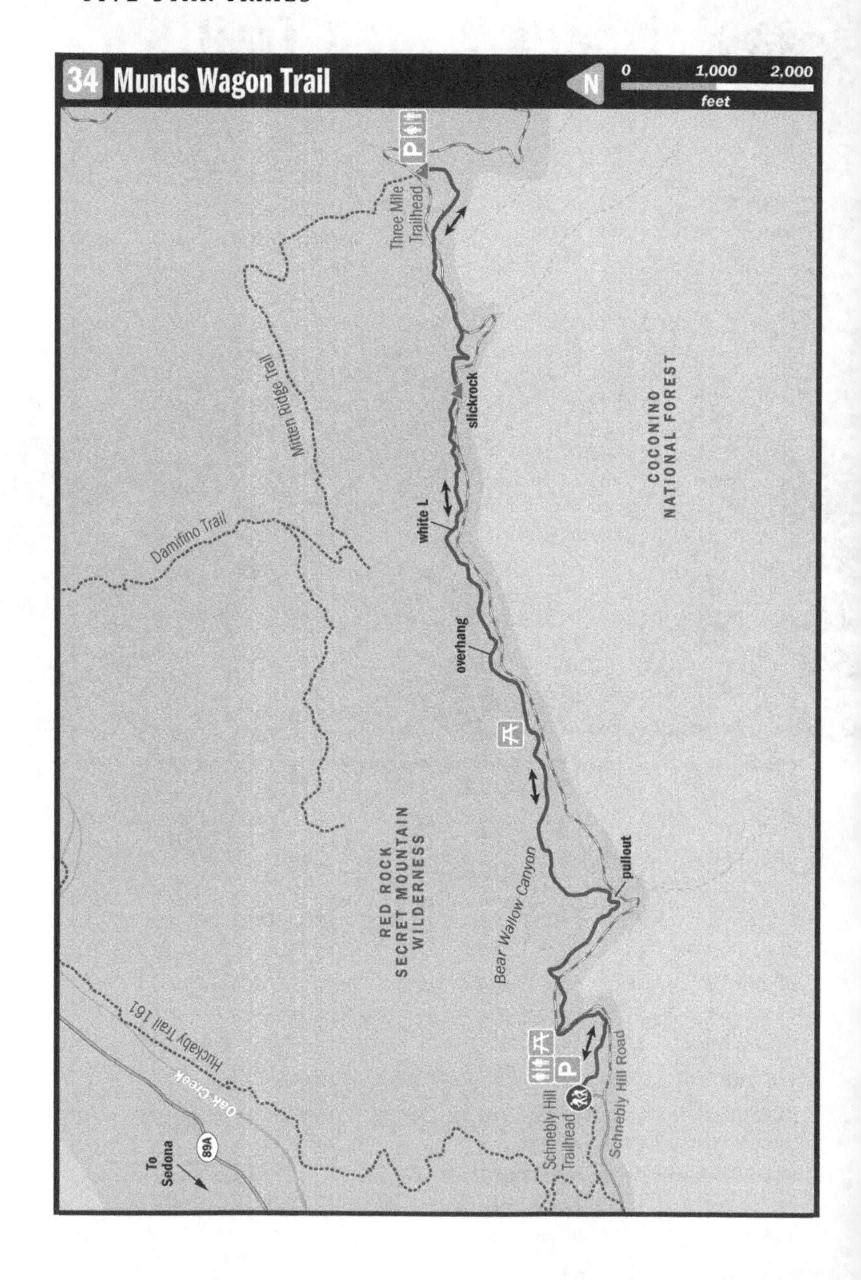
34 Munds Wagon Trail
0
1,000
2,000
feet
N
Three Mile Trailhead
Mitten Ridge Trail
slickrock
COCONINO NATIONAL FOREST
white L
Damifino Trail
overhang
RED ROCK SECRET MOUNTAIN WILDERNESS
Bear Wallow Canyon
pullout
Huckaby Trail 161
Oak Creek
89A
To Sedona
Schnebly Hill Trailhead
Schnebly Hill Road

be combined with other trails to form an 11-mile loop; see adventure option following "Route Details."

CONTACTS: Red Rock Ranger District, P.O. Box 20249, Sedona, AZ 86341; (928) 282-4119; **www.fs.fed.us/r3/coconino/recreation/red_rock/munds-wagon-tr.shtml**

Overview

Munds Wagon Road, once the main cattle route north out of town, is now a recreational trail following Bear Wallow Canyon as it cuts between Schnebly Hill and Mitten Ridge. It closely follows both Bear Wallow Creek and Schnebly Hill Road, the route's more modern replacement. Along the way, the trail features scenic vistas and exposed geology as the canyon cuts through the various layers of the Schnebly Hill formation. The top of the trail provides nearby access to two local landmarks: Merry-Go-Round Rock and the Cow Pies.

Route Details

Munds Wagon Trail 78, also known as Old Munds Trail, starts from the east side of the parking area at the Schnebly Hill Trailhead. The wide dirt track winds around a drainage, and soon crosses the road. This bend in Schnebly Hill Road is also a fine vantage point for views of uptown Sedona and Brins Mesa beyond. Do not follow the deer trail; obey the fiberglass signs leading you across the road and then straight up the ridge. Within 1,000 feet, though, you cross the road

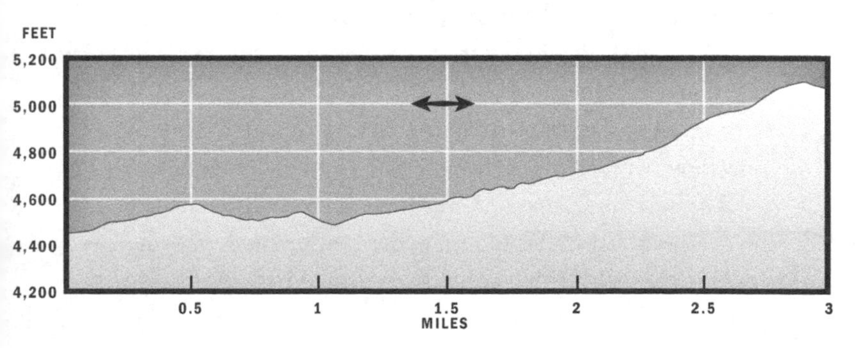

again to descend back into the canyon.

Munds Wagon Road will follow Schnebly Hill Road for most of its length, never more than 0.5 mile away and most of the time within sight. From its origins as an informal cattle route in the late 1800s, the road was first upgraded to accommodate wagons by local pioneer J. J. Thompson (with funds from Coconino County), who completed the task in 1902.

The old trail sinks below the modern road into the canyon, passing through tall junipers as a dirt singletrack. Munds Road follows the canyon more closely than its more modern counterpart, and from a pedestrian standpoint that is a good thing.

At 0.75 mile, the trail makes its first crossing of Bear Wallow Creek, which is normally dry. If the creek is running, there are many cool little waterfalls, as Bear Wallow is really a series of sandstone shelves that look like giant, poorly stacked dishes.

Shortly thereafter, the trail draws near the road at a small pullout—a tiny, unmarked secondary trailhead. Just past the 1-mile mark, the trail crosses the creek again.

The third crossing, at 1.25 miles, hugs a steep red cliff. On the other side, the trail passes two concrete picnic tables set near a sizable pullout from Schnebly Hill Road. A maze of little trails runs through here, so look for the caged cairns that have marked the trail throughout. As if to make certain, one cairn will have a wooden sign wired to it. Past this little sub-trailhead, the trail continues up the drainage.

The old road climbs out of the canyon on the north side next to a large sandstone overhang. At 1.5 miles, this is the halfway mark. After one of the few steep climbs on this hike, the trail wanders across a low ridge, with tall junipers providing scattered shade and startling views of the rock formations crowning Mitten Ridge immediately to the north. In just under 0.5 mile, the trail reunites with the creek, crossing it again. At this crossing, someone has painted a white L upon the rocks in the drainage.

At 0.1 mile farther, follow the cairns across the wide sandstone shelf. This is foreshadowing, for you come to a sign warning of

DANGEROUS SLICKROCK AHEAD and pointing to an equestrian bypass (which is really a spur to Schnebly Hill Road). The sandstone canyon that lies beyond is not really treacherous if you have dry boots. It is hazardous to hooves, though, and worth considering cautiously if it's raining. On the far side of this passage, the trail bends sharply to meet with the equestrian bypass spur, and then climbs through the tall junipers beneath the road.

In 0.5 mile, about 2.6 miles in, the trail has climbed to meet the road, and it crosses that road to keep climbing. You crest the top of the ridge and wind down, crossing a wide rock shelf before reuniting with the road at nearly 3 miles. There may be vehicles parked here because the rock slab is Three Mile Trailhead.

Across the road, a short spur leads to the Cow Pies, a well-known rock formation. Just north up the road is Merry-Go-Round Rock. These are worth exploring if you have the time. When you're ready, return the way you came.

Adventure option: To form a loop, you may combine Munds Wagon Trail 78 with the Huckaby Trail 161 and the Mitten Ridge Trail (see pages 220 and 225) and a few other short trails. This loop is best started from either the Midgely Bridge Trailhead or from Three Mile Trailhead. From either spot, proceed counterclockwise. Plan on hiking 11 miles over 6–7 hours for the entire loop.

From Midgely Bridge (the easiest to reach), take the Huckaby Trail 161 southeast (opposite of how it is described in this book) to Schnebly Hill Trailhead. From there, follow Munds Wagon Trail 78 to the Three Mile Trailhead, where you shift to the Mitten Ridge Trail. At the western terminus of the Mitten Ridge Trail, take the Casner Canyon Trail 11 west to Oak Creek, cross the creek, and then follow Allen's Bend Trail to the Grasshopper Point Day Use Area, which charges $2 a head for pedestrian access. At the south end of the day-use area, a spur trail leads south to meet up with the Huckaby Trail 161 just below the bridge. Do not try to cross Oak Creek at high water levels.

Directions

To Schnebly Hill Trailhead: Schnebly Hill Road is within Sedona on AZ 179 on the roundabout just south of the creek crossing, or 0.3 mile south of the Y—the intersection of AZ 179 and AZ 89A. Turn left onto Schnebly Hill Road and go 0.8 mile to the trailhead on the left side. The pavement ends immediately past the trailhead, so if your tires hit dirt, you've just missed it. The trailhead has vault toilets, several picnic tables, and parking for a couple dozen vehicles.

To Three Mile Trailhead: From the Schnebly Hill Trailhead, continue up the road, now a rough dirt track with a lot of jeep traffic, about 3 miles until you encounter the rock shelf on the left.

35 West Fork Trail

SCENERY: ★★★★★
TRAIL CONDITION: ★★★★★
CHILDREN: ★★★★★
DIFFICULTY: ★★
SOLITUDE: ★

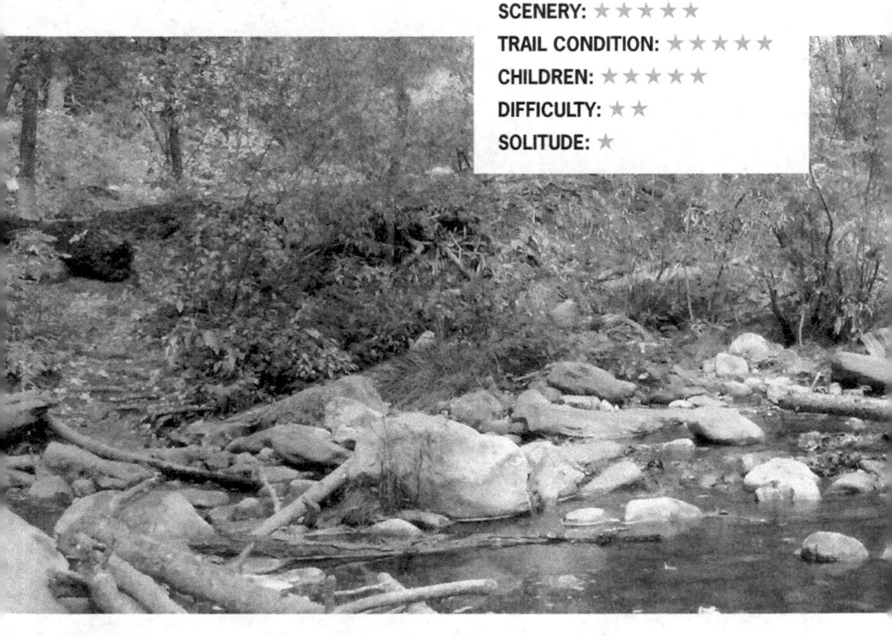

ONE OF MANY CROSSINGS OF THE WEST FORK OF OAK CREEK

GPS TRAILHEAD COORDINATES: *Call of the Canyon Day Use Area:* N34° 59.444' W111° 44.528'

DISTANCE & CONFIGURATION: 8 miles; 6 miles for easy hike; adventure option is 14 miles of serious (and wet) canyoneering

HIKING TIME: 4 hours for the full hike; 3 hours for the easy version; 2 full days for adventure option

HIGHLIGHTS: Riparian forests, old homestead, rapids and pools, wildlife, and seasonal wildflowers or fall leaves

ELEVATION: 5,300 feet at trailhead to 5,530 feet at end of trail

ACCESS: $10 per vehicle fee at Call of the Canyon Day Use Area. They accept a few passes, but those details change, and many of the passes they accept are no longer actually issued. Just bring $10.

MAPS: USGS Dutton Hill, Mountainaire, Wilson Mountain, and Munds Park. Wilson Mountain will actually cover most of the hike.

FACILITIES: Restrooms, picnic tables, and trash cans at Call of the Canyon

WHEELCHAIR ACCESS: The first part of this hike is paved sidewalk.

COMMENTS: Hike has an easy alternative. Up to 15 creek crossings. Poison ivy and

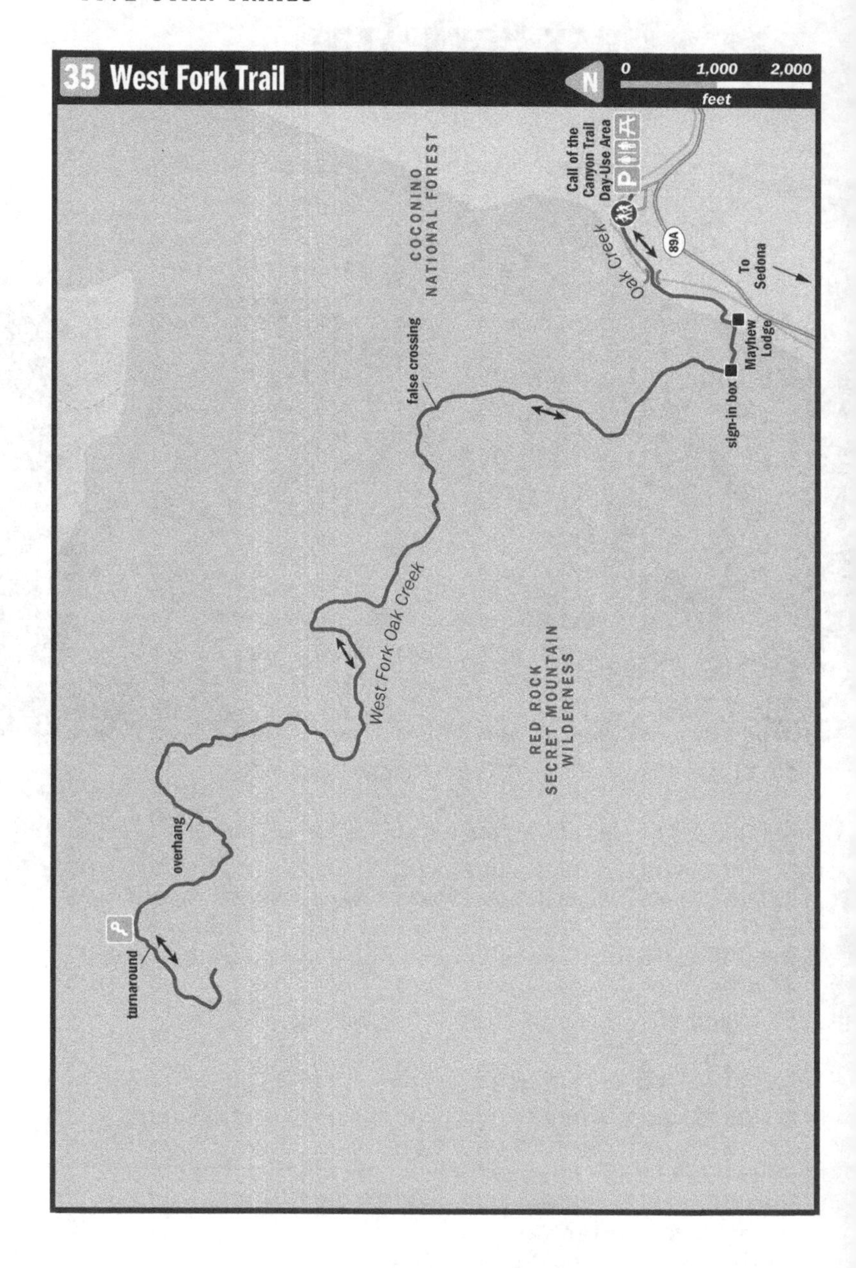
35 West Fork Trail
0
1,000
2,000
feet
N
Call of the Canyon Trail Day-Use Area
COCONINO NATIONAL FOREST
Oak Creek
89A
To Sedona
Mayhew Lodge
sign-in box
false crossing
West Fork Oak Creek
RED ROCK SECRET MOUNTAIN WILDERNESS
overhang
turnaround

poison oak grow in the area. Water from the creek should be treated before drinking. Past the 4-mile mark, you *will* get wet. This is one of the most heavily hiked trails in the state.

CONTACTS: Red Rock Ranger District, P.O. Box 20249, Sedona, AZ 86341; (928) 282-4119; **www.fs.fed.us/r3/coconino/recreation/red_rock/westfork-tr.shtml**

Overview

West Fork Trail 108 follows the West Fork of Oak Creek as it carves its way down through the Mogollon Rim to join Oak Creek at the bottom of the canyon. Before the creek, it passes the ruins of the Mayhew Lodge. This is considered (and publicized as) one of the best hikes in the state, if not the country. It is correspondingly popular.

Route Details

A sight-by-sight account of everything that's cool to see on this hike would occupy a fourth of this volume and exhaust the reader besides. You will see and experience all of the following on this hike:

- Ancient fruit trees full of songbirds;
- Riparian forests;
- Towering sandstone cliffs;
- Burbling rapids and deep pools;
- Towering old-growth trees;

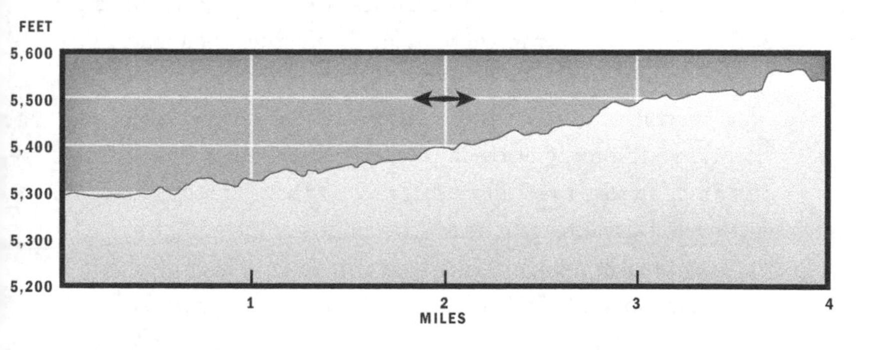

- Weeds, rushes, and thick green moss that you would expect in an area with three times the rainfall;
- Brick-red boulders that tumbled into the canyon from the cliffs above in house-sized chunks;
- Piles of driftwood large enough for building villages;
- And blazing colors from wildflowers in the spring or leaves in the fall.

And you will experience most of these things numerous times.

It all begins with a sidewalk. Follow the Call of the Canyon Nature Trail from the signed trailhead to the left of the restrooms. This is solid concrete for 0.2 mile until the arching bridge spanning Oak Creek. Cross the bridge.

The wide dirt path, once a road, wanders through the old fruit orchards—apple, pear, and plum—of the Mayhew Lodge, a homestead that evolved into a resort. Within 0.2 mile, you come to the ruins of that establishment, the foundations and remnant walls of the main house and outbuildings in various states of decay. The chicken coop, for some reason, is almost completely intact.

Originally homesteaded by "Bear" Howard in the 1870s and John Thomas in the 1880s, the area was acquired by the Mayhew family in 1925 and developed into a commercial lodge. In 1968 they sold the property to the U.S. Forest Service, which had intentions of renovating it, but it burned to the ground in 1980.

Toward the creek, vines cover nearly everything. Within sight of these remains you can see the signed wilderness boundary and a sign-in station. Sign in.

West Fork Trail 108 is not just full of wonders—it is also easy. There are a few rocky places, but for the first 3 miles it is 96% soft dirt. There are also a few ups and downs, but none are sustained, and your overall elevation gain up the canyon is less than 500 feet.

This makes it popular. Very popular. You will have company.

Bring your camera. The hard part lies not in capturing the beauty of the canyon but in finding an angle that isn't full of other hikers.

From the sign, the trail winds quickly to the first creek

crossing. You may have to cross up to 15 times depending on water level and how far you choose to hike. Happily, unless water levels are unusually high, all of these crossings will be easy. Nature, or more likely your fellow hikers, has placed rocks and logs in convenient spots. At most points the creek rarely flows above ankle-height in any case. Just the same, don't wear shoes that you can't get wet. The trail will follow the creek closely most of the way. Early on, that way is to the north.

The West Fork of Oak Creek shifts around from time to time, and the U.S. Forest Service shifts the trail in response. (The crossings on the map are from 2010.) At 1.2 miles in, just before the canyon bends to the west, the trail seems to cross, but that is the old crossing. Look instead for stone steps heading back up the bluff to your right (north and upstream).

The creek heads west, then northwest, and then bends northward around a towering stone butte at 1.75 miles. Past that bend it heads due west, winding among house-sized boulders at about 2 miles. It soon twists sharply north, and here you will pass large piles of logs and deadwood.

For the next mile the creek zigzags roughly northwest. Right around 3 miles, the banks become marshy, with reeds poking out of the mud and moss covering the stones. A few seeps and springs feed the creek through here, forming pools on either side of the trail. Shortly beyond this, before the next creek crossing, the U.S. Forest Service trail officially ends. This is the turnaround for the easy hike.

But if you cross the creek, you'll find the trail continues, now climbing a steep bank away from the creek. This unofficial trail is as obvious as the trail that preceded it as it snakes through the trees. In 0.33 mile, it drops back down to the creek side. At 0.1 mile later, at 3.4 miles, the trail ends at a sandbar facing a slot canyon. Water typically fills this canyon wall-to-wall, so the trail as such really does end here.

If you don't mind getting wet up to the knees, you can continue past the slot canyon (which only goes a few hundred feet) to continue up the creek. You can go at least 2 miles before encountering any serious hazards, but you would be on your own with that. Return the way you came.

Adventure option: It is possible to continue along the canyon for 10 miles until it finally tops the Mogollon Rim at FR 231 near Casner Cabin Draw. This involves real canyoneering: wading, swimming (at least three long stretches), bouldering (and boulder-hopping for miles), and pushing through the trackless brush. The U.S. Forest Service recommends planning 2 days for such an expedition and going equipped for serious canyoneering. Local wisdom recommends starting at the top and heading down. Officially, you are not allowed to build campfires or camp within 6 miles of the confluence with Oak Creek. Also, the upper reaches of the canyon are normally dry, so bring some water.

Directions

Take AZ 89A about 9.5 miles north from Sedona. Call of the Canyon is on the left (west) side of the road between mile markers 384 and 385, but you will also see signs. There may be a line during weekends with good weather.

36 Wilson Mountain

SCENERY: ★★★★
TRAIL CONDITION: ★★★★
CHILDREN: ★★★
DIFFICULTY: ★★★
SOLITUDE: ★★

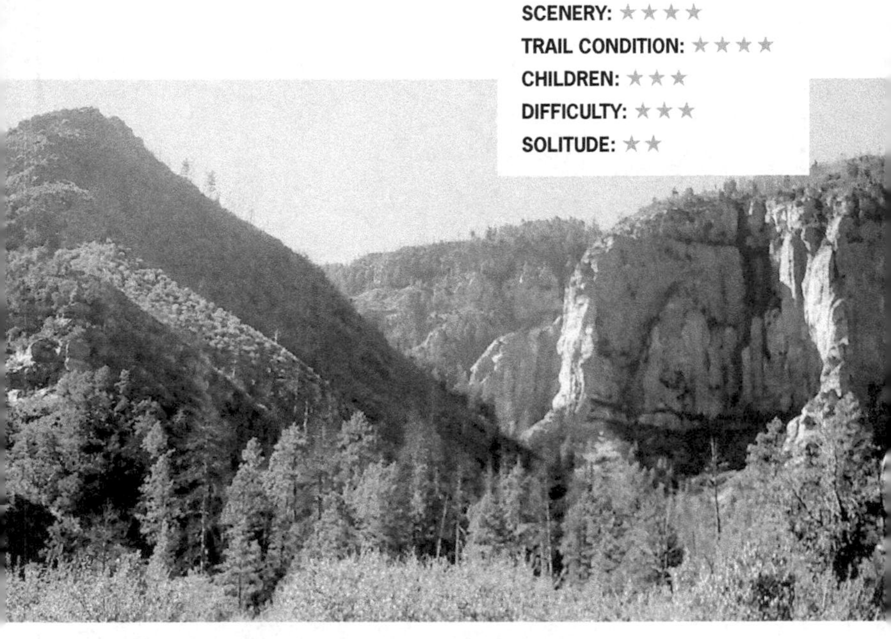

NORTH SLOPES OF WILSON MOUNTAIN—THE TASK AHEAD

GPS TRAILHEAD COORDINATES: *Encinoso Trailhead:* N34° 55.534' W111° 44.126'
Midgely Bridge Trailhead: N34° 53.133' W111° 44.494'

DISTANCE & CONFIGURATION: 10.5 miles as either an out-and-back (from the turn-around point at the top) or a car shuttle to Midgely Bridge. The easy version is 5.3 miles out-and-back.

HIKING TIME: 6 hours; 3 hours for easy hike

HIGHLIGHTS: Scenic vistas and geology

ELEVATION: 4,727 feet at Encinoso Trailhead to 7,004 feet at the peak to 4,514 feet at Midgely Bridge

ACCESS: Requires a Red Rock Pass for both trailheads

MAPS: USGS Wilson Mountain

FACILITIES: The Encinoso Trailhead has restrooms and trash cans; both trailheads have picnic tables

WHEELCHAIR ACCESS: None

COMMENTS: Limited shade; this could be a hot climb on a summer day. On the mountain-top, deadfall could be a hazard during windy conditions. No water available on the hike.

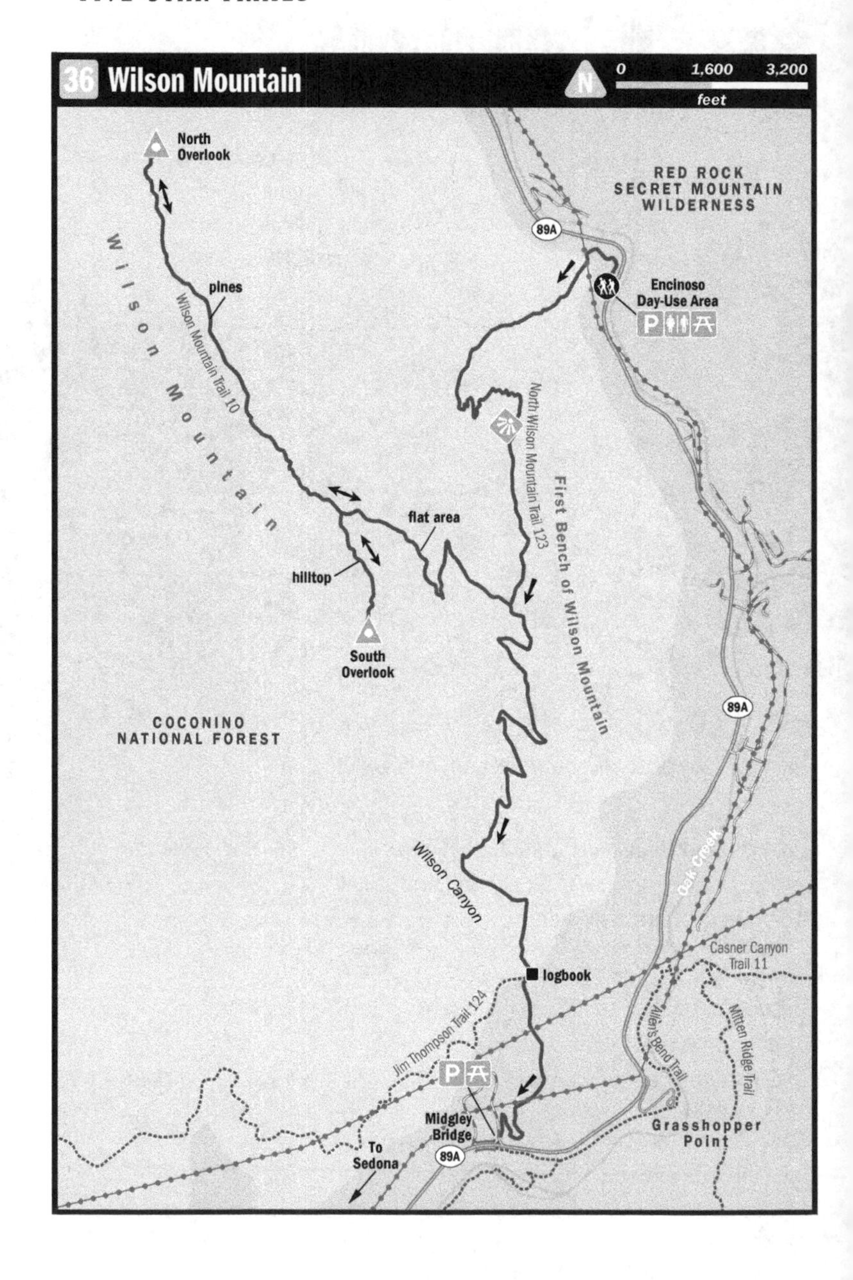
36 Wilson Mountain
N
0
1,600
3,200
feet
North Overlook
RED ROCK SECRET MOUNTAIN WILDERNESS
89A
Encinoso Day-Use Area
Wilson Mountain
pines
Wilson Mountain Trail 10
North Wilson Mountain Trail 123
First Bench of Wilson Mountain
flat area
hilltop
South Overlook
COCONINO NATIONAL FOREST
Oak Creek
Wilson Canyon
Casner Canyon Trail 11
logbook
Jim Thompson Trail 124
Allens Bend Trail
Mitten Ridge Trail
Midgley Bridge
Grasshopper Point
To Sedona

CONTACTS: Red Rock Ranger District, P.O. Box 20249, Sedona, AZ 86341; (928) 282-4119; **www.fs.fed.us/r3/coconino/recreation/red_rock/wilson-mtn-tr.shtml**

Overview

This hike climbs up and down Wilson Mountain, the dominant formation north of Sedona. The "Route Details" are written as a car shuttle, but the hike can be done from either direction as an out-and-back. The route follows the North Wilson Mountain Trail 123 up to the First Bench of Wilson Mountain, where it intersects with Wilson Mountain Trail 10. From there it climbs to the top of Wilson Mountain, splitting off to the distant North Overlook or the closer South Overlook. Wilson Mountain Trail 10 continues south down the mountain to Midgely Bridge.

Route Details

NORTH WILSON: North Wilson Mountain Trail 123 starts north along AZ 89A but quickly switches back south, winding steeply up the ridge through the pines and the oaks. You pass beneath some power lines, and then cross onto an open ridgetop at about 0.25 mile. Here, the task before you, Wilson Mountain, looms dead ahead, an imposing mesa guarded by thousand-foot sandstone cliffs. Not to worry—the

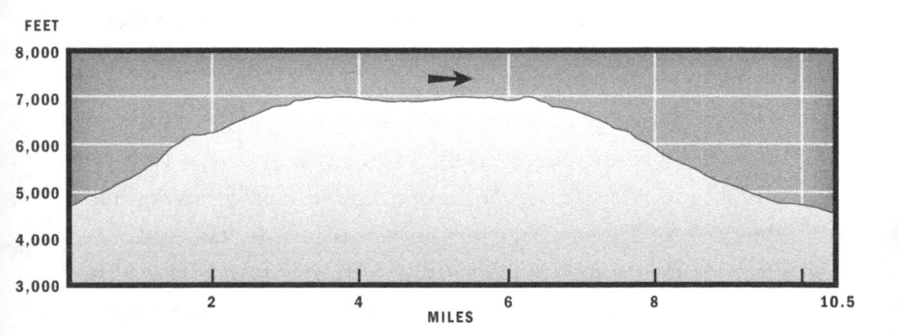

trail finds an easier way up the mountain.

At 0.3 mile in, you cross the wilderness boundary and reenter the woods—or what's left of them. The 2006 Brins Fire torched parts of the forest lining this ravine. At the boundary, though, healthy piñons and ponderosas greet you, for the moment.

As you climb the ravine, you reenter the ghost forest, at least above your head. Lower down, 5 years of brush growth—Gambel oak saplings, wild grape, and chokecherries—now grow around the blackened pines.

After 0.75 mile, the trail crosses the ravine, crosses back, and then starts switching back steeply up the northwestern flank of Wilson Bench. The switchbacks climb about 900 feet in just under 1 mile up the exposed slope. At the top, about 6,000 feet in elevation, you can see Oak Creek Canyon yawning to the north. The trail continues winding through the brush and boulders farther south. It climbs past a little knob to reach the top of the bench proper, where the gray hardpack now wanders through juniper scrub.

The Oak Creek Fault separated this broad bench from the rest of Wilson Mountain several million years ago. The gaping canyon to the east is Munds Canyon, with Schnebly Hill forming its south wall.

At 2.15 miles, North Wilson Mountain Trail 123 forms a T with Wilson Mountain Trail 10. This trail goes up the mountain to the right (west) and down the mountain to the south and east (straight). For the easy hike or car shuttle, you skip going up the mountain.

UP NORTH WILSON MOUNTAIN: Past the junction, the trail climbs gently through the junipers, crossing the Oak Creek Fault, to the base of the higher mesa. From here, leisurely (both in grade and frequency) switchbacks crowded with thickets of Gambel and live oaks wind up the slope for 0.5 mile, straightening across a small, grassy flat.

At about 1 mile past the junction, or 3 miles past the trailhead, the trail comes to a Y near the top of the mesa. As the sign indicates, the trail to the right goes to the North Overlook, while the trail to the left goes to the South or Sedona Overlook.

The listed mileage for this hike accounts for both overlook spurs, out-and-back. Individually, the South Overlook is just under a mile from this Y round-trip, while the more distant North Overlook is 3 miles out-and-back.

The peak of Wilson Mountain is the prominence to the north. Getting there is a bushwhack adventure, and you'd be on your own with that.

THE SOUTH OVERLOOK: This spur starts as a maze of deadfall immediately south of the Y. The way forward is marked by wooden posts and rock cairns, or just head for the metal U.S. Forest Service locker chained to a tree that you can see in the distance—it's right by the trail. Beyond that, the trail climbs steeply up the pine-covered hill to emerge on top of the southern portion of the mesa, an open, windswept prairie. On the far side of the prairie, the thin track leads you to a rocky overlook where Sedona and points south and west stretch before you.

What can you see of Sedona from here? All of it. Return the way you came.

THE NORTH OVERLOOK: The north spur continues as a singletrack across the relatively level top of the mesa, through ghost forests left by fire, interrupted by a few surviving stands of healthy trees. On a windy day—and there are a lot of them up here—these trees will groan and crack all around you, which can be a bit unnerving.

The stands of pines and a few open meadows provide periodic relief from the groaning corpse of the woods. Keep an eye out for any of several large, twisted alligator junipers growing alongside the piñon pines.

Toward the northern terminus, at about 4.5 miles total, the trail seems to end in a pile of deadfall, but despair not: You are less than a hundred yards away. Pick a path through the fallen logs to the rocky lookout you can see beyond.

From here, the rock formations below surround Sterling Pass (see the Vultee Arch & Sterling Pass hike, page 211). The high ridge in the mid-distance is the Mogollon Rim. On a clear day, the San Francisco Peaks rise above it all at the horizon line.

Beware of hedgehog cacti hiding in the rock crevices. Return the way you came.

WILSON MOUNTAIN TRAIL GOING DOWN (AND SOUTH): Back at the Wilson Bench junction, continue south (right) along Wilson Mountain Trail 10 across the bench. After you come to the end of the bench, long switchbacks take you down the brush-choked southern slopes. The gray dirt is as hard as concrete and frequently filled with stumble-rocks. Scrub oaks and other brush crowd the trail, often in an explosion of wildflowers. When you can look up from the rocks, you'll get big views of Oak Creek Canyon.

Just under 1 mile past the junction, the trail crosses the ravine and then crosses back. Soon after, you wind down into juniper-scrub country, with a lot of prickly pear cacti lining the trail. At 0.5 mile down, you cross a third time, where the wash is lined with orange sandstone, and past this point orange gravel replaces the gray hardpack.

The trail winds down the ridge toward Midgely Bridge. At 2.2 miles past the bench junction (or 9.5 miles if you've done the whole hike), you encounter a logbook at the wilderness boundary. A few hundred feet later, the trail comes to a Y. To the right (west) is the Wilson Canyon Trail 49, which also leads to the Jim Thompson Trail 124. Wilson Mountain Trail 10 continues straight (south).

The trail follows the north bank of Wilson Canyon for 0.2 mile before cutting back toward the center of the ridge. You pass beneath two sets of power lines, the second set indicating that you are almost there. Soon the trail wanders down the end of the finger ridge to terminate at Midgely Bridge.

Notes on routing: The north–south route was chosen because Wilson North receives some shade, as opposed to nearly none on the southern approach. Both climbs are actually equally difficult, and in cooler weather they would be interchangeable in terms of preference.

The car-shuttle approach was chosen in order to include both trails. Hiking out-and-back on either trail does not alter the distance beyond 0.5 mile or so.

Directions

To Encinoso Picnic Area: From Sedona, drive north on AZ 89A for about 5 miles (about 3 miles past the bridge). Look for the signed driveway on the left side. If you reach Manzanita Campground, you've gone too far. There is parking for about 16 vehicles. Encinoso has vault toilets, picnic benches, and limited trash service. The water fountain, sadly, was nonfunctional as this guidebook went to press.

To Midgely Bridge Trailhead: Take AZ 89A north from Sedona for 1.9 miles until you cross Midgely Bridge, the first bridge you will come to. The trailhead is on the left side immediately north of the bridge. There are parking spaces for about eight vehicles, but people routinely and creatively cram many more vehicles into this turnout. There are a couple of picnic tables but no other conveniences.

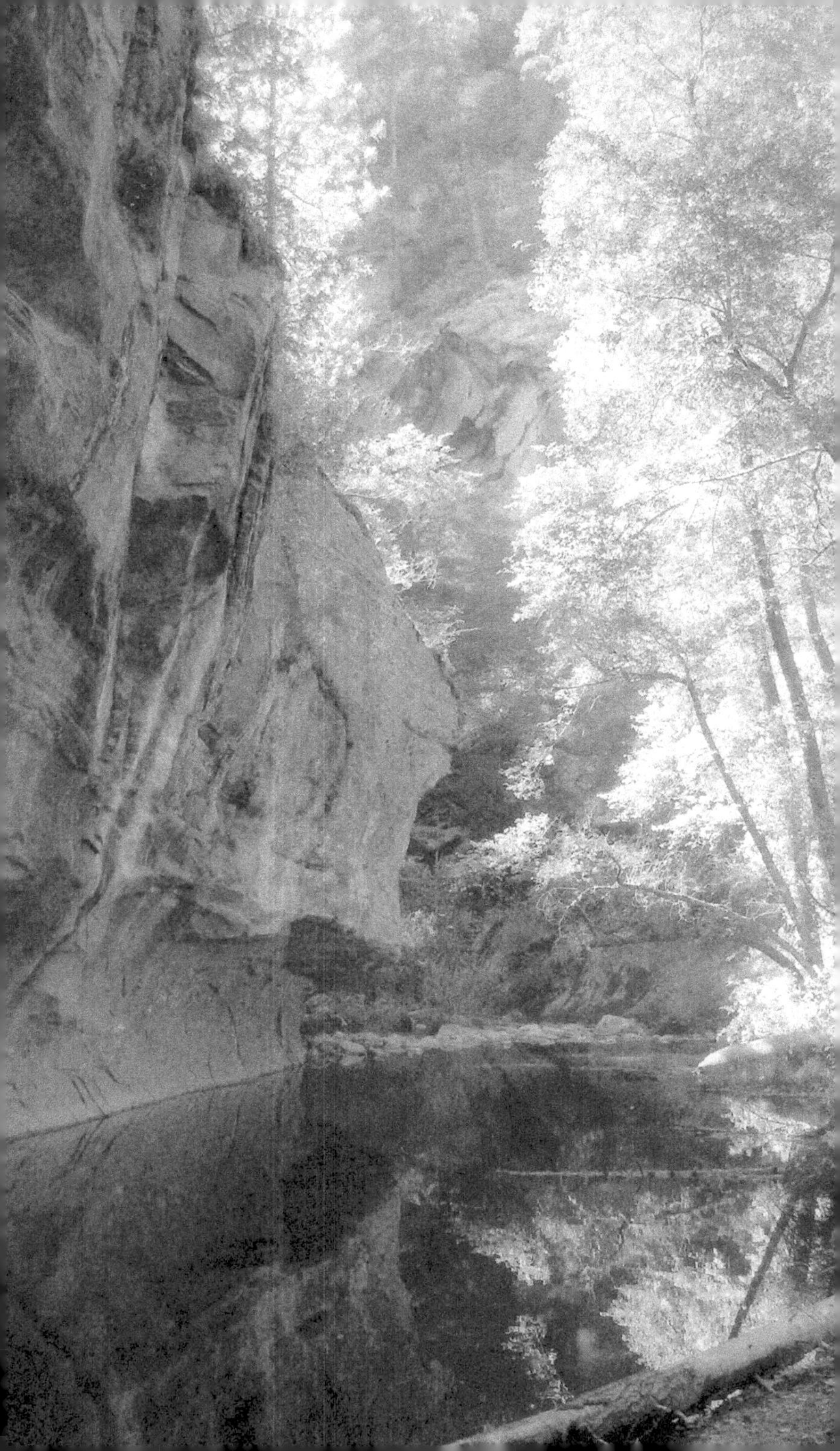

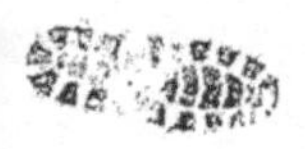

Appendixes & Index

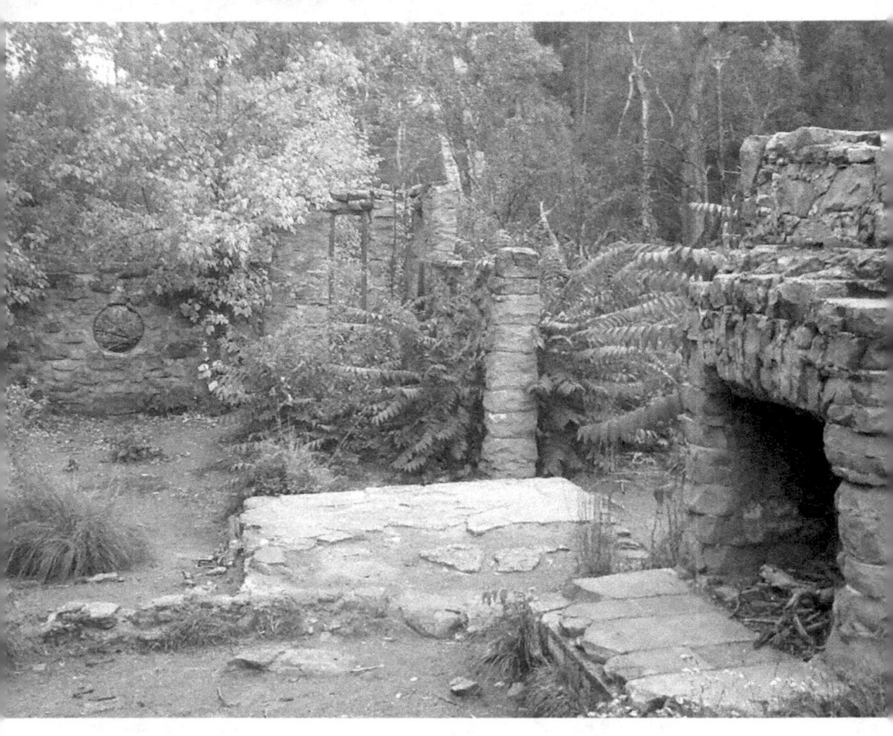

SOME REMAINS OF THE MAYHEW LODGE NEAR WEST FORK OF OAK CREEK

THE WEST FORK OF OAK CREEK FLOWS AROUND A CLIFF. (OPPOSITE)

Appendix A: Outdoor Retailers

While many outlets—from drugstores to supercenters—carry items that would be useful on the trail, the following retailers cater to hikers' needs.

Flagstaff Area

ASPEN SPORTS
15 N. San Francisco St.
Flagstaff, AZ 86001
(928) 779-1935
flagstaffsportinggoods.com

BABBITT'S BACKCOUNTRY OUTFITTERS
12 E. Aspen Ave.
Flagstaff, AZ 86001
(928) 774-4775
babbittsbackcountry.com

FOUR SEASON OUTFITTERS
1051 S. Milton Rd., Ste. F
Flagstaff, AZ 86001
(928) 779-6224
fsguides.com

MOUNTAIN SPORTS
24 N. San Francisco St.
Flagstaff, AZ 86001
(928) 226-2885
mountainsportsflagstaff.com

PEACE SURPLUS
14 W. US 66
Flagstaff, AZ 86001
(928) 779-4521
peacesurplus.com

Sedona Area

MOUNTAIN BIKE HEAVEN
1695 W. AZ 89A
Sedona, AZ 86336
(928) 282-1312
mountainbikeheaven.com

THRIFTY MOUNTAIN SUPPLY
2020 Contractors Rd.
Sedona, AZ 86336
(928) 282-1110

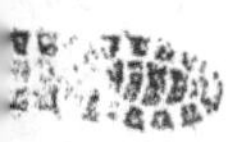

Appendix B: Places to Buy Maps

All of the stores listed in Appendix A (opposite) carry outdoor maps, as do visitor centers. The latter often have free maps of U.S. Forest Service trails.

Flagstaff Area

FLAGSTAFF VISITOR CENTER
1 E. US 66
Flagstaff, AZ 86001
(928) 774-9541
flagstaffarizona.org

HASTINGS ENTERTAINMENT
1540 S. Riordan Rd.
Flagstaff, AZ 86004
(928) 779-1880
gohastings.com

MUSEUM OF NORTHERN ARIZONA
3101 N. Fort Valley Rd.
Flagstaff, AZ 86001
(928) 779-1703
musnaz.org

NEW FRONTIERS NATURAL MARKETPLACE
320 S. Cambridge Ln.
Flagstaff, AZ 86001
(928) 774-5747

NORTHERN ARIZONA UNIVERSITY BOOKSTORE
1014 S. Beaver St., Bldg. 35
(NAU campus)
Flagstaff, AZ 86001
(928) 523-4041
nau.bkstr.com

RIORDAN MANSION STATE HISTORIC PARK
409 W. Riordan Rd.
Flagstaff, AZ 86001
(928) 779-4395
pr.state.az.us/parks/rima

STARRLIGHT BOOKS
15 N. Leroux St.
Flagstaff, AZ 86001
(928) 774-6813

WILLIAMS VISITOR INFORMATION CENTER
200 W. Railroad Ave.
Williams, AZ 86046
(800) 863-0546
experiencewilliams.com

Sedona Area

ENCHANTMENT RESORT GIFT SHOP
525 Boynton Canyon Rd.
Sedona, AZ 86336
(928) 282-2900
enchantmentresort.com

GOLDEN WORD BOOKS & MUSIC
1575 W. AZ 89A, Ste. D
Sedona, AZ 86336
(928) 282-2688
goldenwordbooksandmusic.com

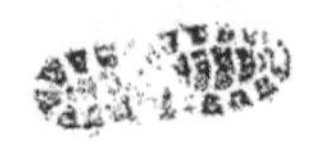

Appendix B: Places to Buy Maps (continued)

Sedona Area *(continued)*

JUNIPINE RESORT
8351 N. AZ 89A
Sedona, AZ 86336
(928) 282-3375
junipine.com

RED ROCK VISITOR CONTACT CENTER
8375 AZ 179
Sedona, AZ 86351
(928) 203-7500
redrockcountry.org/about-us/south-gateway.shtml

SEDONA BIKE & BEAN
6020 AZ 179
Village of Oak Creek
Sedona, AZ 86336
(928) 284-0210
bike-bean.com

SEDONA WORM BOOKSTORE
6645 AZ 179, Ste. C-1
Sedona, AZ 86336
(928) 282-3471
sedonaworm.com

THE WELL RED COYOTE
3190 W. AZ 89A, Ste. 400
Sedona, AZ 86336
(928) 282-2284
wellredcoyote2.com

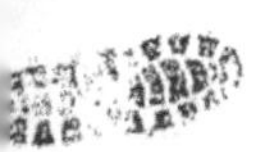

Appendix C: Hiking Clubs

Dozens of hiking clubs function at any given time within or around Sedona and Flagstaff. The clubs selected below have long, stable histories. Contact information given below was accurate as of this guide's 2011 publication date.

Flagstaff Area

FLAGSTAFF HIKING CLUB

P.O. Box 423
Flagstaff, AZ 86002
(928) 774-4560
flagstaffhikingclub.com
Annual dues: $10
Contact Jack Johnson: **jjohnson1241@gmail.com**
This group does not hold actual meetings other than the hikes themselves.

THE SIERRA CLUB–PLATEAU CHAPTER

(For correspondence, use the address on the following page for the Sierra Club–Grand Canyon.)
arizona.sierraclub.org/plateau
Contact Tom Martin: **tomhazel@grand-canyon.az.us;** or Jim McCarthy: (928) 779-3748; **jm436mc@gmail.com**

Sedona Area

SEDONA WESTERNERS
JEWISH COMMUNITY CENTER

Jewish Community Center
100 Meadowlark Dr.
Sedona, AZ 86336
(The above address is for the regular meeting venue and not a mailing address.)
sedonawesterners.org
Annual dues: $20
Contact Alan Gore: **pr0spector@sedonawesterners.org**
Founded in 1961, Sedona Westerners helped establish many of the trails around Sedona. The group is highly organized and has many rules.

THE SIERRA CLUB–SEDONA/VERDE VALLEY CHAPTER

70 Whitetail Ln.
Sedona, AZ 86336
arizona.sierraclub.org/sedona
Contact Marlene Rayner: (928) 203-0340; **marlenerayner@yahoo.com**

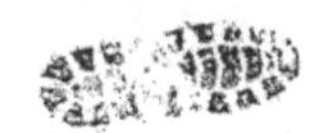

Appendix C: Hiking Clubs (continued)

Statewide

FRIENDS HIKING CLUB

Boulders on Broadway *(sports pub)*
530 W. Broadway Rd.
Tempe, AZ 85282
friendshiking.com
Annual dues: $15
Contact Kurt Sedler: 50 E. Myrna, Tempe, AZ 85284; **mail@friendshiking.com**
Friends Hiking Club typically meets the first Monday of every month and organizes hikes across the Southwest—from day hikes to serious adventures.

HIKE ARIZONA

hikearizona.com
Contact **traildex@gmailcom**
Free registration
This online-only group not only provides a forum for organizing hikes but also maintains one of the most comprehensive hike databases available online.

THE SIERRA CLUB–GRAND CANYON CHAPTER

202 E. McDowell Rd., Ste. 277
Phoenix, AZ 85004
arizona.sierraclub.org
Annual dues: $39 and up
The main Arizona arm of this environmental advocacy organization, the Grand Canyon chapter organizes hikes for members and has groups in both Flagstaff and Sedona (see previous listings).

For information on other groups, visit Internet sources such as **meetup.com** *or Yahoo Groups (***groups.yahoo.com***).*

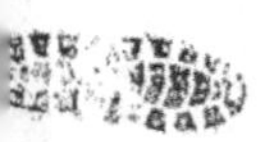

Index

D

E

F

G

H

M *(continued)*

N

O

P

R

S

T

U

V

W

Y

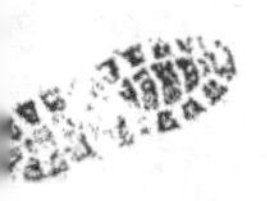

About the Author

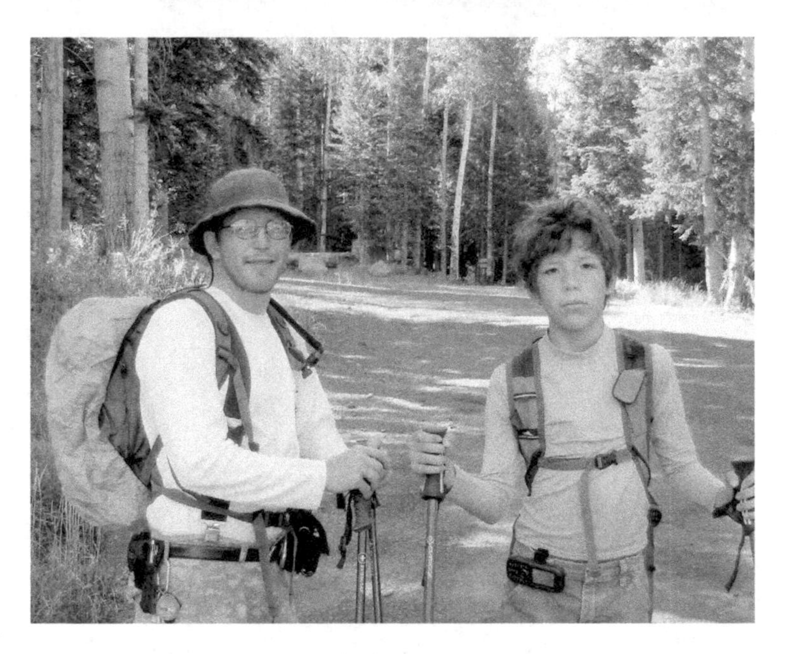

TONY PADEGIMAS is, among many other things, a freelance writer who spends as much time as possible in his hammock slung in some random part of a national forest. His wife, two children, and two dogs join him on occasion but report mixed feelings about whether these endeavors are really worthwhile. The cats have no doubts: They prefer to remain at home in Phoenix.

In addition to his wanderings in the wilderness, Padegimas chronicles sports, fitness, historical curiosities, technical theater (his day job), the inside guts of buildings, and other random topics by assignment. From time to time, he writes over-the-top space opera and other strange fiction.

His work has appeared in numerous local and regional magazines and in a handful of national publications. This is his second book for Menasha Ridge Press: *Five-Star Trails: Flagstaff & Sedona* follows *Day & Overnight Hikes: Tonto National Forest,* published in 2008.

Day & Overnight Hikes: Tonto National Forest

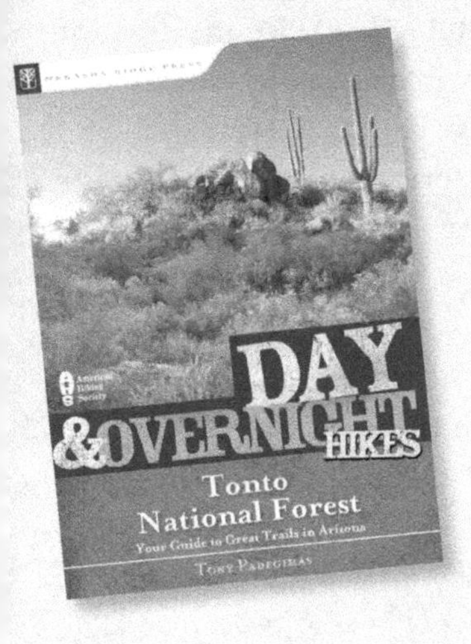

by Tony Padegimas
ISBN: 978-0-89732-639-1
5x7, paperback, $14.95
240 pages
maps, photographs, index

Without this book, Arizona's Tonto National Forest, the fifth-largest national forest in the U.S., might overwhelm even intrepid hikers.

But with the expert guidance of local author Tony Padegimas, you'll easily explore Tonto's 3 million acres of high peaks, deep gorges, babbling rivers, near-silent deserts, and thousand-year-old Native American settlements.

Tony details the 34 best day and overnight hikes so you can save time and make the most of your hiking adventure, gaining the full experience of Tonto's natural wonders.

This guide includes:

- **GPS-based trail maps and elevation profiles**
- **Detailed directions to trailheads**
- **GPS trailhead coordinates**

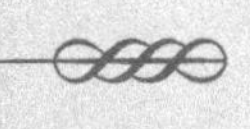
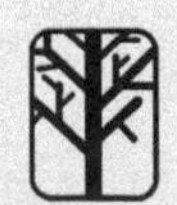
MENASHA RIDGE PRESS
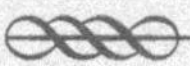
www.menasharidge.com

DEAR CUSTOMERS AND FRIENDS,

SUPPORTING YOUR INTEREST IN OUTDOOR ADVENTURE, travel, and an active lifestyle is central to our operations, from the authors we choose to the locations we detail to the way we design our books. Menasha Ridge Press was incorporated in 1982 by a group of veteran outdoorsmen and professional outfitters. For many years now, we've specialized in creating books that benefit the outdoors enthusiast.

Almost immediately, Menasha Ridge Press earned a reputation for revolutionizing outdoors- and travel-guidebook publishing. For such activities as canoeing, kayaking, hiking, backpacking, and mountain biking, we established new standards of quality that transformed the whole genre, resulting in outdoor-recreation guides of great sophistication and solid content. Menasha Ridge continues to be outdoor publishing's greatest innovator.

The folks at Menasha Ridge Press are as at home on a white-water river or mountain trail as they are editing a manuscript. The books we build for you are the best they can be, because we're responding to your needs. Plus, we use and depend on them ourselves.

We look forward to seeing you on the river or the trail. If you'd like to contact us directly, join in at www.trekalong.com or visit us at www.menasharidge.com. We thank you for your interest in our books and the natural world around us all.

SAFE TRAVELS,

Bob Sehlinger

BOB SEHLINGER
PUBLISHER

Printed in the USA
CPSIA information can be obtained
at www.ICGtesting.com
JSHW012021140824
68134JS00033B/2815